Orthobiologics *for* Fractures *and* Nonunion Management

Orthobiologics *for* Fractures *and* Nonunion Management

EDITORS

J. Tracy Watson, MD
Professor
The CORE Institute for Orthopaedics
University of Arizona College
of Medicine
Phoenix, Arizona

Hassan R. Mir, MD, MBA
Professor of Orthopaedic Surgery
and Medical Education
Director of Orthopaedic Trauma
Research
Past Chief Financial Officer of the
Orthopaedic Trauma Association
Florida Orthopaedic Institute
University of South Florida
Tampa, Florida

Wolters Kluwer

Philadelphia • Baltimore • New York • London
Buenos Aires • Hong Kong • Sydney • Tokyo

Acquisitions Editor: Keith Donnellan
Development Editor: Stacey Sebring
Editorial Coordinator: Ann Francis
Marketing Manager: Kirsten Watrud
Production Project Manager: Matthew West
Manager, Graphic Arts & Design: Stephen Druding
Manufacturing Coordinator: Lisa Bowling
Prepress Vendor: Straive

9 8 7 6 5 4 3 2 1

Printed in the United States of America

Cataloging in Publication Data available on request from publisher

ISBN: 978-1-9751-8295-3

shop.lww.com

MPP0625

Contributors

Mike T. Archdeacon, MD, MSE
CEO, UC Physicians
Senior Associate Dean of Clinical Affairs
Peter J. Stern Professor and Chair
Department of Orthopaedic Surgery
University of Cincinnati College of Medicine
Cincinnati, Ohio

Michael Beebe, MD
Assistant Professor of Orthopaedic Trauma
Department of Orthopaedics
University of Tennessee
Campbell Clinic
Memphis, Tennessee

Michael J. Beltran, MD
Orthopaedic Trauma Surgeon
Department of Orthopaedics and Sports Medicine
University of Cincinnati
Cincinnati, Ohio

Taco J. Blokhuis, MD, PhD
Trauma Surgeon
Department of Surgery
Maastricht University Medical Center
Maastricht, Limburg, The Netherlands

Mark Cinque, MD, MS
Orthopaedic Sports Medicine Surgeon
The Steadman Clinic
Vail, Colorado

William Doss, DO
Orthopaedic Trauma Surgeon
Integris Health Baptist Medical Center
Oklahoma City, Oklahoma

Luke Farrow, MBChB, MRCS, BSc
Clinical Lecturer
Grampian Orthopaedics
University of Aberdeen
Aberdeen, Scotland, United Kingdom

Henry Goodnough, MD, PhD
Assistant Professor
Department of Orthopaedic Surgery
Stanford University
Stanford, California

Varun Gudapati, MD
Orthopaedic Surgery Resident
Department of Orthopaedic Surgery
UCLA David Geffen School of Medicine
Los Angeles, California

David J. Hak, MD
Orthopedic Trauma Surgeon
Department of Orthopedic Surgery
Hughston Clinic
University of Central Florida
Sanford, Florida

Kelly Krohn, MD
Director of Bone Health
Department of Orthopaedics
University of Arizona
Phoenix, Arizona

Christopher M. LaPrade, MD
Orthopaedic Surgeon
Twin Cities Orthopedics
Eagan, Minnesota

Christopher Lee, MD
Assistant Professor of Orthopaedic Trauma
Department of Orthopaedic Surgery
University of California, Los Angeles
Los Angeles, California

Philipp Leucht, MD, PhD
Raj-Sobti-Menon Associate Professor
Department of Orthopedic Surgery
NYU Grossman School of Medicine
New York, New York

Anna J. L. Lodewijks, MD
PhD Candidate
Department of Trauma Surgery
Maastricht University Medical Center
Maastricht, Limburg, The Netherlands

Gregory Lupica, MD
Orthopaedic Surgery Resident
Department of Orthopaedic Surgery
Harbor-UCLA Medical Center
Torrance, California

Tristan McMillan, MBCHB, FRCS
Consultant Orthopaedic Surgeon
Leeds Teaching Hospital Trust
Leeds, West Yorkshire, United Kingdom

Devan D. Mehta, MD
Clinical Instructor
Department of Orthopaedic Surgery
Stanford University
Palo Alto, California

Brent Norris, MD
Professor
Department of Orthopaedic Surgery
Oklahoma State University
Tulsa, Oklahoma

Martijn Poeze, MD, PhD, MSc
Professor of Trauma Surgery and Orthopedic Traumatology
Department of Trauma Surgery
Maastricht University Medical Center
Maastricht, The Netherlands

Benjamin C. Schaffler, MD
Resident Physician, PGY-3
Clinician Scientist Training Program
Department of Orthopaedic Surgery
NYU Langone Health
New York, New York

Emil Schemitsch, MD, FRCS
Richard Ivey Professor and Chair
Department of Surgery
University of Western Ontario
London, Ontario, Canada

Iain Stevenson, FRCS, Tr & ORTH
Consultant Orthopaedic Surgeon
Aberdeen Royal Infirmary
NHS Grampian
Aberdeen, Scotland, United Kingdom

J. Tracy Watson, MD
Professor
The CORE Institute for Orthopaedics
University of Arizona College of Medicine
Phoenix, Arizona

John Michael Yingling, MD, DO
Orthopedic Trauma Surgeon, Assistant Professor
Department of Orthopedics and Sports Medicine
University of Michigan Health-Sparrow
Lansing, Michigan

Jack Zhong, MD
Resident
Orthopaedic Surgery
NYU Langone Health
New York, New York

Contents

1 Fracture Healing Response

J. Tracy Watson

INTRODUCTION

With the development of new bone graft substitutes and bone inductive factors, the correct use of these materials is dependent on the clinician fully understanding the fracture healing cascade. This chapter will review the fracture healing response as it relates to those factors that can affect the remodeling response. This sequence is controlled by various local hormonal responses, specific cellular and substrate requirements, presence of growth factors, and expression and release of regulatory factors in a well-organized manner.

INFLAMMATORY PHASE OF FRACTURE HEALING

Following initial trauma, the common pathway for union of most fractures occurs by secondary healing, which is also described as endochondral bone formation. This usually occurs under the biomechanical conditions of fracture instability with micromotion at the site of the injury. This begins with cartilage formation and an intervening soft tissue conversion to endochondral bone. As well, committed osteoprogenitor cells and undifferentiated mesenchymal cells (MSCs) derived from the intact periosteum can also contribute to the healing process via intramembranous bone formation that occurs on either side of the fracture.[1] Intramembranous ossification occurs at the periphery of the fracture ends and forms bone without an intervening cartilage phase.

Fractures heal by a combination of intramembranous and endochondral ossification and demonstrate a series of distinct stages that comprise four temporally defined phases of repair response: the **inflammatory phase, early callus phase, mature callus phase, and remodeling phase** (Table 1.1).

The initial response to the injury is known as the **inflammatory phase of fracture healing**. This phase begins immediately after fracture with clot formation and hematoma development. This is accompanied by the invasion of macrophages, polymorphonuclear leukocytes, and lymphocytic cells.[2]

Platelets found in the hematoma degranulate releasing various signaling molecules, and cytokines involve in the processes of chemotaxis and angiogenesis. They also regulate cell proliferation and differentiation of the cells that have migrated to the site of the fracture.[3] The inflammatory phase is characterized by neovascularization and ingrowth of proliferative blood vessels. This neovascularization response brings with it migrating pericytes that convert into undifferentiated mesenchymal stem cells. This oxygen-rich environment is vitally important to the MSCs that have migrated to the site of injury under the influence of the platelet-derived cytokine factors. The attachment of undifferentiated MSCs to the extracellular matrix and conductive substrates takes place through the formation of cell adhesion complexes, which consist of integrins and cytoplasmic proteins such as alpha-actinin.[4] Cellular binding to conductive substrates is necessary for circulating inductive factors to stimulate the differentiation of these cells into an osteoblastic lineage.[4] Thus, any material that induces this process to cause the direct differentiation of cells should be considered osteoinductive. This is the locale of action of the true inductive factors known as the bone morphogenetic proteins (BMPs). BMPs are members

TABLE 1.1 Fracture Healing Response

	Inflammatory Phase	Early Callus Phase	Mature Callus Phase	Remodeling Phase
Primary Biologic Event	• Neo vascularization • Migration of undifferentiated mesenchymal cells That bind to conductive substrate • Differentiation of cells to osteoblastic lineage	• Development of cartilage anlage • Migration/proliferation chondrocytes • Early mineralization • Primary spongiosa	• Mineralization of cartilaginous matrix • Release of matrix vesicles • Osteoblast secret collagen • Chondrocyte apoptosis • Chondroclast removal early calcific matrix and chondrocytes • Secondary spongiosa	Six stages of remodeling • Quiescence • Activation • Resorption • Reversal • Formation • Termination
Biologic requirements	• Vascular bed • Conductive substrate • Viable cells • PDGF • BMPs	• PDGF • TGF-β	• Collagen fibrils • Noncollagenous proteins • Perivascular infiltration continues • Osteoblast osteoid deposition	• Hormonal stimuli • Inductive growth factors • Glucocorticoids • Vitamin D • Thyroid/parathyroid • Osteoclast • Osteoblast
Increasing Biologic Activity (ability to form bone) →				

of the transforming growth factor-β (TGF-β) superfamily and regulate differentiation of MSCs into components of bone, cartilage, or adipose tissue. BMP-2, -4, -5, -6, and -7 all have strong osteogenic capabilities and that their signaling is essential for bone remodeling and maintenance of bone mass through activation of BMP receptors.[2,5]

There is considerable interest in creating osteoconductive matrices using nonbiological porous structures that mimic the cancellous bony architecture that have very specific surface kinetics to facilitate the migration, attachment, and proliferation of mesenchymal stem cells.[6] Cellular elements and conductive substrates require each other's presence to actively function as a viable component for the healing of skeletal tissues. Similarly, osteoconductive materials alone work well when filling non–critical-size defects in subchondral locations, but these materials do require the migration of osteoprogenitor cells into these matrices in order to incorporate and support the subchondral surfaces. For challenging critical-size defects, all three types of these materials are necessary to achieve efficacy equivalent to autograft.[7,8]

FACTORS INFLUENCING THE INFLAMMATORY RESPONSE PHASE

Arachidonic Acid Metabolism

Arachidonic acid metabolism exerts complex control over many bodily systems, mainly involved in inflammation and immunity. These actions include a direct role in the stimulation of platelet aggregation and vasoconstriction, both important for the activation and degranulation of platelets. As well, leukocyte chemotaxis is activated, and these factors may directly activate gene transcription of the attached mesenchymal stem cells. The **classical cyclooxygenase (COX) inhibitors** are the nonsteroidal anti-inflammatory drugs and prevent the production of prostaglandin products. They are not selective and inhibit all phases of the inflammatory process, including fracture healing. Because COX-2 is specific to inflamed tissue, there is much less gastric irritation associated with COX-2 inhibitors. The selectivity of COX-2 is specific to inflamed tissue but does not seem to negate the other fracture healing side effects of nonsteroidal anti-inflammatory drugs and should be avoided in patients at risk for delayed fracture healing.[9]

Wnt Pathway

Wnt signaling pathways are a group of signal transduction pathways made of proteins that pass signals from outside of a cell through cell surface receptors to the inside of the cell. These pathways are activated by the binding of a Wnt-protein ligand to a Frizzled cell surface receptor. This leads to regulation of gene transcription and conversion of undifferentiated mesenchymal stem cells into an osteoblastic lineage.[10] Potential therapeutic approaches attempt to stimulate the Wnt pathway by upregulating the intracellular mediators of the Wnt cascade and inhibiting the antagonists of the pathway. Sclerostin is produced by the osteocyte and binds to a co-receptor group inhibiting the Wnt signaling pathway.[11] Inhibition of the Wnt pathway leads to decreased bone formation. Antibodies against sclerostin have demonstrated promising results in promoting bone formation and increased callus size.[12] An antibody for sclerostin (romosozumab) is available and in clinical use. Its use has demonstrated increased bone growth and increased bone mineral density (BMD) of the hip and spine,[13,14] but its effect on fresh fractures and nonunions is not known.

Early Callus Phase

Early callus formation is located adjacent to the fracture site and is initially a cartilage anlage developed from undifferentiated MSCs in the peripheral soft tissues that are recruited, proliferate, and differentiate into cartilage-forming cells.[15] These cells gradually become calcified and are replaced by bone (see Table 1.1). The *early callus phase* response of chondrogenesis begins approximately 7 to 10 days after injury. The migration and proliferation of chondroprogenitor MSCs and differentiation into chondrocytes with the expression of cartilage-specific matrix occurs at this time. The formation of a malleable cartilage callus provides some limited mechanical stability to the bone ends and delivers a specific architecture to provide sites of attachment for additional cells to facilitate new bone formation. Within 2 weeks of injury, protein synthesis is complete and hypertrophic chondrocytes release calcium into the extracellular matrix in order to precipitate with phosphate ions[16] and begins to calcify. The presence of proteoglycans in this early callus prevents mineralization; however, once a critical threshold of cartilaginous callus is formed, mineralization will then take place by the removal of the proteoglycan inhibitors.[17]

Factors Effecting the Early Callus Phase

Platelet concentrate contains alpha-granules, which contain more than 30 bioactive proteins, many of which have a fundamental role in hemostasis and/or tissue healing. Of these, platelet-derived growth factor (PDGF) and TGF-β appear to have the most potent effect on the soft callus stage of healing.[18]

TGF-β has a broad range of effect on tissues found in the soft callus and activates fibroblasts to induce collagen formation, endothelial cells to promote further angiogenesis, stimulates chondroprogenitor cells for cartilage formation, and acts on MSCs in an effort to increase the population of factors all crucial to the propagation of the soft callus phase.

The main function of PDGF is stimulating cellular replication (mitogenesis). This increases cell populations of mesenchymal stem cells and osteoprogenitor cells. PDGF also activates macrophages, resulting in the débridement of the traumatic site, which then triggers a second source of growth factors released from the host tissues.[19,20]

Mature Callus Phase

The mature callus phase is characterized by mineralization of the cartilaginous callus matrix (Table 1.1). This occurs as hypertrophic chondrocytes develop budding of their membrane structures to form vesicularized bodies. Matrix vesicles (MVs) are released from hypertrophic chondrocytes and from mature osteoblasts. MVs are extracellular vesicles enveloped by a plasma membrane (ranging 30-1,000 nm in diameter). MVs bear several membrane transporters and enzymes on their membranes and in their interior, providing a nurturing microenvironment *for* calcium phosphate nucleation and subsequent crystal growth.[21] Primary mineralization is orchestrated by osteoblasts; osteoblasts secret a large amount of collagen fibrils, noncollagenous proteins, and their own MV membranes. The degree of the primary mineralization is controlled by fine-tuning bone formation and mineral apposition rates as the MVs bind to the collagen. Simultaneously the chondrocytes then undergo apoptosis, and mineral is laid down on the callus surfaces.[17]

Chondroclasts invade, and the removal of calcified cartilage includes not only resorption of the mineralized matrix but also removes the chondrocytes themselves. As chondroclasts remove the calcified cartilage, the ongoing process of neovascularization brings in additional perivascular cells and osteoblast progenitors, which infiltrate the calcified matrix surfaces.[20] The osteoblast progenitors then continue with osteoid deposition and subsequent mineralization. This is the remodeling of the primary spongiosa (early calcified cartilage) to secondary spongiosa (woven bone), resulting in early fracture union by approximately 4 to 5 weeks (see Table 1.1).

Remodeling Phase

As osteoblastic formation of woven bone takes place, it remodels to form mature lamellar bone and restores the original cortical end plates and cortical structure.[22] **The remodeling phase** is composed of six sequential stages, namely quiescence, activation, resorption, reversal, formation, and termination (see Tables 1.1 and 1.2).[23] The first stage of bone remodeling involves resorption

TABLE 1.2 Biologic Characteristics of the Bone Remodeling Phase Sequence

Phase of Remodeling	Conductive Scaffold	Hormones and Regulatory Factors	Inductive Growth Factors	Living Cells
Activation Phase	• Soft callus • Vascularized fibrous tissue	• +PTH • +IGF-1 • +PGE_2 • +Calcitriol • +TNG-α • −Estrogen		• Pluripotential mesenchymal stem cells
Osteoclast Recruitment Resorption Phase	• Mineralized cartilage • Hard callus	• +RANKL • −OPG • +Retinoic • −Estrogen • Acid • −Calcitonin • +TNF-α • +αvβ3 Integrins	• −TGF-β	• Osteoblasts respond to signals generated by osteocytes or direct endocrine activation, recruiting osteoclast precursors
Reversal Phase	• Early membranous bone • Endochondral bone		• TGF-β • IGF-1, IGF-2 • BMPs • PDGF • FGF	• Preosteoblasts • Disappearance of almost all Osteoclasts
Osteoblast Recruitment Formation Phase	• Early membranous bone • Endochondral bone	• +PTH • −PDGFs • +1,25$(OH)_2$ • −Steroids • Vitamin D_3 • −$PyroPO_4$ • +WNTs • −Leptin • +Runx2	• BMPs • IGF-1 • FGF-2 • FGF-18 • PDGFs • TGF-β	• Complete replacement of osteoclastic cells with osteoblastic cells and osteoblast differentiation
Termination Phase	• Lamellar bone • Cortical end plates • Resting bone surface environment is maintained until the next wave of remodeling is initiated	• Feedback signal of normal sclerostin expression		• Final differentiation to osteoblastic lineage only

+ Facilitates process.
− Inhibits process.
Biologic characteristics of the bone remodeling phase sequence.
The bone remodeling process is controlled by various local hormonal response, specific cellular and substrate requirements, presence of growth factors, and expression and release of regulatory factors in a well-organized manner.

of bone by osteoclasts. In the resorption phase, osteoblasts respond to signals generated by osteocytes or direct endocrine activation signals, recruiting osteoclast precursors to the remodeling site. To initiate the initial resorption phase, **multinucleated osteoclasts** are formed by cell-cell fusion of mononuclear preosteoclasts in the blood. Although most osteoclasts contain only 2 to 12 nuclei (chromosome-containing organelles), some may have as many as 200 nuclei. The osteoclast's job is to then secrete a high concentration of hydrochloric acid and enzymes from their cell membrane to dissolve a small area of the old bone forming a pit, called **Howship's lacunae**.

The resorption phase is of limited duration depending on level of the stimuli responsible for osteoclast differentiation and activity. It is followed by the reversal phase that is characterized by disappearance of almost all osteoclasts. Once a resorption pit has been created, new bone needs to form in order to maintain bone mass. To initiate the growth of new bone, osteoclasts secrete growth factors that instruct circulating mesenchymal stem cells in the bone marrow to form into osteoblasts.

The osteoblasts migrate to the resorption site so they can proliferate and begin laying down new bone. This is called the "reversal" phase. The formation phase is distinct by complete replacement of osteoclastic cells with osteoblastic cells. The termination signals of bone remodeling include the terminal differentiation of the osteoblast. The resting bone surface environment is maintained until the next wave of remodeling is initiated.

After the osteoblasts form new bone, they die, become osteoblastic lining cells in the periosteum, or become mature osteocytes ("mineralization phase"). These osteocytes can "awaken" at a later date to restart these remodeling phases. As a result, the five phases are a cycle, not a linear process. In humans, the cycle is variable in time but takes approximately 120 to 200 days to complete. Thus, typical fracture healing is complete within approximately 3 months.

Bone remodeling literally cuts "tunnels" into the bone to accomplish normal physiological bone remodeling; the proper coupling of bone formation and bone resorption requires direct communication among different bone cells. Cells of the osteoblast lineage (osteoblasts, osteocytes, and bone-lining cells) and bone-resorbing cells (osteoclasts), together with their precursor cells, are organized in specialized units called bone multicellular units (BMU).[24]

Factors Effecting the Remodeling Phase

Osteoblastic cells secrete factors that induce fully differentiated osteoblasts to express ligands that regulate the activity of osteoclasts. Receptor activator of NF-κB ligand (RANKL) is essential for the development of osteoclast precursors. This surface-bound molecule RANKL found on osteoblasts serves to activate osteoclasts, which are critically involved in bone resorption,[22] as osteoclasts and osteoblasts play a vital role in normal bone remodeling. RANKL is strongly induced by a fracture to increase its activity[22] and demonstrates a peak in expression just before calcified cartilage removal begins (remodeling phase) (see Table 1.1).

Factors Effecting the Remodeling Phase

Estrogen inhibits the osteoclast recruitment and resorption phase of remodeling by the formation and activation of the bone-resorbing osteoclasts via suppression of RANKL signaling within the osteoclast. Estrogen has also been shown to modulate the production of a number of bone-resorbing cytokines, including IL-1, IL-6, TNF-α, M-CSF, and prostaglandins.[25-28] T cells are an essential mediator of the bone-wasting effects of estrogen deficiency in vivo, and estrogen prevents osteoclastic bone resorption through suppressing the production of TNF-α from T cells.[29]

Selective estrogen receptor modulators are ligands for estrogen receptors that induce these receptors to affect intracellular transcriptional modulators. Raloxifene is such a class of SERM, mimics estrogen's suppression of RANKL and thus can also inhibit osteoclast formation.

Denosumab is the first RANKL inhibitor to be approved by the Food and Drug Administration. Denosumab inhibits this maturation of osteoclasts by binding to and inhibiting RANKL thus preventing the binding to receptor activator of NF-κB (RANK).

Parathyroid hormone (PTH) is a polypeptide involved in the regulation of calcium and phosphate metabolism. Bone resorption is caused by osteoclasts, which are indirectly stimulated by PTH. PTH has no direct effect on osteoclasts, since osteoclasts do not have a receptor for PTH. PTH binds to the osteoblasts stimulating osteoblasts to increase their expression of RANKL. PTH inhibits their expression of osteoprotegerin (OPG) mRNA. OPG functions to bind to RANKL and block it from interacting with RANK. The binding of RANKL to RANK stimulates these osteoclast precursors to fuse, forming new osteoclasts.[30] While continual exposure to PTH leads to an increase in osteoclast activity and density, intermittent exposure stimulates osteoblasts more than osteoclasts and results in increased bone formation. PTH's anabolic actions are thought to be via its effects to increase the proliferation and differentiation of osteoblasts in vitro and in vivo decrease osteoblast apoptosis and activate bone-lining cells.[30-35]

Teriparatide is a recombinant form of PTH identical to a portion of human PTH. It is an effective anabolic (ie, bone growing) agent[30] used in the treatment of some forms of osteoporosis. Clinically, recombinant PTH has been approved by the Food and Drug Administration for its use in the treatment of osteoporosis, and several recent clinical trials have demonstrated that daily systemic treatment with PTH increases BMD and reduces fracture risk in osteoporotic patients. It is also used off-label to speed fracture healing and treat nonunions and has demonstrated increased fracture callus volume, enhanced mechanical properties, as well as increased BMD, bone mineral content, and total osseous tissue volume.[31-34]

Vitamin D affects the osteoblast recruitment and formation phase of remodeling. It promotes osteoblast proliferation and maturation in human osteoblasts and appears to promote osteoclast differentiation, ameliorate osteoclast activity, and promote coupling of bone resorption to formation.[36,37]

It has been recently shown that $1,25(OH)_2D_3$ treatment enhances mineralization of the osteoblast function and suggests that $1,25(OH)_2D_3$ is a potent promoter of the osteoblast to osteocyte transition further enhancing the remodeling phase of fracture healing.

Glucocorticoids (GCs) also affect the osteoblast recruitment and formation phase. GCs stimulate osteoclast numbers by suppressing synthesis of OPG and stimulating RANKL synthesis by preosteoblast/stromal cells, with the decrease in the OPG to RANKL ratio supporting osteoclast differentiation and net bone resorption.[38,39] The long-term use of GCs reduces bone formation either via direct inhibition of osteoblast proliferation and differentiation (suppression of Runx2 and type I collagen) or by the augmentation of apoptosis rates of mature osteoblasts and osteocytes.[40-42] In addition, GCs negatively regulate secretion of androgens and estrogens by inhibiting gonadotropin secretion and finally increase bone resorption.[43] GCs also induce negative calcium balance by decreasing intestinal calcium absorption and increasing urinary calcium excretion.[44] In adult bone, glucocorticoid receptors (GR) are mainly found in pre-osteoblast/stromal cells and osteoblasts. Thus, the negative effects of GCs on bone formation are mediated through osteoblastic GR. Taken together, direct GC-GR (glucocorticoid-glucocorticoid receptors) signaling in bone can reduce bone mass as well as through indirectly affecting systemic regulators of bone remodeling.

Fracture healing and thus bone remodeling occur continuously to repair skeletal damage. Bone is continually resorbed by osteoclasts and replaced by osteoblasts even without fracture repair; this close coordination between resorption and formation ensures that structural integrity is maintained while allowing up to 10% of the skeleton to be replaced each year.[45] As has been demonstrated, healing and remodeling are regulated by both systemic and local factors and the key signaling pathways have been identified in this review.

References

1. Gerstenfeld LC, Cullinane DM, Barnes GL, Graves DT, Einhorn TA. Fracture healing as a post-natal development process: molecular, spatial and temporal aspects of its regulation. *J Cell Biochem.* 2003;88:873-884.
2. Kudo TA, Kanetaka H, Watanabe A, et al. Investigating bone morphogenetic protein (BMP) signaling in a newly established human cell line expressing BMP receptor type II Tohoku. *J Exp Med.* 2010;222:121-129.
3. Casati L, Celotti F, Negri-Cesi P, Sacchi MC, Castano P, Colciago A. Platelet derived growth factor (PDGF) contained in platelet rich plasma (PRP) stimulates migration of osteoblasts by reorganizing actin cytoskeleton. *Cell Adh Migr.* 2014;8(6):595-602.
4. Triplett JW, Pavalko FM. Disruption of alpha-actinin-integrin interactions at focal adhesions renders osteoblasts susceptible to apoptosis. *J Physiol Cell Physiol.* 2006;291(5):C909-C921.
5. Mishina Y, Starbuck MW, Gentile MA, et al. Bone morphogenetic protein type IA receptor signaling regulates post-natal osteoblast function and bone remodeling. *J Biol Chem.* 2004;279:27560-27566.
6. Holmes RE, Bucholz RW, Mooney V. Porous hydroxyapatite as a bone-graft substitute in metaphyseal defects. A histometric study. *J Bone Joint Surg Am.* 1986;68(6):904-911.
7. Patterson TE, Kumagai K, Griffith L, Muschler GF. Cellular strategies for enhancement of fracture repair. *J Bone Joint Surg Am.* 2008;90(Suppl 1):111-119.
8. Goodman SB. Cell-based therapies for regenerating bone. *Minerva Ortop Traumatol.* 2013;64(2):107-113.
9. Geusens P, Emans PJ, de Jong JJ, van den Bergh J. NSAIDs and fracture healing. *Curr Opin Rheumatol.* 2013;25(4):524-531.
10. Kim JH, Liu X, Wang J, Chen X. Wnt signaling in bone formation and its therapeutic potential for bone diseases. *Ther Adv Musculoskelet Dis.* 2013;5(1):13-31.
11. Li X, Zhang Y, Kang H, Liu W. Sclerostin binds to LRP5/6 and antagonizes canonical Wnt signaling. *J Biol Chem.* 2005;280(20):19883-19887.
12. Bellido T, Saini V, Pajevic PD. Effects of PTH on osteocyte function. *Bone.* 2013;54(2):250-257.
13. Ominsky MS, Vlasseros F, Jolette J, Smith SY. Two doses of sclerostin antibody in cynomolgus monkeys increases bone formation, bone mineral density, and bone strength. *J Bone Miner Res.* 2010;25(5):948-959.
14. Recker RR, Benson CT, Matsumoto T, Bolognese MA. A randomized, double-blind phase 2 clinical trial of blosozumab, a sclerostin antibody, in postmenopausal women with low bone mineral density. *J Bone Miner Res.* 2015;30(2):216-224.
15. Nakahara H, Bruder SP, Haynesworth SE, et al. Bone and cartilage formation in diffusion chambers by subcultured cells derived from the periosteum. *Bone.* 1990;11:181-188.
16. Einhorn TA. The cell and molecular biology of fracture healing. *Clin Orthop.* 1998;355:S7-S21.
17. Einhorn TA, Hirschman A, Kaplan C, Nashed R, Devlin VJ, Warman J. Neutral protein-degrading enzymes in experimental fracture callus: a preliminary report. *J Orthop Res.* 1989;7:792-805.
18. Mehta S, Watson JT. Platelet rich concentrate: basic science and current clinical applications. *J Orthop Trauma.* 2008;22(6):432-438.
19. Cho T-J, Gerstenfeld LC, Einhorn TA. Differential temporal expression of members of the TGF-B superfamily during murine fracture healing. *J Bone Miner Res.* 2002;17:513-520.
20. Goldring MB, Tsuchimochi K, Ijiri K. The control of chondrogenesis. *J Cell Biochem.* 2006;97(1):33-44.
21. Anderson HC. Vesicles associated with calcification in the matrix of epiphyseal cartilage. *J Cell Biol.* 1969;41:59-72.
22. Einhorn TA, Gerstenfeld LC. Fracture healing: mechanisms and interventions. *Nat Rev Rheumatol.* 2015;11(1):45-54. PMC. Web. 8 Nov. 2015.
23. Siddiqui JA, Partridge NC. Physiological bone remodeling: systemic regulation and growth factor involvement. *Physiology.* 2016;31:233-245.
24. Courpron P, Meunier P, Vignon G. Dynamics of bone remodeling explained by Harold Frost. Theory of the BMU (basic multicellular unit). *Nouv Presse Med.* 1975;4:421-424.
25. Ammann P, Rizzoli R, Bonjour JP, et al. Transgenic mice expressing soluble tumor necrosis factor-receptor are protected against bone loss caused by estrogen deficiency. *J Clin Invest.* 1997;99:1699-1703.
26. Kimble RB, Srivastava S, Ross FP, Matayoshi A, Pacifici R. Estrogen deficiency increases the ability of stromal cells to support murine osteoclastogenesis via an interleukin-1 and tumor necrosis factor-mediated stimulation of macrophage colony-stimulating factor production. *J Biol Chem.* 1996;271:28890-28897.
27. Manolagas SC, Jilka RL. Bone marrow, cytokines, and bone remodeling. Emerging insights into the pathophysiology of osteoporosis. *N Engl J Med.* 1995;332:305-311.
28. Pacifici R, Brown C, Puscheck E, et al. Effect of surgical menopause and estrogen replacement on cytokine release from human blood mononuclear cells. *Proc Natl Acad Sci USA.* 1991;88:5134-5138.
29. Cenci S, Weitzmann MN, Roggia C, et al. Estrogen deficiency induces bone loss by enhancing T-cell production of TNF-alpha. *J Clin Invest.* 2000;106:1229-1237.
30. Juppner H, Kronenberg HM. Parathyroid hormone. In: Favus MJ, ed. *Primer on the Metabolic Bone Diseases and Disorders of Mineral Metabolism.* 5th ed. American Society for Bone and Mineral Research; 2003:117-124.77.

31. Agholme F, Macias B, Hamang M, Lucchesi J, Adrian MD. Efficacy of a sclerostin antibody compared to a low dose of PTH on metaphyseal bone healing. *J Orthop Res.* 2014;32(3):471-476.
32. Ellegaard M, Kringelbach T, Syberg S, Petersen S. The effect of PTH (1-34) on fracture healing during different loading conditions. *J Bone Miner Res.* 2013;28(10):2145-2155.
33. Zhang D, Potty A, Vyas P, Lane J. The role of recombinant PTH in human fracture healing: a systematic review. *J Orthop Trauma.* 2014;28(1):57-62.
34. Barnes GL, Kakar S, Vora S, Morgan EF, Gerstenfeld LC, Einhorn TA. Stimulation of fracture-healing with systemic intermittent parathyroid hormone treatment. *J Bone Joint Surg Am.* 2008;90(Suppl 1):120-127.
35. Li YF, Zhou CC, Li JH, Luo E, Zhu SS. The effects of combined human parathyroid hormone (1-34) and zoledronic acid treatment on fracture healing in osteoporotic rats. *Osteoporos Int.* 2012;23(4):1463-1474.
36. Kogawa M, Anderson PH, Findlay DM, Morris HA, Atkins GJ. The metabolism of 25-(OH)vitamin D3 by osteoclasts and their precursors regulates the differentiation of osteoclasts. *J Steroid Biochem Mol Biol.* 2010;121:277-280.
37. Kogawa M, Findlay DM, Anderson PH, et al. Osteoclastic metabolism of 25(OH)-vitamin D3: a potential mechanism for optimization of bone resorption. *Endocrinology.* 2010;151:4613-4625.
38. Hofbauer LC, Gori F, Riggs BL, et al. Stimulation of osteoprotegerin ligand and inhibition of osteoprotegerin production by glucocorticoids in human osteoblastic lineage cells: potential paracrine mechanisms of glucocorticoid-induced osteoporosis. *Endocrinology.* 1999;140:4382-4389.
39. Ishida Y, Heersche JN. Glucocorticoid-induced osteoporosis: both in vivo and in vitro concentrations of glucocorticoids higher than physiological levels attenuate osteoblast differentiation. *J Bone Miner Res.* 1998;13:1822-1826.
40. Pereira RM, Carvalho JF, Canalis E. Glucocorticoid-induced osteoporosis in rheumatic diseases. *Clinics (Sao Paulo).* 2010;65:1197-1205.
41. Pereira RM, Delany AM, Canalis E. Cortisol inhibits the differentiation and apoptosis of osteoblasts in culture. *Bone.* 2001;28:484-490.
42. Weinstein RS. Clinical practice. Glucocorticoid induced bone disease. *N Engl J Med.* 2011;365:62-70.
43. Pearce G, Tabensky DA, Delmas PD, Baker HW, Seeman E. Corticosteroid-induced bone loss in men. *J Clin Endocrinol Metab.* 1998;83:801-806.
44. Gennari C. Differential effect of glucocorticoids on calcium absorption and bone mass. *Br J Rheumatol.* 1993;32(Suppl 2):11-14.
45. Kenkre JS, Bassett J. The bone remodelling cycle. *Ann Clin Biochem.* 2018;55(3):308-327.

2 Impairments to Fracture Repair

Varun Gudapati, Gregory Lupica, and Christopher Lee

KEY POINTS

- The goal of any fracture fixation is to provide the necessary interim stability to allow the biology of bone regeneration to heal the fracture.
- The general principle defining a fracture nonunion is a total time elapsed of 9 months since the injury with no radiographical sign of healing progression at the fracture site for the last 3 months. This can be clinically defined as a fracture that will not heal without further intervention.
- Nonunion rates vary across the literature and depend on multiple factors including patient characteristics, mechanism of injury, the bone fractured, and the location of the fracture.
- Higher-energy long bone fractures have the highest rates of nonunion.
- The economic burden of fracture nonunions in the United States correlates anywhere between $35,000 and $186,000 per nonunion.
- Independently, increased age is generally considered to be a risk factor for higher likelihood of nonunions.
- The role of smoking and nicotine in nonunions is of some debate, but it is generally accepted by physicians and practice guidelines that smoking impairs fracture healing.
- Obesity might lead to longer time to union secondary to increased fracture strain. However, increased leptin concentration in obesity theoretically has opposing effects on bone density.
- Diabetes is a clear risk factor that delays fracture healing, increases the risk of nonunion, and creates susceptibilities to infection.
- Although controversial, inhibition of cyclooxygenase (COX)-2 and prostaglandin pathways secondary to nonsteroidal anti-inflammatory drug (NSAID) use is generally regarded as having a minimal effect on nonunion rates while improving postoperative pain management. Theoretical impairment of fracture healing depends on which type of NSAID is being utilized.
- Corticosteroids directly affect osteoblasts and osteocytes, leading to decreased bone density along with higher rates of fractures, nonunions, and infections.
- Bisphosphonates have not been found to significantly affect fracture healing.
- Teriparatide, a parathyroid hormone analog, has been found to promote callus formation and accelerate fracture healing.
- Warfarin and heparin reduce bone density and impair fracture healing, while direct oral anticoagulants (DOACs) are not associated with significant changes to bone quality.
- Higher-energy injuries are associated with significant periosteal and soft tissue injury, leading to higher rates of nonunion. If the injury is open, this also carries an increased risk for infection, furthering the risk for a nonunion.
- Fracture location predisposes certain bones to higher rates of nonunion secondary to factors such as limited vascularity or typical injuries associated with higher-energy mechanisms.
- While stability is generally beneficial in the fracture healing process, some degree of interfragmentary motion is normal and facilitates appropriate callus formation.

- Critical size bone defects around 1 to 3 cm reduce strain and impair nutrient and cellular supply to fracture sites, increasing the risk of nonunion.
- Infection is a major and multifactorial cause of impaired fracture healing that requires significant surgical consideration.

INTRODUCTION

Bone regeneration is an integral process to the management of all fractures. Inherent to the treatment of any fracture is the race between the biology of bone regeneration and the failure of hardware or immobilization. When the biology of fracture repair loses, the result can lead to a fracture nonunion. The U.S. Food and Drug Administration defines a nonunion as a fracture that is at least 9 months old and has not shown any signs of healing for 3 consecutive months.[1] Although generally accepted, this definition relies solely on a time frame when in reality, there are many other factors that lead to fracture healing. For instance, the relative energy of the mechanism of injury, if the fracture is an open or closed injury, and fracture location can greatly affect the time to union of any fracture. In general, lower-energy closed fractures can be expected to progress to union in much shorter time than high-energy open long bone fractures.[2] It has been proposed that rather than relying solely on a specific time frame to define a nonunion, a more clinical and relevant definition would correlate to a fracture that will not heal without further intervention.

Classification of nonunions relies on infectious processes, physical examination, and radiographic appearance of the fracture site. Until proven otherwise, infection should always be considered as a principal factor leading to fracture nonunion. Known as **septic nonunions**, the most sensitive and easily available lab marker to detect infection is C-reactive protein. This acute phase reactant rises sharply in accordance with onset of clinical infection or tissue damage with peak elevation around 2 to 3 days and resolution to baseline between 5 to 21 days after initial insult when treated. While more sensitive and specific to IL-6 in detecting infections, C-reactive protein can be completely normal in more chronic infections where bacteria have formed a biofilm over implants, effectively helping to evade the body's immune response.[3,4] Thus, detection of infections can be clinically and serologically difficult.

Radiographic examination of the fracture site is also utilized to determine the extent or lack of callus formation. **Hypertrophic nonunions** are noted to have abundant callus formation and, thus, great biologic potential for healing. However, due to inadequate stability and substantial motion at the fracture site, these fractures go on to nonunion. **Oligotrophic nonunions** have poor callus formation on radiographs secondary to excessive motion, fracture fragment displacement, and impaired biology at the fracture site. Finally, **atrophic nonunions** have no radiographic callus formation with impaired vascularity and increased strain over the fracture site secondary to inadequate stabilization.[2,4,5] Classification of the types of nonunion allows the surgeon to determine necessary methods to improve fracture healing, whether it be improved stabilization, local and/or systemic antibiotics, or biologic adjuvants.

Nonunion Rates

Nonunion rates vary significantly in literature but are influenced by multiple factors including patient characteristics, the bone fractured, location of the fracture, age of the patient, and type of fracture. Mills et al[6] examined the rate of nonunions occurring in Scotland over a 5-year period in patients aged 15 years or more and found that an overall risk of nonunion per fracture was 1.9% with a slightly higher risk in men. The more commonly cited nonunion rate is estimated between 5% and 10% of all fractures, but certain diaphyseal fractures can have as high as 20% for certain injuries.[2,7,8] Interestingly, the age distribution was bimodal in males with the highest being in men aged 25 to 34 years while a unimodal distribution was noted in females aged 65 to 74 years.

Certain bones have higher nonunion rates than others. Current literature has documented high rates of nonunion in the scaphoid, femur, clavicle, humerus, and tibia fractures with 15% of scaphoid fractures, 8% to 13.9% of femur fractures,[7,9] 2% to 13.4% of humerus fractures,[9,10] 8.6% of clavicle fractures,[7] and 2.6% to 7.6% of tibial fractures,[7,9] whereas pelvic fractures have a rate around 1.3% to 5%.[6,11,12] It is important to recognize the factors that play into these nonunion rates as patients are subjected to substantial physical and mental burdens, chronic pain, and significant economic burden due to medical costs and lost income from delayed return to work.

Cost of Nonunions

Medical treatment costs for patients with nonunions are significantly elevated from that of fractures that heal without complication. A retrospective database study in 2023 in the United States found that the baseline increased cost of medical care for long bone nonunions varied between $33,000 and $46,000. With the additions of reoperation cost and nonunions secondary to infection, there was an added increase of $16,000 to $34,000 and $46,000 to $86,000, respectively, for a total of $95,000 to $186,000.[13,14] Nonunion treatments for single bone fractures within the United Kingdom were estimated between £7,000 and £79,000. Based upon a previously studied nonunion rate of 3.6%, this study estimated the annual cost for treatment on nonunions to be £320 million.[15] Per bone fractured, these estimates are greater than at least twice the cost of a normal fracture that goes on to union.[14,16] This substantial increase in medical expenditures along with the opportunity cost of lost wages poses a large financial burden to patients and their families.

RISK FACTORS

Risk factors of nonunion provide a framework for understanding impairments to fracture healing. They are multifactorial and often difficult to characterize. Several cohort, case-control, and randomized controlled studies have attempted to study the nature of these risk factors with conflicting results. Major challenges in studying these variables include the presence of confounding factors and the fact that these impairments exist on a spectrum without a clear threshold for clinical significance. Despite these barriers, they provide key insights both into predicting the incidence of nonunion and into targets for treatment intervention.

Patient Characteristics

Age

Older patients have decreased regeneration potential, which translates to a reduced capacity for bone healing.[17] Aging is associated with an increase in osteoclastogenesis and a relative increase of osteoclasts relative to osteoblasts.[18] Older patients experience a reduction in mesenchymal stem cell activity and poorer vascularity that impairs their ability to heal fractures. Additionally, aging is associated with the presence of other comorbidities that are independent impairments to fracture healing. While the theoretical framework suggests that age increases the risk of nonunion, clinical results are variable. A slight majority of clinical studies identify older age as a risk factor of nonunion, influenced by fracture site.[17,19] However, in some populations, aging is associated with a decreased rate of nonunion, potentially explained by the presence of lower-energy injury mechanisms in the geriatric population.[7] Independently, aging is considered to increase the risk of nonunion, but this relationship may amplify or diminish depending on other confounding risk factors.

Sex

Sex hormones modulate the bone healing response and create theoretical differences in fracture healing between males and females.[20] Notably, estrogen plays a role in bone development of both males and females and inhibits bone resorption by inducing apoptosis of osteoclasts.[21] Traditionally, this mechanism is considered to be protective for bone density and explains some of the vulnerability to osteoporosis in postmenopausal females. A study of femoral shaft fractures in mice found that female mice were dependent on estrogen for skeletal stem cell regeneration, which was not the case in male mice.[22] This tissue-specific sexual dimorphism explains differences in fracture healing rates observed in animal studies. A second study of femoral shaft fractures in mice noted more rapid and robust callus formation in male mice as compared to female mice, potentially modulated by increased osteoanabolic Wnt/β-catenin signaling and decreased estrogen receptor expression.[23]

Clinical studies have found variable results. For example, a cohort study of over 200,000 pediatric fractures found nonunion rates to increase in males.[24] In contrast, hip fracture rates and rates of nonunion following hip fracture have been found to be greater in females.[25] Multiple studies across fracture types have not found a significant difference in nonunion between males and females.[17] Ultimately, literature suggests that age and estrogen deficiency are major mediators in determining the specific effect sex has on fracture healing.

Smoking

Smoking is widely considered to create environments unfavorable to wound healing. Nicotine produces a vasoconstrictive and microthrombotic environment that disrupts cellular processes important for tissue healing.[26] Early study of smoking on tibial shaft fractures found a significantly high rate of nonunion in smokers.[27] However, more recent studies have provided conflicting evidence, with some even finding decreased rates of nonunion among smoking populations, and even biological studies provide sources of controversy.[17,19] Nicotine receptors promote angiogenesis, and the application of nicotine to wounds in the setting of diabetes in animal models has been found to improve wound healing.[28] Despite the inconsistent clinical findings, there is a general consensus among physicians and practice guidelines that smoking impairs fracture healing and that smoking cessation is an important intervention in the setting of an orthopedic injury.[29]

Obesity

Obesity has multifactorial and sometimes contrasting theoretical effects on fracture healing. Adipocytes arise from the same mesenchymal stem cell origin as osteoblasts, and it is hypothesized that in the setting of obesity, there are fewer mesenchymal stem cells available for the osteoblastic lineage.[30] These stem cells also have a reduced osteogenic response in the presence of increased leptin, as found in obesity, and increased inflammatory cytokines from excessive adiposity may stimulate bone resorption.[31-33] Increased body mass also increases fracture strain following stabilization, which can reduce the ability to form osseous bridging across a fracture site.

However, obesity also confers theoretically beneficial effects with regard to bone strength. Wolff's law suggests that the greater loading of bones stimulates the development of increased bone density.[34,35] At a molecular level, leptin has also been found to stimulate osteoblastogenesis and inhibit osteoclastogenesis, perhaps as an adaptive response to facilitate increased bone density in the setting of increased body weight.[36] This is in contrast to leptin's aforementioned reduction of mesenchymal stem cell osteogenic potential. Obesity has historically been considered a protective effect against fracture, which has been challenged in recent years by a growing body of conflicting clinical studies demonstrating increased or variable effects on fracture risk.[37] Studies assessing healing largely conclude that obesity causes a longer time to union and is an impairment to fracture healing.

Diabetes

The domestic and global incidence of diabetes has risen steadily over the past decades and is projected to continue to rise in the future.[38] Diabetes is a well-known impairment to fracture healing that merits increased or prolonged stabilization of fractures. The effects of diabetes on union are multifactorial but more clearly and consistently detrimental to fracture healing compared to smoking or obesity. The compromised microvascular supply impairs delivery of nutrients and progenitor cells to fracture sites; the proinflammatory environment delays progression into regenerative stages of healing; and hyperglycemia reduces osteoblast and increases osteoclast function.[17,19,39] Diabetes also indirectly increases the risk of nonunion via a concomitant increase in the risk of infection. Animal and human clinical studies consistently demonstrate delayed and decreased bone formation following a fracture and are thought to prolong time to union by over 80% and may double the risk of nonunion in certain fractures.[39,40] Some of the impairments caused by diabetes including effects on osteoblasts are mediated by hyperglycemia and suggest that strict glycemic control is an important measure to take in the setting of a fracture that may mitigate some of the nonunion risk associated with diabetes.[41,42]

Nutritional Status

Diet and nutrition are important factors in fracture healing that can be modified and monitored in the setting of a fracture. Amino acids, notably arginine, contribute to the bone healing process.[43] Increased dietary protein has been correlated with improved bone density at the hip and spine, though this relationship is contested, with some studies demonstrating an increased fracture risk in female populations with high protein intake.[44,45] In rats, increased protein intake was associated with more robust callus formation of femoral shaft fractures. Malnutrition is thought to impair fracture healing, and low albumin, which is a marker of poor nutritional status, has inconsistently been correlated with nonunion risk.[46]

While various micronutrients such as calcium, vitamin C, vitamin B_{12}, zinc, and magnesium have been identified as contributors to bone development and maintenance, vitamin D is of particular interest. Vitamin D plays a role in osteoblastogenesis, and some animal studies have noted improved fracture healing with administration of vitamin D, though this finding has not consistently replicated in humans.[47] Clinical studies often find that vitamin D deficiency is a significant risk factor for nonunion, and vitamin D levels are routinely included in the workup of nonunions.[46]

Genetic Disorders

Genetic skeletal disorders create clear disruptions in bone development and remodeling pathways that can impair fracture healing. Osteogenesis imperfecta (OI) has an incidence of up to 1 in 10,000 and is caused by mutations in the COL1A1 or COL1A2 genes that lead to defective type I collagen synthesis.[48] OI is characterized by impaired bone density with a high predisposition to fractures. A study of tibia fractures in mice noted that this collagen impairment resulted in reduced fracture callus size and strength and subsequently, biomechanical weakness at healed fracture sites compared to unfractured bones.[49] However, clinical studies have overall noted predictable fracture healing in patients with OI. A database study of over 40 tibial fractures in OI patients noted a 5% nonunion rate and concluded that while rates of fracture were significantly higher, union rates were comparable to patients without OI.[50] This may be attributed to the high vascularity and cellularity of bone in OI, which increases the rate of bone turnover and thus drives fracture remodeling.[51] Given this, treatment of fractures in OI is tailored more toward preventing or preparing for future fractures rather than toward mitigating nonunion risk.

Neurofibromatosis type 1 (NF1) has an incidence of up to 1 in 2,500 and is characterized by optic gliomas, cutaneous manifestations such as neurofibromas or cafe au lait spots, and skeletal dysplasia.[52] Mutations in the NF1 gene impair production of the tumor suppressor gene neurofibromin, leading to the development of the tumor sequelae described above. Neurofibromin regulates RAS, which may play a role in osseous development, and altered RAS signaling is thought to compromise fracture healing.[53,54] NF1 is associated with the presence of dysplasia and decreased bone density as well as an increased fracture risk that is less remarkable than that seen with OI.[55] The long bone dysplasia seen in NF1 creates focal defects with poor bone healing and risk of progression to pseudoarthrosis. Animal studies have noted premature apoptosis of osteoprogenitor cells in the setting of NF1 as well as impaired osteoblast differentiation with discordant phenotypes.[56] A clinical study of over 50 NF1 tibial pseudoarthrosis noted a postoperative nonunion rate of 13% as compared to 5% in non-NF1 patients.[57] Overall, both theoretical frameworks and clinical studies suggest that NF1 impairs fracture healing.

Osteopetrosis is associated with impaired osteoclast function, leading to hyperplastic and brittle bone. The defective osteoclast function results in impaired remodeling of the callous, delaying fracture healing and predisposing patients to nonunion.[58,59] Similarly, hypophosphatasia, which is characterized by decreased alkaline phosphatase activity, is associated with reduced bone quality, prolonged healing time, and nonunion risk.[60] Connective tissue disorders like Marfan syndrome and Ehlers-Danlos have been associated with a decreased bone density and increased fracture risk, but their effects on fracture healing have not been clearly defined.[61-63] While genetic skeletal disorders compromise bone quality in some way, they have nuanced effects on fracture healing. The different effects on healing time, nonunion risk, and recurrent fracture risk necessitate tailored treatment regimens.

Medications

The landscape of medications is ever changing as new drugs come to market and existing drugs fall in and out of favor. Medications are therefore the most dynamic category of risk factors. Perhaps the most studied and controversial are NSAIDs, given their widespread use for analgesia following orthopedic injury or surgery.

Nonsteroidal Anti-inflammatory Drugs

NSAIDs are among the most frequently used analgesics, available in both prescription and over the counter forms. Following orthopedic trauma, they can effectively reduce pain scores and opioid consumption.[64] NSAIDs act by inhibiting the COX enzymes. COX-1 is constitutively expressed and modulates thromboxane, prostacyclin, and prostaglandin function to facilitate a variety of functions including platelet aggregation, gastric protection, and renal function. COX-2 is inducible and primarily serves to mediate the inflammatory response via prostaglandin pathways.[65,66] The majority of NSAIDs are nonselective or partially selective and differentially inhibit both COX-1 and COX-2 expression, in contrast to celecoxib, a selective COX-2 inhibitor.

COX pathways also mediate bone healing, primarily through COX-2–mediated PGE2 expression, which plays a critical role in osteoblast differentiation and osteogenesis.[67] Mouse studies using COX-2 knockout mice reveal increased rates of undifferentiated mesenchyme and fibrous nonunion following stabilized tibia fractures, which could be reversed with the administration of PGE2.[68,69] This pathway establishes the clear theoretical framework as to how NSAIDs can disrupt osteogenesis and forms the basis for NSAID use as prophylaxis for heterotopic ossification. Given their high efficacy for postfracture pain control and the theoretical impairment to fracture healing, NSAIDs have been extensively studied in the context of nonunions.

In the 1970s, multiple studies were conducted to investigate the impact of indomethacin on fracture healing in rats and rabbits. Across both immobilized and nonimmobilized lower extremity fractures, these experiments convincingly found that daily administration of indomethacin was associated with reduced radiographic callous formation, decreased mechanical stability, and diminished histological osteogenesis.[70-74] These effects were amplified with dosage and nullified when cortical drill holes were used in the place of complete fractures. These studies established that indomethacin produced an observable reduction in osteogenesis, and on that basis, it remains a common choice for heterotopic ossification prophylaxis. However, they raised questions about how variables including type of NSAID, dose, duration, and fracture characteristics alter this effect.

Follow-up studies revealed that other NSAIDs may be less disruptive to bone healing pathways. Ketorolac, a commonly used intraoperative NSAID, was found to not impair osteotomy healing in rats, in direct comparison to indomethacin, which did.[75] Clinical studies have found both no significant increase in nonunion and some degree of increase in nonunions depending on dosages used. Celecoxib, a selective COX-2 inhibitor, yielded similar results; early animal studies showed no significant differences on fracture healing, but later investigation revealed dose-dependent impairment of fracture healing and increase in nonunions.[68,76]

While there is consensus regarding the theoretical impairment of fracture healing by NSAIDs via inhibition of COX-2 and prostaglandin pathways, the clinical significance of this impairment remains controversial. Variations in parameters including specific medication, dosage, treatment duration, and fracture characteristics has made it difficult to conclusively determine the consequence of NSAID use with regard to nonunion.

Current understanding guides and agreement that while NSAIDs cause some degree of suppression of the osteogenic response, a short course of NSAIDs has minimal consequences on nonunion rates while offering benefits of improved pain control and reduction of opioid usage.[17,74] Practices regarding the use of NSAIDs following fracture continue to vary dramatically based on differences in the perceived risk of nonunions.

Corticosteroids

Corticosteroids are potent anti-inflammatory medications with a variety of cellular targets. They are a mainstay of treatment in many autoimmune or inflammatory disease processes.[74] One of many effects of corticosteroids is to inhibit the conversion of phospholipids to arachidonic acid, a precursor to COX enzymes. Additionally, they have widespread direct cellular targets including osteoblasts and osteocytes. They inhibit the differentiation of osteoblasts and induce apoptosis of osteoblasts and osteocytes.[77,78] The imbalance between osteoblasts and osteoclasts in the setting of chronic corticosteroid use leads to noticeable decreases in bone density. Consequently, corticosteroids are the most common cause of secondary osteoporosis and even the most common nontraumatic cause of osteonecrosis.[79]

Similar to NSAIDs, early animal models demonstrated decreased callous formation and compromised histological osteogenesis with administration of cortisone in a dose-dependent fashion.[80] Clinical studies have supported these findings, widely demonstrating both an increased rate of fractures and of nonunions in chronic corticosteroid users.[81,82]

In addition to direct biologic effects, steroids are known to be associated with an increased risk of infections and can thus indirectly increase the incidence of nonunions.[83] Chronic corticosteroid use are mainstays of treatment in autoimmune or inflammatory disease processes that may themselves independently impair the fracture healing response.

Cessation of chronic corticosteroids may improve bone quality and healing, but frequently they are critical to management of systemic illnesses and may not be viable to stop in the setting of a fracture. Bisphosphonate use has been shown to improve bone density and improve secondary osteoporosis, reducing fracture risk, but its ability to alter fracture healing in patients using corticosteroids is not clear.[84]

Anti-osteoporotic Drugs

Osteoporosis is associated with a compromise of bony architecture and increased fracture risk, as well as a delayed and diminished cellular response and healing following fracture. Medications used in the treatment of osteoporosis are of interest because they directly affect anabolic and catabolic osseous pathways and address a pathology that itself is an impairment to fracture healing.[35,74]

Bisphosphonates inhibit osteoclast-mediated bony resorption. Nitrogen-containing bisphosphonates inhibit the mevalonate pathway in osteoclasts, disrupting the prenylation pathway downstream, and non–nitrogen-containing bisphosphonates induce cytotoxic metabolites and subsequently apoptosis in osteoclasts.[85] While this has been found to improve bone density and reduce fracture risk, the disruption of osteoclast pathways may reduce the efficacy of bony remodeling following a fracture. The theoretical impact of bisphosphonates on fracture healing is unclear, but clinical studies have shown that bisphosphonate use in osteoporosis does not significantly alter fracture healing.[74,86]

Denosumab and selective estrogen receptor modulators similarly do not appear to noticeably delay union time.[87,88] Other osteoporotic treatment medications may have more dramatic effects. Most recently, teriparatide is a parathyroid hormone analog that has been found to promote callus formation and accelerate endochondral ossification.[89,90] Current clinical understanding suggests that the most important role of medications that treat osteoporosis such as bisphosphonates is to reduce the risk of fracture, rather than to significantly alter the course of fracture healing.

Anticoagulants

Anticoagulant therapy is used in orthopedic and nonorthopedic contexts to prevent thromboembolic events.

Warfarin inhibits the enzyme vitamin K epoxide reductase, preventing vitamin K activation and thus impairing the production and function of vitamin K–dependent clotting factors.[91] Osteocalcin is a vitamin K–dependent peptide produced by osteoblasts to aid in bone mineralization whose function is impaired directly by the effects of warfarin and by the reduced dietary vitamin K intake recommended for patients on warfarin.[92] While the magnitude of osteocalcin's impact is controversial, case-control studies have found a decreased bone mineral density in patients on warfarin, suggesting that warfarin increases fracture risk and impairs fracture healing.[93]

Heparin is available as unfractionated heparin (UFH) and low molecular weight heparin (LMWH). Heparins binds to and activates antithrombin III, reducing the downstream conversion of fibrinogen to fibrin in the coagulation cascade.[94] Animal models suggest that UFH reduces osteoblast and promotes osteoclast function, leading to a loss of trabecular bone volume. LMWH similarly reduces osteoblast function as evidenced by a dose-dependent decrease in serum alkaline phosphatase but may not significantly promote osteoclast function.[95-97] However, LMWH may suppress vascular endothelial growth factor (VEGF)-mediated angiogenesis to a greater degree, which is a theoretical impairment of fracture healing, given VEGF's role as a mediator of ossification.[98,99] Though the relative impairment of fracture healing between UFH and LMWH is not clear, LMWH has been found to reduce bone density to a lesser degree compared to UFH. Seminal animal studies found that both warfarin and heparin comparably delayed fracture healing, with warfarin impairing fracture healing to a greater extent when started early.[100]

DOACs may not significantly impair fracture healing. While the effects of DOACs on fracture healing have not been clearly studied, they are associated with a more favorable effect with regard to bone density and a lower risk of fracture when compared to other anticoagulants.[101] Current conceptions of anticoagulants suggest that the use of particular anticoagulants such as warfarin, heparin, and aspirin and early initiation of anticoagulation following injury or surgery do impair fracture healing.[95] Though the timely initiation of anticoagulation is often crucial for appropriate thromboembolic prophylaxis following fracture, selection of certain agents may mitigate risks of nonunion or delayed union in vulnerable populations.

Fracture Characteristics

Fracture characteristics including the location, degree of injury, bone quality, and stabilization greatly affect their healing potential. The studies of other risk factors consistently demonstrate that fracture characteristics are also a modulator of vulnerability to other known risk factors of nonunion.

Degree of Injury

Higher degrees of injury are associated with a greater risk of nonunions. Animal models found that degree of injury, for example, comparing displaced fractures to drill holes, significantly modulated fracture healing compromise seen with medication administration. In the clinical setting, high-energy injury mechanisms and more severe injuries are associated with periosteal damage, which compromises the effective mobilization of stem cells and nutrients necessary for fracture healing and predisposes to other independent risk factors such as infection and use of analgesics.[19,102] Open fractures are inherently associated with significant periosteal and soft tissue injury as well as an elevated risk of infection. A large database cohort study found a nonunion rate of over 10% following open fractures, compared to less than 5% for closed fractures.[19] Similarly, a case-control study of operative fractures found a nonunion rate of 34% in open fractures, compared to less than 7% in closed fractures.[103]

Location

Fracture location correlates strongly with robustness of vasculature and thus fracture healing potential. A database cohort study of over 300,000 fractures found an overall nonunion rate of 5%, with a nonunion rate for scaphoid just above 15%, and nonunion rates for the tibia and femur around 14%.[19] Injuries associated with tenuous vascular supply including scaphoid fractures and fifth metatarsal metaphyseal fractures are predisposed to nonunion. Femur and tibia fractures are associated with high-energy mechanisms with periosteal and soft tissue injury that inherently harm healing potential. One contradictory observation is that patients with concomitant traumatic brain injury frequently have earlier and larger callous formation following femoral shaft fractures.[104,105] In contrast, metacarpal and distal radius fractures, commonly low-energy mechanisms are associated with some of the lowest rates of nonunion at 2% or below.[19] Various database studies incorporating different patient populations have found different overall rates of nonunion but similar trends regarding the impact of fracture types on nonunion risk.[6,106,107]

Stabilization

Inadequate immobilization is a known risk factor for nonunion and malunion and the primary motivator for surgical fixation of certain fractures. Perren strain theory explains that fracture healing is related to interfragmentary stability. High strain environments promote soft callus formation in an attempt to reduce the strain and allow for bony bridging. With excessive interfragmentary movement, the high strain environment prevents effective bony healing and results in a hypertrophic nonunion. Conversely, environments with excessive stiffness can cause a low strain environment without callus development, leading to an atrophic nonunion.[108-110] While stability is generally beneficial in the fracture healing process, some degree of interfragmentary motion is normal and facilitates appropriate callus formation. The 2% to 10% strain rule associated with Perren strain theory hypothesized that strains below 2% were conducive to primary bone healing, 2% to 10% conducive to secondary bone healing, and greater than 10% leading to nonunion. Though strain is widely agreed to influence fracture healing and nonunion risk, the particular quantitative thresholds of strain remain controversial and unclear.[111,112]

Mechanical considerations also guide risk profiles of fixation constructs. The two most commonly employed strategies for definitive fixation of long bones are plate and intramedullary nail fixation. Compression plating can offer rigid fixation and a path for absolute stability, and bridge plating can offer effective control over alignment in fractures with gaps or comminution.[108,113] Single-plate constructs are subject to cantilever stresses that asymmetrically load the fracture and may eventually lead to implant failure via cantilever bending or screw pull-out.[114] Asymmetrical strain environments can be a source of impaired fracture healing in the setting of plating, as can overly rigid constructs. In contrast, intramedullary nails are typically load sharing constructs that experience axial stresses and facilitate secondary healing. The axial compression and micromotion of fracture fragments stabilized by a nail promotes callous formation and thus fracture healing.[115] Consequently, fracture gaps can create significant vulnerabilities in nail constructs by forcing the nail to become entirely load bearing and compromising the axial interactions between fracture fragments. Clinical studies do not demonstrate a clear advantage between plating or nailing with regard to nonunion risk, but foundational biomechanical principles suggest that appropriate implant selection influences effective fracture healing.[116,117]

Fracture Gap

Large fracture gaps reduce strain and impair nutrient and cellular supply to a fracture site, increasing the risk of nonunion. Critical size bone defects are gaps that will not heal spontaneously despite appropriate surgical stabilization. There is no clear number that constitutes a critical size bone defect, but current understanding estimates 1 to 3 cm.[118] A retrospective study of open tibia fractures found that fractures with a radiographic gap above 2.5 cm did not achieve union and fractures around 2 cm had a high rate of nonunion.[119] The quantifiable understanding of how fracture gaps affect fracture healing is primarily associated with tibia fractures, but the general principle that a larger defect will impair bone healing can be applied broadly.

Infection

Fracture-related infections are a significant cause of nonunion that impair fracture healing via multiple mechanisms that have been found to occur in up to 5% of closed fractures and over 20% of open fractures.[120,121] The inflammatory response associated with infection is considered to be detrimental to bone healing. Osteoblasts share reciprocal interactions with the immune system, and a mouse model has demonstrated a reduction in osteoblastic bone formation in the setting of sepsis.[122,123] Additionally, chronic infections are associated with necrotic bone, which may present as a sequestrum. Necrotic bone impairs fracture healing processes and can serve as substrate for continued infection.[124] Another significant complication of certain infections is the formation of biofilm. Open fractures often sustain polymicrobial contamination, but *Staphylococcus aureus* is the most common causative pathogen of osteomyelitis and of infected nonunions. *S aureus* can induce apoptosis of osteoblasts and stimulation of osteoclasts, resulting in destruction of bone and facilitates biofilm formation on bone and implants, which reduces the efficacy of antibiotic and immune responses.[121] The presence of biofilm frequently necessitates additional surgical intervention, including the removal or exchange of implants, which subjects the fracture to additional instability. Fracture-related infections impair bone healing from a biomarker, cellular, and tissue standpoint, and clinical data supports this notion. Around 30% of femoral or tibial shaft fracture nonunions following intramedullary nailing are attributable to infection, and across clinical studies and surgeon consensus, infection is reliably identified as a risk factor for nonunion.[17,125]

CONCLUSION

Fracture healing is a complex and multifactorial process that relies on a stable macroenvironment and multiple molecular pathways. Nonunions are morbid complications of impaired fracture healing that result in significant detriment to physical and mental patient outcomes and lasting financial strain on patients and the health care system. Understanding impairments to fracture healing provides key insights into how nonunions risk can be mitigated at an individual or systems level.

The conflicting published clinical and biological data surrounding these impairments to fracture healing suggests that there is a greater nuance to the etiology of nonunions than surgeon consensus would suggest. Challenges begin with the diagnosis of nonunion, where practical radiographic and clinical ambiguity make it difficult to rely on the straightforward time frame–based definition proposed by the U.S. Food and Drug Administration. Incorporation of additional diagnostic tools and laboratory markers allow for a more holistic assessment that reflects that diverse array of variables that contribute to nonunions.

Additionally, available data makes it nearly impossible to understand the exact overall effect or relative importance of each etiology of nonunion, but considering them from a framework of theoretical mechanisms of action, laboratory studies, and clinical studies provides an effective basis for understanding risk factors.

Some variables including medical comorbidities, such as diabetes, and fracture characteristics—degree of injury, location, stabilization, infection—are strongly and consistently demonstrated to contribute to impaired fracture healing. Other widely studied risk factors such as NSAID, corticosteroid, and anticoagulation use have clear theoretical impairments to fracture healing but ambiguous clinical significance, which reflects the lack of clear consensus regarding medication use in the setting of fracture. Finally, while smoking and obesity do have theoretical and practical evidence to suggest that they impair fracture healing, in some regards, they also have subtle protective mechanisms that may partially mitigate this effect.

Clinical care should incorporate patient and fracture-specific risk factors and fracture characteristics. Many patient characteristics such as age, sex, obesity, and chronic comorbidities are either nonmodifiable or cannot be drastically altered within the time frame of a fracture healing event. Other characteristics such as smoking, nutritional status, and glycemic control can be addressed and optimized in the acute setting. In contrast, medication administration can typically be altered on a short-term basis. NSAIDs and anticoagulants are of particular interest because they are also frequently deployed in the care of fracture patients for analgesia and thromboembolic prophylaxis, respectively. Surgeons can select specific medications and dosages within these classes that maintain their clinical benefits while reducing deleterious effects on fracture healing. Finally, fracture characteristics are dictated by the nature of the injury and guide surgical techniques and management.

In conclusion, the successful management of nonunions requires a comprehensive understanding of multifactorial impairments to fracture healing. As clinical and biological models for fracture healing develop, future multivariate research approaches will continue to clarify the interdependent impairments to fracture healing.

References

1. Food and Drug Administration. Guidance document for industry and CDRH staff for the preparation of investigational device exemptions and premarket approval applications for bone growth stimulator devices. *Federal Register.* 1998;63(81).
2. Nicholson J, Makaram N, Simpson A, Keating J. Fracture nonunion in long bones: a literature review of risk factors and surgical management. *Injury.* 2021;52:S3-S11. doi:10.1016/j.injury.2020.11.029
3. Wang S, Yin P, Quan C, et al. Evaluating the use of serum inflammatory markers for preoperative diagnosis of infection in patients with nonunions. *BioMed Res Int.* 2017;2017:1-5. doi:10.1155/2017/9146317
4. Simpson AHRW, Robiati L, Jalal MMK, Tsang STJ. Non-union: indications for external fixation. *Injury.* 2019;50:S73-S78. doi:10.1016/j.injury.2019.03.053
5. Andrzejowski P, Giannoudis PV. The 'diamond concept' for long bone non-union management. *J Orthop Traumatol.* 2019;20(1):21. doi:10.1186/s10195-019-0528-0
6. Mills LA, Aitken SA, Simpson AHRW. The risk of non-union per fracture: current myths and revised figures from a population of over 4 million adults. *Acta Orthop.* 2017;88(4):434-439. doi:10.1080/17453674.2017.1321351
   Mills et al. performed a retrospective cohort study evaluating data from a population of over 4 million adults in Scotland. It found that the overall risk of nonunion is lower than previously reported, and that certain fracture types and patient factors (such as age and comorbidities) are more predictive of nonunion than traditionally thought.
7. Zura R, Braid-Forbes MJ, Jeray K, et al. Bone fracture nonunion rate decreases with increasing age: a prospective inception cohort study. *Bone.* 2017;95:26-32. doi:10.1016/j.bone.2016.11.006
8. Wolinsky PR, McCarty E, Shyr Y, Johnson K. Reamed intramedullary nailing of the femur: 551 cases. *J Trauma Inj Infect Crit Care.* 1999;46(3):392-399. doi:10.1097/00005373-199903000-00007
9. Tzioupis C, Giannoudis PV. Prevalence of long-bone non-unions. *Injury.* 2007;38:S3-S9. doi:10.1016/S0020-1383(07)80003-9
10. Sarmiento A, Horowitch A, Aboulafia A, Vangsness CT. Functional bracing for comminuted extra-articular fractures of the distal third of the humerus. *J Bone Joint Surg Br.* 1990;72-B(2):283-287. doi:10.1302/0301-620X.72B2.2312570
11. Lee KJ, Min BW, Oh GM, Lee SW. Surgical correction of pelvic malunion and nonunion. *Clin Orthop Surg.* 2015;7(3):396. doi:10.4055/cios.2015.7.3.396
12. Ekegren CL, Edwards ER, De Steiger R, Gabbe BJ. Incidence, costs and predictors of non-union, delayed union and mal-union following long bone fracture. *Int J Environ Res Public Health.* 2018;15(12):2845. doi:10.3390/ijerph15122845

13. Vanderkarr MF, Ruppenkamp JW, Vanderkarr M, Holy CE, Blauth M. Risk factors and healthcare costs associated with long bone fracture non-union: a retrospective US claims database analysis. *J Orthop Surg*. 2023;18(1):745. doi:10.1186/s13018-023-04232-3
Vanderkarr et al performed a retrospective database study evaluating additional treatment costs related to fracture nonunions. Marginal cost was found to be baseline ranging from $33K to $45K at 2 years post-index. When patients had undergone a reoperation, those costs further increased by $16K to $34K, and a concurrent fracture-related infection diagnosis further increased those costs by $46K to $86K.
14. Dunlop S, McCormack M, Zigler J, Neher R. PIT23 The cost burden of nonunion following long bone fracture in a commercially insured population in the United States. *Value Health*. 2019;22:S215.
15. Stewart S. Fracture non-union: a review of clinical challenges and future research needs. *Malays Orthop J*. 2019;13(2):1-10. doi:10.5704/MOJ.1907.001
16. Flores MJ, Brown KE, O'Marr JM, et al. The economic impact of infection and/or nonunion on long-bone shaft fractures: a systematic review. *OTA Int*. 2024;7(3). doi:10.1097/OI9.0000000000000337
17. Zura R, Mehta S, Della Rocca GJ, Steen RG. Biological risk factors for nonunion of bone fracture. *JBJS Rev*. 2016;4(1). doi:10.2106/JBJS.RVW.O.00008
Zura et al performed a systematic review of all referenced publications related to risk factors for nonunion over a 20-year period. They found a progressive increase in the annual publication of studies regarding nonunion and discussed conflicting outcomes seen with risk factors such as smoking, obesity, and medications.
18. Cao JJ, Wronski TJ, Iwaniec U, et al. Aging increases stromal/osteoblastic cell-induced osteoclastogenesis and alters the osteoclast precursor pool in the mouse. *J Bone Miner Res Off J Am Soc Bone Miner Res*. 2005;20(9):1659-1668. doi:10.1359/JBMR.050503
19. Zura R, Xiong Z, Einhorn T, et al. Epidemiology of fracture nonunion in 18 human bones. *JAMA Surg*. 2016;151(11):e162775. doi:10.1001/jamasurg.2016.2775
Zura et al performed a database cohort study of over 300,000 fractures across 18 bones and found an overall nonunion rate of 4.9%. OR for nonunion was increased with degree of injury, NSAID use, anticoagulant use, anticonvulsant use, opioid use, osteoporosis medication use, rheumatoid arthritis, and diabetes as well as other comorbidities.
20. Ortona E, Pagano MT, Capossela L, Malorni W. The role of sex differences in bone health and healing. *Biology*. 2023;12(7):993. doi:10.3390/biology12070993
21. Kameda T, Mano H, Yuasa T, et al. Estrogen inhibits bone resorption by directly inducing apoptosis of the bone-resorbing osteoclasts. *J Exp Med*. 1997;186(4):489-495.
22. Andrew TW, Koepke LS, Wang Y, et al. Sexually dimorphic estrogen sensing in skeletal stem cells controls skeletal regeneration. *Nat Commun*. 2022;13:6491. doi:10.1038/s41467-022-34063-5
23. Haffner-Luntzer M, Fischer V, Ignatius A. Differences in fracture healing between female and male C57BL/6J mice. *Front Physiol*. 2021;12. doi:10.3389/fphys.2021.712494
24. Zura R, Kaste SC, Heffernan MJ, et al. Risk factors for nonunion of bone fracture in pediatric patients. *Medicine (Baltimore)*. 2018;97(31):e11691. doi:10.1097/MD.0000000000011691
25. Endo Y, Aharonoff GB, Zuckerman JD, Egol KA, Koval KJ. Gender differences in patients with hip fracture: a greater risk of morbidity and mortality in men. *J Orthop Trauma*. 2005;19(1):29-35. doi:10.1097/00005131-200501000-00006
26. Silverstein P. Smoking and wound healing. *Am J Med*. 1992;93(1A):22S-24S. doi:10.1016/0002-9343(92)90623-j
27. Schmitz MA, Finnegan M, Natarajan R, Champine J. Effect of smoking on tibial shaft fracture healing. *Clin Orthop*. 1999;365:184-200. doi:10.1097/00003086-199908000-00024
28. Martin JW, Mousa SS, Shaker O, Mousa SA. The multiple faces of nicotine and its implications in tissue and wound repair. *Exp Dermatol*. 2009;18(6):497-505. doi:10.1111/j.1600-0625.2009.00854.x
29. Scolaro JA, Schenker ML, Yannascoli S, Baldwin K, Mehta S, Ahn J. Cigarette smoking increases complications following fracture: a systematic review. *J Bone Joint Surg Am*. 2014;96(8):674-681. doi:10.2106/JBJS.M.00081
30. Zaidi M, Buettner C, Sun L, Iqbal J. Minireview: the link between fat and bone: does mass beget mass? *Endocrinology*. 2012;153(5):2070-2075. doi:10.1210/en.2012-1022
31. Ke KX, Gao X, Liu L, et al. Leptin attenuates the osteogenic induction potential of BMP9 by increasing β-catenin malonylation modification via Sirt5 down-regulation. *Aging*. 2024;16(9):7870-7888. doi:10.18632/aging.205790
32. Yue R, Zhou BO, Shimada IS, Zhao Z, Morrison SJ. Leptin receptor promotes adipogenesis and reduces osteogenesis by regulating mesenchymal stromal cells in adult bone marrow. *Cell Stem Cell*. 2016;18(6):782-796. doi:10.1016/j.stem.2016.02.015
33. Rinonapoli G, Pace V, Ruggiero C, et al. Obesity and bone: a complex relationship. *Int J Mol Sci*. 2021;22(24):13662. doi:10.3390/ijms222413662
34. Frost HM. Obesity, and bone strength and "mass": a tutorial based on insights from a new paradigm. *Bone*. 1997;21(3):211-214. doi:10.1016/S8756-3282(97)00124-5
35. Gkastaris K, Goulis DG, Potoupnis M, Anastasilakis AD, Kapetanos G. Obesity, osteoporosis and bone metabolism. *J Musculoskelet Neuronal Interact*. 2020;20(3):372-381.
36. Thomas T, Gori F, Khosla S, Jensen MD, Burguera B, Riggs BL. Leptin acts on human marrow stromal cells to enhance differentiation to osteoblasts and to inhibit differentiation to adipocytes. *Endocrinology*. 1999;140(4):1630-1638. doi:10.1210/endo.140.4.6637

37. Turcotte AF, O'Connor S, Morin SN, et al. Association between obesity and risk of fracture, bone mineral density and bone quality in adults: a systematic review and meta-analysis. *PLoS One.* 2021;16(6):e0252487. doi:10.1371/journal.pone.0252487
38. National diabetes statistics report. *Diabetes.* July 23, 2024. Accessed January 5, 2025. https://www.cdc.gov/diabetes/php/data-research/index.html
39. Jiao H, Xiao E, Graves DT. Diabetes and its effect on bone and fracture healing. *Curr Osteoporos Rep.* 2015;13(5):327-335. doi:10.1007/s11914-015-0286-8
40. Loder RT. The influence of diabetes mellitus on the healing of closed fractures. *Clin Orthop.* 1988;232:210-216.
41. Medeiros C, Wallace JM. High glucose-induced inhibition of osteoblast like MC3T3-E1 differentiation promotes mitochondrial perturbations. *PLoS One.* 2022;17(6):e0270001. doi:10.1371/journal.pone.0270001
42. Yang L, Liu J, Shan Q, Geng G, Shao P. High glucose inhibits proliferation and differentiation of osteoblast in alveolar bone by inducing pyroptosis. *Biochem Biophys Res Commun.* 2020;522(2):471-478. doi:10.1016/j.bbrc.2019.11.080
43. Meesters DM, Wijnands KAP, Brink PRG, Poeze M. Malnutrition and fracture healing: are specific deficiencies in amino acids important in nonunion development? *Nutrients.* 2018;10(11):1597. doi:10.3390/nu10111597
44. Weaver AA, Tooze JA, Cauley JA, et al. Effect of dietary protein intake on bone mineral density and fracture incidence in older adults in the health, aging, and body composition study. *J Gerontol A Biol Sci Med Sci.* 2021;76(12):2213-2222. doi:10.1093/gerona/glab068
45. Karpouzos A, Diamantis E, Farmaki P, Savvanis S, Troupis T. Nutritional aspects of bone health and fracture healing. *J Osteoporos.* 2017;2017:4218472. doi:10.1155/2017/4218472
46. Christianson E, Thomas M, Sprague S, Rivera J, Chapple A, Zura R. Nutritional indicators of bone nonunion: a systematic review. *J Clin Med.* 2024;13(21):6553. doi:10.3390/jcm13216553
47. van Driel M, van Leeuwen JPTM. Vitamin D and bone: a story of endocrine and auto/paracrine action in osteoblasts. *Nutrients.* 2023;15(3):480. doi:10.3390/nu15030480
48. Marini JC, Dang Do AN. Osteogenesis imperfecta. In: Feingold KR, Anawalt B, Blackman MR, et al., eds. *Endotext.* MDText.com, Inc.; 2000. Accessed January 26, 2025. http://www.ncbi.nlm.nih.gov/books/NBK279109/
49. Zieba J, Munivez E, Castellon A, et al. Fracture healing in collagen-related preclinical models of osteogenesis imperfecta. *J Bone Miner Res.* 2020;35(6):1132-1148. doi:10.1002/jbmr.3979
50. Munk SA, Harsevoort GJ, Gooijer K, Edens MA, Franken AA, Janus GJM. Incidence and nonunion rates of tibial fractures in adults with osteogenesis imperfecta: a retrospective cohort study of 402 patients with 42 fractures at an expert clinic. *BMC Musculoskelet Disord.* 2022;23(1):1077. doi:10.1186/s12891-022-05966-7
51. Nijhuis W, Verhoef M, van Bergen C, Weinans H, Sakkers R. Fractures in osteogenesis imperfecta: pathogenesis, treatment, rehabilitation and prevention. *Children.* 2022;9(2):268. doi:10.3390/children9020268
52. Lee TSJ, Chopra M, Kim RH, Parkin PC, Barnett-Tapia C. Incidence and prevalence of neurofibromatosis type 1 and 2: a systematic review and meta-analysis. *Orphanet J Rare Dis.* 2023;18:292. doi:10.1186/s13023-023-02911-2
53. Anastasaki C, Orozco P, Gutmann DH. RAS and beyond: the many faces of the neurofibromatosis type 1 protein. *Dis Model Mech.* 2022;15(2):dmm049362. doi:10.1242/dmm.049362
54. Stevenson DA, Schwarz EL, Viskochil DH, et al. Evidence of increased bone resorption in neurofibromatosis type 1 using urinary pyridinium crosslink analysis. *Pediatr Res.* 2008;63(6):697-701. doi:10.1203/PDR.0b013e31816fee45
55. Heervä E, Koffert A, Jokinen E, et al. A controlled register-based study of 460 neurofibromatosis 1 patients: increased fracture risk in children and adults over 41 years of age. *J Bone Miner Res Off J Am Soc Bone Miner Res.* 2012;27(11):2333-2337. doi:10.1002/jbmr.1685
56. Yu X, Chen S, Potter OL, et al. Neurofibromin and its inactivation of Ras are prerequisites for osteoblast functioning. *Bone.* 2005;36(5):793-802. doi:10.1016/j.bone.2005.01.022
57. Zhu G, Zheng Y, Liu Y, et al. Identification and characterization of NF1 and non-NF1 congenital pseudarthrosis of the tibia based on germline NF1 variants: genetic and clinical analysis of 75 patients. *Orphanet J Rare Dis.* 2019;14(1):221. doi:10.1186/s13023-019-1196-0
58. Bhargava A, Vagela M, Lennox CME. "Challenges in the management of fractures in osteopetrosis"! Review of literature and technical tips learned from long-term management of seven patients. *Injury.* 2009;40(11):1167-1171. doi:10.1016/j.injury.2009.02.009
59. Bailey JR, Tapscott DC. Osteopetrosis. In: *StatPearls.* StatPearls Publishing; 2025. Accessed January 27, 2025. http://www.ncbi.nlm.nih.gov/books/NBK557529/
60. Stürznickel J, Schmidt FN, von Vopelius E, et al. Bone healing and reactivation of remodeling under asfotase alfa therapy in adult patients with pediatric-onset hypophosphatasia. *Bone.* 2021;143:115794. doi:10.1016/j.bone.2020.115794
61. Dolan A, Arden N, Grahame R, Spector T. Assessment of bone in Ehlers Danlos syndrome by ultrasound and densitometry. *Ann Rheum Dis.* 1998;57(10):630-633.
62. Coussens M, Banica T, Lapauw B, et al. Bone parameters in hypermobile Ehlers-Danlos syndrome and hypermobility spectrum disorder: a comparative cross-sectional study. *Bone.* 2023;166:116583. doi:10.1016/j.bone.2022.116583
63. Folkestad L, Stochholm K, Groth K, Hove H, Andersen NH, Gravholt CH. Fracture rates and fracture risk in patients with Marfan syndrome: a nationwide register-based cohort study. *J Bone Miner Res.* 2020;36(5):901-909. doi:10.1002/jbmr.4258

64. Murphy PB, Kasotakis G, Haut ER, et al. Efficacy and safety of non-steroidal anti-inflammatory drugs (NSAIDs) for the treatment of acute pain after orthopedic trauma: a practice management guideline from the Eastern Association for the Surgery of Trauma and the Orthopedic Trauma Association. *Trauma Surg Acute Care Open.* 2023;8(1). doi:10.1136/tsaco-2022-001056
65. Rouzer CA, Marnett LJ. Cyclooxygenases: structural and functional insights. *J Lipid Res.* 2009;50:S29-S34. doi:10.1194/jlr.R800042-JLR200
66. Ghlichloo I, Gerriets V. Nonsteroidal anti-inflammatory drugs (NSAIDs). In: *StatPearls.* StatPearls Publishing; 2024. Accessed December 25, 2024. http://www.ncbi.nlm.nih.gov/books/NBK547742/
67. Zhang X, Schwarz EM, Young DA, Puzas JE, Rosier RN, O'Keefe RJ. Cyclooxygenase-2 regulates mesenchymal cell differentiation into the osteoblast lineage and is critically involved in bone repair. *J Clin Invest.* 2002;109(11):1405-1415. doi:10.1172/JCI15681
68. Simon AM, O'Connor JP. Dose and time-dependent effects of cyclooxygenase-2 inhibition on fracture-healing. *J Bone Joint Surg Am.* 2007;89(3):500-511. doi:10.2106/JBJS.F.00127
69. Paralkar VM, Borovecki F, Ke HZ, et al. An EP2 receptor-selective prostaglandin E_2 agonist induces bone healing. *Proc Natl Acad Sci.* 2003;100(11):6736-6740. doi:10.1073/pnas.1037343100
70. Bo J, Sudmann E, Marton PF. Effect of indomethacin on fracture healing in rats. *Acta Orthop Scand.* 1976;47(6):588-599. doi:10.3109/17453677608988744
71. Elves MW, Bayley I, Roylance PJ. The effect of indomethacin upon experimental fractures in the rat. *Acta Orthop Scand.* 1982;53(1):35-41. doi:10.3109/17453678208992176
72. Keller J, Bayer-Kristensen I, Bak B, et al. Indomethacin and bone remodeling. Effect on cortical bone after osteotomy in rabbits. *Acta Orthop Scand.* 1989;60(1):119-121. doi:10.3109/17453678909150109
73. Keller J, Kjaersgaard-Andersen P, Bayer-Kristensen I, Melsen F. Indomethacin and bone trauma. Effects on remodeling of rabbit bone. *Acta Orthop Scand.* 1990;61(1):66-69. doi:10.3109/17453679008993070
74. Pountos I, Georgouli T, Blokhuis TJ, Pape HC, Giannoudis PV. Pharmacological agents and impairment of fracture healing: what is the evidence? *Injury.* 2008;39(4):384-394. doi:10.1016/j.injury.2007.10.035
Pountos et al summarized historical literature studying fracture healing associated with use of chemotherapy, corticosteroids, antibiotics, NSAIDs, anticoagulants, and bisphosphonates. All medications aside from bisphosphonates have some degree of evidence suggesting impairment of fracture healing with administration.
75. Reikeraas O, Engebretsen L. Effects of ketorolac tromethamine and indomethacin on primary and secondary bone healing. An experimental study in rats. *Arch Orthop Trauma Surg.* 1998;118(1-2):50-52. doi:10.1007/s004020050310
76. Brown KM, Saunders MM, Kirsch T, Donahue HJ, Reid JS. Effect of COX-2-specific inhibition on fracture-healing in the rat femur. *J Bone Joint Surg Am.* 2004;86(1):116-123. doi:10.2106/00004623-200401000-00017
77. Gado M, Baschant U, Hofbauer LC, Henneicke H. Bad to the bone: the effects of therapeutic glucocorticoids on osteoblasts and osteocytes. *Front Endocrinol.* 2022;13:835720. doi:10.3389/fendo.2022.835720
78. Jia D, O'Brien CA, Stewart SA, Manolagas SC, Weinstein RS. Glucocorticoids act directly on osteoclasts to increase their life span and reduce bone density. *Endocrinology.* 2006;147(12):5592-5599. doi:10.1210/en.2006-0459
79. Weinstein RS. Glucocorticoid-induced osteonecrosis. *Endocrine.* 2012;41(2):183-190. doi:10.1007/s12020-011-9580-0
80. Blunt JW, Plotz CM, Lattes R, Howes EL, Meyer K, Ragan C. Effect of cortisone on experimental fractures in the rabbit. *Proc Soc Exp Biol Med Soc Exp Biol Med N Y N.* 1950;73(4):678-681. doi:10.3181/00379727-73-17785
81. Sytsma TT, Thomas S, Fischer KM, Greenlund LS. Corticosteroid injections and risk of fracture. *JAMA Netw Open.* 2024;7(5):e2414316. doi:10.1001/jamanetworkopen.2024.14316
82. Liu SH, Cerri-Droz P, Ling K, et al. Chronic steroid use, complications, and readmission following open reduction internal fixation of distal radius fracture. *J Hand Surg Glob Online.* 2023;5(6):757-762. doi:10.1016/j.jhsg.2023.07.007
83. Youssef J, Novosad S, Winthrop K. Infection risk and safety of corticosteroid use. *Rheum Dis Clin North Am.* 2016;42(1):157-176. doi:10.1016/j.rdc.2015.08.004
84. Saag KG, Emkey R, Schnitzer TJ, et al. Alendronate for the prevention and treatment of glucocorticoid-induced osteoporosis. *N Engl J Med.* 1998;339(5):292-299. doi:10.1056/NEJM199807303390502
85. Drake MT, Clarke BL, Khosla S. Bisphosphonates: mechanism of action and role in clinical practice. *Mayo Clin Proc Mayo Clin.* 2008;83(9):1032-1045.
86. Gao Y, Liu X, Gu Y, et al. The effect of bisphosphonates on fracture healing time and changes in bone mass density: a meta-analysis. *Front Endocrinol.* 2021;12:688269. doi:10.3389/fendo.2021.688269
87. Shin YH, Shin WC, Kim JW. Effect of osteoporosis medication on fracture healing: an evidence based review. *J Bone Metab.* 2020;27(1):15-26. doi:10.11005/jbm.2020.27.1.15
88. Hino M, Tanaka M, Kamoi F, et al. Does early administration of denosumab delay bone healing after intertrochanteric femoral fractures? *J Orthop Sci.* 2025;30(1):136-141. doi:10.1016/j.jos.2024.03.005
89. Puvvada CS, Soomro FH, Osman HA, et al. Efficacy and safety of teriparatide in improving fracture healing and callus formation: a systematic review. *Cureus.* 2023;15(4):e37478. doi:10.7759/cureus.37478
90. Babu S, Sandiford NA, Vrahas M. Use of Teriparatide to improve fracture healing: what is the evidence? *World J Orthop.* 2015;6(6):457-461. doi:10.5312/wjo.v6.i6.457
91. Warfarin—an overview | sciencedirect topics. Accessed January 5, 2025. https://www.sciencedirect.com/topics/agricultural-and-biological-sciences/warfarin

92. Fawzy AM, Lip GYH. Warfarin and increased fracture risk? Answering the big question. *Age Ageing.* 2022;51(2):afab263. doi:10.1093/ageing/afab263
93. Osteocalcin—an overview | sciencedirect topics. Accessed January 5, 2025. https://www.sciencedirect.com/topics/agricultural-and-biological-sciences/osteocalcin#:~:text=Osteocalcin%20is%20a%2049%2Damino,vitamin%20K%20as%20a%20cofactor
94. Gray E, Hogwood J, Mulloy B. The anticoagulant and antithrombotic mechanisms of heparin. *Handb Exp Pharmacol.* 2012;207:43-61. doi:10.1007/978-3-642-23056-1_3
95. Lindner T, Cockbain AJ, Masry MAE, et al. The effect of anticoagulant pharmacotherapy on fracture healing. *Expert Opin Pharmacother.* 2008;9(7):1169-1187. doi:10.1517/14656566.9.7.1169
96. Muir JM, Andrew M, Hirsh J, et al. Histomorphometric analysis of the effects of standard heparin on trabecular bone in vivo. *Blood.* 1996;88(4):1314-1320.
97. Muir JM, Hirsh J, Weitz JI, Andrew M, Young E, Shaughnessy SG. A histomorphometric comparison of the effects of heparin and low-molecular-weight heparin on cancellous bone in rats. *Blood.* 1997;89(9):3236-3242.
98. Norrby K. Low-molecular-weight heparins and angiogenesis. *APMIS.* 2006;114(2):79-102. doi:10.1111/j.1600-0463.2006.apm_235.x
99. Hu K, Olsen BR. The roles of vascular endothelial growth factor in bone repair and regeneration. *Bone.* 2016;91:30-38. doi:10.1016/j.bone.2016.06.013
100. Stinchfield F, Sankaran B, Samilson R. The effect of anticoagulant therapy on bone repair. *J Bone Jt Surg.* 1956;38(2):270-282.
101. Tsai SHL, Hu CW, Shao SC, et al. Comparative risks of fracture among direct oral anticoagulants and warfarin: a systematic review and network meta-analysis. *Front Cardiovasc Med.* 2022;9:896952. doi:10.3389/fcvm.2022.896952
102. Ono N. The mechanism of bone repair: stem cells in the periosteum dedicated to bridging a large gap. *Cell Rep Med.* 2022;3(11):100807. doi:10.1016/j.xcrm.2022.100807
103. Quan K, Xu Q, Zhu M, Liu X, Dai M. Analysis of risk factors for non-union after surgery for limb fractures: a case-control study of 669 subjects. *Front Surg.* 2021;8:754150. doi:10.3389/fsurg.2021.754150
104. Giannoudis PV, Mushtaq S, Harwood P, et al. Accelerated bone healing and excessive callus formation in patients with femoral fracture and head injury. *Injury.* 2006;37(Suppl 3):S18-S24. doi:10.1016/j.injury.2006.08.020
105. Yang TY, Wang TC, Tsai YH, Huang KC. The effects of an injury to the brain on bone healing and callus formation in young adults with fractures of the femoral shaft. *J Bone Joint Surg Br.* 2012;94(2):227-230. doi:10.1302/0301-620X.94B2.28193
106. Calori GM, Albisetti W, Agus A, Iori S, Tagliabue L. Risk factors contributing to fracture non-unions. *Injury.* 2007;38(Suppl 2):S11-S18. doi:10.1016/s0020-1383(07)80004-0
107. Copuroglu C, Calori GM, Giannoudis PV. Fracture non-union: who is at risk? *Injury.* 2013;44(11):1379-1382. doi:10.1016/j.injury.2013.08.003
108. Perren SM. Evolution of the internal fixation of long bone fractures: the scientific basis of biological internal fixation: choosing a new balance between stability and biology. *J Bone Joint Surg Br.* 2002;84-B(8):1093-1110. doi:10.1302/0301-620X.84B8.0841093
109. Halvachizadeh S, Pape HC. Perren's strain theory and fracture healing. In: Crist BD, Borrelli Jr. J, Harvey EJ, eds. *Essential Biomechanics for Orthopedic Trauma: A Case-Based Guide.* Springer International Publishing; 2020:17-25. doi:10.1007/978-3-030-36990-3_2
110. Foster AL, Moriarty TF, Zalavras C, et al. The influence of biomechanical stability on bone healing and fracture-related infection: the legacy of Stephan Perren. *Injury.* 2021;52(1):43-52. doi:10.1016/j.injury.2020.06.044
111. Tanveer M, Klein K, von Rechenberg B, Darwiche S, Dailey HL. Don't mind the gap: reframing the Perren strain rule for fracture healing using insights from virtual mechanical testing. *Bone Jt Res.* 2025;14(1):5-15. doi:10.1302/2046-3758.141.BJR-2024-0191.R2
112. Inacio JV, Schwarzenberg P, Kantzos A, Malige A, Nwachuku CO, Dailey HL. Rethinking the 10% strain rule in fracture healing: a distal femur fracture case series. *J Orthop Res.* 2023;41(5):1049-1059. doi:10.1002/jor.25446
113. Stoffel K, Dieter U, Stachowiak G, Gächter A, Kuster MS. Biomechanical testing of the LCP—how can stability in locked internal fixators be controlled? *Injury.* 2003;34:11-19. doi:10.1016/j.injury.2003.09.021
114. Le T. *Biomechanics of Fractures and Fixation.* Presented at: October 2009. Accessed January 27, 2025. https://ota.org/sites/files/2018-06/G08_Biomechanics-%20Edited%20with%20Questions%20%5BCompatibility%20Mode%5D.pdf
115. *Intramedullary Nailing. AO Surgery Reference.* https://surgeryreference.aofoundation.org/orthopedic-trauma/adult-trauma/basic-technique/basic-principles-of-im-nailing
116. Li X, Chen K, Xue H, Cheng J, Yu X. Efficacy comparison between intramedullary nail fixation and plate fixation in distal tibia fractures: a meta-analysis of randomized controlled trials. *J Orthop Surg.* 2024;19:403. doi:10.1186/s13018-024-04900-y
117. Shah JK, Szukics P, Gianakos AL, Liporace FA, Yoon RS. Equivalent union rates between intramedullary nail and locked plate fixation for distal femur periprosthetic fractures—a systematic review. *Injury.* 2020;51(4):1062-1068. doi:10.1016/j.injury.2020.02.043
118. Schemitsch EH. Size matters: defining critical in bone defect size! *J Orthop Trauma.* 2017;31(Suppl 5):S20-S22. doi:10.1097/BOT.0000000000000978

119. Haines NM, Lack WD, Seymour RB, Bosse MJ. Defining the lower limit of a "critical bone defect" in open diaphyseal tibial fractures. *J Orthop Trauma*. 2016;30(5):e158-e163. doi:10.1097/BOT.0000000000000531
120. Lu V, Zhang J, Patel R, Zhou AK, Thahir A, Krkovic M. Fracture related infections and their risk factors for treatment failure—a major trauma centre perspective. *Diagnostics*. 2022;12(5):1289. doi:10.3390/diagnostics12051289
121. Hellwinkel JE, Working ZM, Certain L, García AJ, Wenke JC, Bahney CS. The intersection of fracture healing and infection: ORS Workshop 2021. *J Orthop Res Off Publ Orthop Res Soc*. 2022;40(3):541-552. doi:10.1002/jor.25261
122. Tsukasaki M, Takayanagi H. Osteoimmunology: evolving concepts in bone-immune interactions in health and disease. *Nat Rev Immunol*. 2019;19(10):626-642. doi:10.1038/s41577-019-0178-8
123. Terashima A, Okamoto K, Nakashima T, Akira S, Ikuta K, Takayanagi H. Sepsis-induced osteoblast ablation causes immunodeficiency. *Immunity*. 2016;44(6):1434-1443. doi:10.1016/j.immuni.2016.05.012
124. Lew DP, Waldvogel FA. Osteomyelitis. *Lancet Lond Engl*. 2004;364(9431):369-379. doi:10.1016/S0140-6736(04)16727-5
125. Simpson AH, Tsang JST. Current treatment of infected non-union after intramedullary nailing. *Injury*. 2017;48:S82-S90. doi:10.1016/j.injury.2017.04.026

3 Biology of Graft Substitutes

Devan D. Mehta and Philipp Leucht

INTRODUCTION

Bone grafting remains the mainstay of surgical treatment of certain complex fractures and atrophic nonunions. More than 500,000 bone grafting procedures are performed yearly in the United States alone, and on a global scale, this number is easily more than doubled.[1-3] Autologous bone graft has been accepted for decades as the gold standard due to its inherent biologic compatibility and excellent regenerative potential. However, the utilization of autograft is not always ideal or possible. Traditionally, bone autograft is harvested from the iliac crest, causing increased morbidity as patients experience significant donor-site pain and are at risk for complications such as infection, bleeding, and nerve damage. The harvest process also increases operative time and cost.[4] Another downside of autograft is that the harvestable volume is limited, and in many cases, it is not enough to address large segmental bone defects.[5] Furthermore, in patients with poor regenerative biology, such as those who have undergone radiation or chemotherapy, the efficacy of autograft would greatly be reduced.[6] In such circumstances, an orthopedic surgeon must be comfortable utilizing bone allograft or bone graft substitutes to augment a patient's inherent healing ability.

Thus, the question arises: what makes an acceptable and effective bone graft or graft substitute? On a superficial level, it is clear that the ideal graft material provides healing bone with increased regenerative potential, fills osseous voids, and provides mechanical support. The deeper, more sophisticated answer to this question is rooted in an understanding of the basic science of fracture healing and how an employed graft or adjuvant influences and augments this process in a given clinical setting. The aim of this chapter is to elucidate the inherent biologic attributes of successful grafting and to discuss how currently available graft materials and substitutes directly impact the bone healing process.

THE PROPERTIES OF IDEAL BONE GRAFT

Three qualities are essential for successful grafting: osteogenesis, osteoinduction, and osteoconduction (Figure 3.1). Osteogenesis is the ability of a graft's cellular elements to differentiate into bone matrix–producing osteoblasts. Osteoinduction is the ability of growth factors to recruit skeletal progenitor cells and induce osteogenic differentiation and osteoid deposition in osteoblasts. Osteoconduction describes the ability of a material to attract bone-forming cells and allow for their attachment and subsequent bone matrix deposition. These three characteristics are crucial for efficacious bone grafting and will be expanded upon below.

Osteogenesis

For a graft material to be considered osteogenic, it must directly provide the cells that produce and sustain bone, including skeletal stem cells (SSCs), osteoblasts, and osteocytes. In the setting of certain osteogenic cues, such as those resulting from an inflammatory response after fracture, SSCs are able to differentiate into osteoprogenitor cells that can further differentiate into osteoblasts, which ultimately lay down bone.[4,7] Endogenously, SSCs with the potential to differentiate along

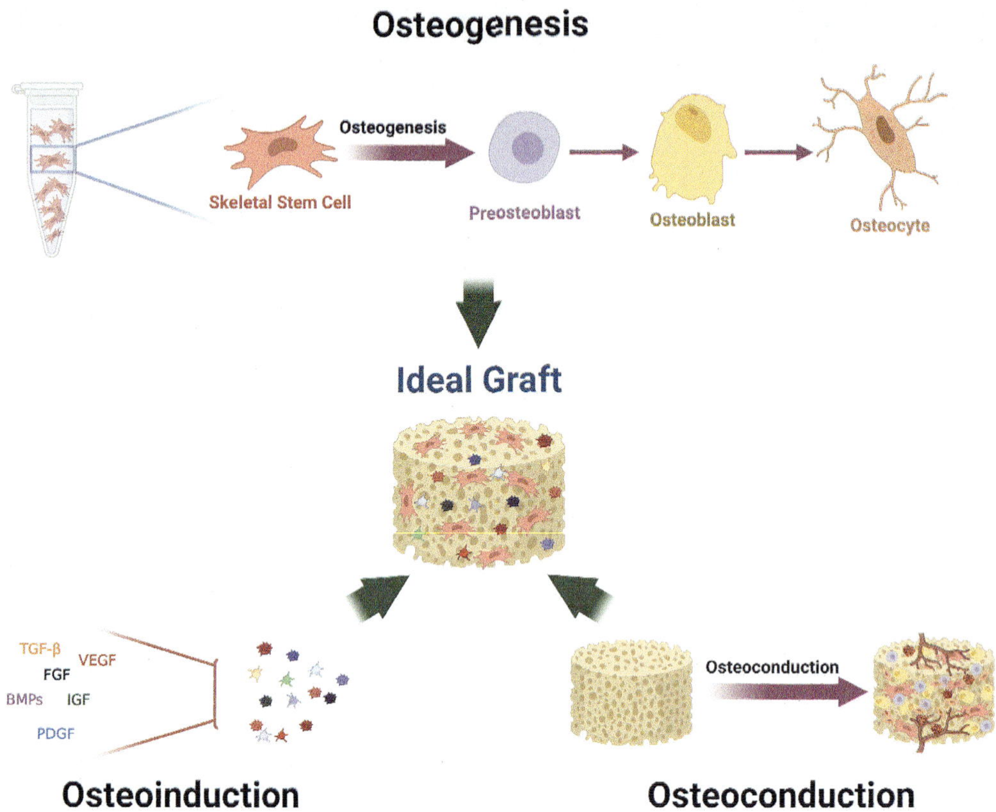

Figure 3.1. Three properties of the ideal bone graft. Osteogenesis is the ability of skeletal progenitor cells to differentiate into osteoblasts and osteocytes. Osteoinduction refers to growth factor effects on recruiting progenitor cells and inducing osteogenesis. Osteoinduction is the property of the graft to act as a scaffold for the cellular, vascular, and matrix elements of forming bone. The ideal graft requires these three characteristics. BMP, morphogenetic protein; FGF, fibroblast growth factor; IGF, insulin-like growth factor; PDGF, platelet-derived growth factor; TGF-β, transforming growth factor-β; VEGF, vascular endothelial growth factor. (Created in BioRender. Mehta, D. (2025) https://BioRender.com/k07s300.)

the osteogenic lineage are not only found in the periosteum, endosteum, and marrow cavity, but may also originate from overlying muscle, adipose tissue, or even from systemic circulation.[8]

In young healthy patients, there is no doubt that fresh bone autograft, most commonly from the iliac crest or from the femur via the use of a reamer-irrigator-aspirator, contains plentiful SSCs and bone-forming cells. These isolates also contain the inductive environment that is vital for osteogenesis. However, while the young skeleton is rich in skeletal progenitor cells, the abundance of bone-forming cells decreases with age.[9-11] In the older population, osteogenesis is limited by progenitor frequency, and thus, the treatment of fractures or nonunions may need to rely on other osteogenic grafts and adjuvants.

Bone marrow aspirate concentrate is obtained by bone marrow aspiration and centrifugal concentration and therefore increases the nucleated cell fraction of bone marrow aspirate. This concentrate has an increased number of progenitor cells in a given volume and can be mixed with cancellous bone chips or freeze-dried allograft and used to aid the healing of a bony defect.[12,13]

More recently, cellular bone allografts (CBAs) have gained significant momentum as an osteogenic autograft alternative. CBAs contain viable, lineage committed bone cells contained in an inductive corticocancellous matrix gel. This can be directly placed in a fracture or nonunion site, and because of its intrinsic osteogenic properties, it can promote bony regeneration with excellent efficacy.[14-16]

Osteoinduction

Historically, the concept of osteoinduction was advanced by Levander in 1938 after he discovered that crude alcoholic extracts of bone were able to induce bone formation when injected into muscle tissue. Over the past century, the authors have come to understand osteoinduction as the process that actively recruits host SSCs from surrounding tissue and promotes the osteogenic differentiation of these cells. In traditional teaching, bone matrix is considered osteoinductive because it contains certain growth factors and immunomodulatory cytokines that can promote osteogenesis. When this matrix is resorbed, as it is during the early stages of fracture healing, the released growth factors recruit SSCs and induce their osteogenic differentiation, leading to bone regeneration and remodeling. It is now known that in addition to growth factors embedded in the matrix, these factors are also secreted directly by reactive cells during bone healing.[17]

The main growth factors that act on the healing skeleton are the numerous bone morphogenetic proteins (BMPs), transforming growth factor-β (TGF-β), fibroblast growth factors (FGFs), platelet-derived growth factors (PDGFs), insulin-like growth factor (IGF), and vascular endothelial growth factor (VEGF). The cellular origin, biologic effect, and direct action on bone are expanded upon in Table 3.1.

After a fracture occurs, a clot is formed at the site of bony injury. Within this clot, platelet granules release TGF-β, PDGF, VEGF, and IGF. Then, during the inflammatory reaction, inflammatory cells such as macrophages secrete FGF, PDGF, and TGF-β. During bone regeneration, cells of the bone microenvironment including inflammatory cells, endothelial cells, fibroblasts, SSCs, and osteoblasts produce BMPs, PDGF, FGF, and VEGF. These factors play a large role in the migration and recruitment of osteoprogenitor cells from surrounding tissue including the

TABLE 3.1 Growth Factors Involved in Osteoinduction

Growth Factor	Cellular Origin	Biologic Action	Action on Bone Healing
Bone morphogenetic proteins (BMPs)	Skeletal stem cells (SSCs), osteoblasts, chondrocyte, endothelial cell	Osteogenesis, chondrogenesis, osteoinduction (BMP-2)	Progenitor cells differentiation toward bone-producing cells, recruitment of osteoprogenitors, matrix synthesis
Transforming growth factor-β	Platelets, osteoblasts, chondrocytes, SSCs, fibroblasts, macrophages	Angiogenesis, stimulation of cell growth, cellular differentiation, synthesis of extracellular matrix, immunosuppression	Proliferation of undifferentiated SSCs, recruitment of osteoprogenitors, differentiation of osteoblasts and chondrocytes, matrix production, osteoclast precursor recruitment
Fibroblast growth factor	Inflammatory cells, osteoblasts, chondrocytes, SSCs, endothelial cells	Proliferation of fibroblast and smooth muscle cells of vessels, angiogenesis	Maturation of chondrocytes, proliferation and differentiation of osteoblast
Platelet-derived growth factor	Platelets, monocytes, endothelial cells	Proliferation of connective tissue cells, collagen formation, angiogenesis, inflammatory cell chemotaxis	Osteoprogenitor recruitment, proliferation, and differentiation
Insulin-like growth factor	Osteoblasts, chondrocytes, endothelial cells	Regulation of effects of growth hormone	Matrix synthesis, osteoblast proliferation, bone resorption
Vascular endothelial growth factor	Platelets, osteoblasts	Angiogenesis	Cartilage conversion to bone, osteoblast proliferation and differentiation

endosteum and periosteum. Certain BMPs (BMP-2, -3, -4, and -7), IGF, and TGF-β are important in the proliferation and differentiation of the recruited osteoprogenitors.[18-20]

Bone grafts and bone graft substitutes contain these growth factors and are considered as osteoinductive. Of course, cancellous and cortical autografts are able to induce bone regeneration. CBAs also contain these active inductive factors. Demineralized bone matrix (DBM), which is prepared by decalcification of cortical bone, is another substitute that is highly osteoinductive. It is believed that DBM is more osteoinductive than regular allograft because the bioavailability of growth factors is enhanced following the demineralization process.[12]

Currently, two recombinant growth factors (rhBMP-2 INFUSE Bone Graft, Medtronic, and rhPDGF Augment Bone Graft, Wright Medical) are approved by the Food and Drug Administration for use as graft alternatives or adjuvants.[17,21,22]

Osteoconduction

Arguably, the easiest graft property to augment is osteoconduction. This is the process by which the graft acts as a scaffold and permits bone cell attachment and matrix deposition. The graft's biology and mechanical environment allow for an ordered, spatial three-dimensional ingrowth of vasculature, perivascular tissue, and SSCs.[4,23] This process of osteoconduction is vital because for bone grafting to be successful, new bone must be distributed evenly throughout the grafted volume and should unite with the local host bone. Without adequate osteoconduction, discontinuous bone formation leads to loss of mechanical strength and decreased function.

Decade-long research has provided a plethora of scaffold options with varying pore sizes, resorption times, mechanical properties, and customizable shapes. Cancellous autograft and allograft are both well-known to be osteoconductive. Commonly employed exclusively osteoconductive graft substitutes include calcium phosphate–based ceramics and cements, calcium sulfate cements, and solid DBM.[23]

Mechanical Support

In certain circumstances, a fourth vital property is needed for ideal bone grafting: mechanical support. For example, in the treatment of complex segmental fractures and nonunions, a graft material needs to be able to support mechanical loads and resist failure (eg, using a fibular strut graft for long bone nonunion). As another example, in treating a tibial plateau fracture with significant depression and bone loss, metaphyseal augmentation needs to be able to resist compressive forces. Cortical autograft and allograft, or vascularized autograft (eg, vascularized fibular struct graft), can provide excellent structural support and promote bone regeneration. In addition, calcium phosphate cements can also provide needed structural support.

AVAILABLE BONE GRAFT AND BONE GRAFT SUBSTITUTES

There are numerous options for bone grafts or bone graft substitutes available to the practicing orthopedic surgeon. Each of these have different properties in terms of osteogenic, osteoinductive, and osteoconductive capability. Table 3.2 expands upon the available bone grafts and graft substitutes. It is important to note that multiple grafts and/or graft substitutes may be combined to create a more efficacious graft. For example, bone marrow aspirate can be combined with allogenic cancellous bone chips to create a graft with the three ideal properties. The types and characteristics of the various available grafts and composites will be discussed in depth in the subsequent chapters.

TABLE 3.2 Properties of Bone Grafts and Bone Graft Substitutes

Graft or Graft Substitute		Osteogenesis	Osteoinduction	Osteoconduction	Mechanical
Autologous	Cortical bone graft	+/–	+	+	+
	Cancellous bone graft	+	+	+	–
	Bone marrow aspirate	+	+	–	–
Allogenic	Cortical bone graft	–	–	+	+
	Cancellous bone graft	–	+	+/–	–
	Cellular bone allograft	+	+	+	–
	Demineralized bone matrix	–	+	+	+/– (if solid)
Xenograft	Coralline hydroxyapatite	–	–	+	–
	Bovine xenograft (calcified matrix)	–	–	+	–
	Porcine xenograft (calcified matrix)	–	–	+	–
Ceramics	Hydroxyapatite	–	–	+	–
	Tricalcium phosphate	–	–	+	–
Cements	Calcium phosphate cement	–	–	+	+
Inorganic Scaffolds	Calcium sulfate	–	–	+	–
	Bioactive glass	–	–	+	–
Recombinant Growth Factors	rhBMP-2	–	+	– (w/o carrier)	–
	rhPDGF	–	+	– (w/o carrier)	–

+ present, – absent, +/– conditional.

REFERENCES

1. Campana V, Milano G, Pagano E, et al. Bone substitutes in orthopaedic surgery: from basic science to clinical practice. *J Mater Sci Mater Med.* 2014;25:2445-2461.
2. McAuliffe JA. Bone graft substitutes. *J Hand Ther.* 2003;16:180-187.
3. Greenwald AS, Boden SD, Barrack RL, et al. The evolving role of bone-graft substitutes. *Am Acad Orthop Surg.* 2010;83:98-103.
4. Khan SN, Cammisa FP, Sandhu HS, Diwan AD, Girardi FP, Lane JM. The biology of bone grafting. *J Am Acad Orthop Surg.* 2005;13:77-86.
5. Sagi HC, Young ML, Gerstenfeld L, Einhorn T, Tornetta P. Qualitative and quantitative differences between bone graft obtained from the medullary canal (with a reamer/irrigator/aspirator) and the iliac crest of the same patient. *J Bone Jt Surg Am.* 2012;94(23):2128-2135.
6. Jegoux F, Malard O, Goyenvalle E, Aguado E, Daculsi G. Radiation effects on bone healing and reconstruction: interpretation of the literature. *Oral Surg Oral Med Oral Pathol Ortal Radiol Endod.* 2010;109:173-184.
7. Fillingham Y, Jacobs J. Bone grafts and their substitutes. *Bone Jt J.* 2016;98B:6-9.
8. Knight MN, Hankenson KD. Mesenchymal stem cells in bone regeneration. *Adv Wound Care.* 2013;2:306-316.
9. Zhou S, Greenberger JS, Epperly MW, et al. Age-related intrinsic changes in human bone-marrow-derived mesenchymal stem cells and their differentiation to osteoblasts. *Aging Cell.* 2008;7:335-343.
10. Nishida S, Endo N, Yamagiwa H, Tanizawa T, Takahashi HE. Number of osteoprogenitor cells in human bone marrow markedly decrease after skeletal maturation. *J Bone Miner Metab.* 1999;17:171-177.
11. Muschler GF, Nitto H, Boehm CA, Easley KA. Age- and gender-related changes in the cellularity of human bone marrow and the prevalence of osteoblastic progenitors. *J Orthop Res.* 2001;19:117-125.

12. Nauth A, Lane J, Watson JT, Giannoudis P. Bone graft substitution and augmentation. *J Orthop Trauma.* 2015;29:S34-S38.
13. Dimitriou R, Jones E, McGonagle D, Giannoudis P. Bone regeneration: current concepts and future directions. *BMC Med.* 2011;9:66.
14. Baboolal TG, Boxall SA, El-sherbiny YM, et al. Multipotential stromal cell abundance in cellular bone allograft: comparison with fresh age-matched iliac crest bone and bone marrow aspirate. *Regen Med.* 2014;9:593-607.
15. Dekker TJ, White P, Adams SB. Efficacy of a cellular bone allograft for foot and ankle arthrodesis and revision non-union procedures. *Foot Ankle Int.* 2017;38:277-282.
16. Marino JT, Ziran BH. Use of solid and cancellous autologous bone graft for fractures and nonunions. *Orthop Clin NA.* 2010;41:15-26.
17. Miron RJ, Zhang YF. Osteoinduction: a review of old concepts with new standards. *J Dent Res.* 2012;91:736-744.
18. Devescovi V, Leonardi E, Ciapetti G, Cenni E. Growth factors in bone repair. *Chir Organi Mov.* 2008;92:161-168.
19. Marx RE. Bone and Bone graft healing. *Oral Maxillofac Surg Clin North Am.* 2007;19:455-466.
20. Albrektsson T, Johansson C. Osteoinduction, osteoconduction and osseointegration. *Eur Spine J.* 2001;10:S96-S101.
21. Baldwin P, Li DJ, Auston DA, Mir HS, Yoon RS, Koval KJ. Autograft, allograft, and bone graft substitutes: clinical evidence and indications for use in the setting of orthopaedic trauma surgery. *J Orthop Trauma.* 2019;33:203-213.
22. Peterson JR, Chen F, Nwankwo E, Dekker TJ, Adams SB. The use of bone grafts, bone graft substitutes, and orthobiologics for osseous healing in foot and ankle surgery. *Foot Ankle Orthop.* 2019;4:247301141984901.
23. Bhatt RA, Rozental TD. Bone graft substitutes. *Hand Clin.* 2012;28:457-468.

4 Basic Science and Use of Autogenous Bone Graft

John Michael Yingling and Mike T. Archdeacon

INTRODUCTION

Autogenous graft or "autograft" is defined as a material originating or derived from within the same individual, as opposed to an allograft that is obtained from a source of the same species but not genetically identical. Autogenous graft has provided the mainstay treatment to address skeletal injuries where bone loss, bone healing, and structural stability augmentation is required due to its osteoconductive, osteoinductive, and osteogenic properties.

As noted in Chapter 3, **osteoinduction** refers to the geometric scaffolding, which provides an environment for new bone apposition by supporting host capillary ingrowth, perivascular tissue, and osteoprogenitor cells. **Osteoinduction** refers to the ability of the graft to recruit pluripotent mesenchymal stem cells that differentiate into bone-forming osteoblasts and chondroblasts. **Osteogenic** material contains viable osteocytes or their precursors which promote primary bone healing.[1,2]

The ideal graft material is one that contains all three properties. The various donor sites have subtly different characteristics of these properties as well as advantages and disadvantages that depend on the patient's specific problem (Table 4.1). This first step requires establishing a proper diagnosis to define what the patient is lacking in order to select the most appropriate graft characteristics and donor site. Autograft is not without limitations, including donor-site morbidity, such as pain, infection, nerve injury; volume limits; accessibility; blood loss; and surgical time. However, it precludes worries of graft rejection, tissue compromise with processing, and graft-induced infection transmission that can occur with allograft.

LEVEL OF EVIDENCE

The literature summarized in this article is evaluated with the use of the levels of evidence ratings for studies addressing clinical care.[3] These levels are summarized with the use of Grades of Recommendation previously published in *The Journal of Bone and Joint Surgery*.[4] Grade A recommendations are based on consistent Level-I studies. Grade B recommendations are based on consistent Level-II or Level-III evidence. Grade C recommendations represent either conflicting evidence or are based on Level-IV or V evidence. A grade of I indicates that there is insufficient evidence to make a treatment recommendation.

TYPES OF AUTOGENOUS BONE GRAFT

Cortical bone graft provides an immediate structural osteoconductive medium with minimal osteoinductive and osteogenic properties. Consequently, it is best suited for defects that require mechanical stability for healing. The dense cortical matrix results in a relatively slow revascularization and incorporation. The limited perfusion and donor osteocytes make this a poorly osteogenic option, as resorption must occur before deposition of new bone. These grafts become weaker within the first 6 months of implantation due to resorption but regain structural integrity by 12 months (grade C).[1,5,6]

TABLE 4.1 A Summary of the Clinical Characteristics for Various Autograft Harvest Sites/Techniques

	Osteoconductive	Osteoinductive	Osteogenic	Cortical	Cancellous	Corticocancellous	Average Volume	Maximum Volume	Complications	Pros	Cons
Iliac crest	Excellent	Excellent	Excellent	Yes	Yes	Yes	13-30 cm^3	90 cm^3	Donor-site morbidity, persistent pain, deep infection, neurovascular injury, fracture	Most effective graft	Morbidity, increased time for harvest
Greater trochanter	Poor	Excellent	Good	No	Yes	No	5-10 cm^3	10 cm^3	Persistent thigh pain	Ease of access	Limited volume, no corticocancellous option
Proximal tibia	Good	Excellent	Good	No	Yes	Yes	25 cm^3	70 cm^3	Iatrogenic joint injury	Ease of access, larger volume	Limited volume, limited corticocancellous option, weight bearing restriction
Distal tibia	Good	Excellent	Good	No	Yes	Yes	2-3 cm^3	3 cm^3	Nonunion, iatrogenic fracture	Ease of access, corticocancellous option	Area prone to nonunion, small volume, weight bearing restriction
Distal radius	Good	Excellent	Good	No	Yes	Yes	3 cm^3	3 cm^3	Adhesions, wound complications	Ease of access	Low volume
RIA	Good	Excellent	Excellent	No	Yes	Yes	33-40 cm^3	90 cm^3	Iatrogenic fracture or joint injury, blood loss	Equal most effective graft, less time for harvest, low morbidity	Cost, blood loss

Cancellous bone graft, while providing less mechanical stability, contains all three characteristics, but most notably is a highly osteogenic substrate due to the porous trabeculae lined with functional osteoblasts.[2,7] The implanted osteocytes, graft porosity, and local cytokines promote angiogenesis and host mesenchymal stem cell recruitment that carry the potential to differentiate into osteoblasts.[2,8] Cancellous bone graft undergoes rapid vascularization within the first 2 days, bone formation within the first few weeks, remodeling by 8 weeks, and complete turnover via creeping substitution by 1 year. Creeping substitution is defined as concomitant osteoclastic resorption of necrotic donor trabeculae and osteoblastic osteoid deposition.[9] These features as well as the large surface area lead to rapid remodeling and incorporation, but no structural stability, making this graft a suitable choice for arthrodesis and nonunion treatment.[9-12]

Corticocancellous bone graft, as expected, provides osteoconductive structural properties from the cortical portion and osteoinductive and osteogenic from the cancellous portion. Usually harvested from the iliac crest as either unicortical, bicortical, or tricortical graft, it can be used to treat conditions that need mechanical stability and biologically active properties.

Vascularized bone grafts are cortical or corticocancellous grafts harvested with a vascular pedicle and therefore carry an immediate blood supply. Although there are technical aspects of graft harvest that make procurement more complex, this graft contains all three components and is highly osteogenic, as more than 90% of the original osteocytes typically survive. Vascularized bone grafts are often used to treat large segmental defects with voids over 12 cm (grade B).[1,5,6,13,14] Common donor sites for vascularized grafts include the iliac crest with its deep circumflex iliac artery, the fibular shaft with its peroneal branches, the distal radius with the supraretinacular artery, or the ribs with the posterior intercostal artery.

ILIAC CREST

Indications

Anterior or posterior iliac crest autogenous bone graft (IC-ABG) is the most common donor site for cancellous and corticocancellous graft. Depending on the patient's treatment requirements, unicortical, bicortical, tricortical, or purely cancellous segments can be harvested.[15] Average volumes for anterior iliac crest harvest are 27 cm^3, though there are reports of yields reaching 90 cm^3 with the acetabular reamer technique (grade B).[16,17] The posterior approach offers up to 30 cm^3, and a combination of anterior and posterior approaches can be utilized if inadequate volumes are obtained.[18]

Technique

Anterior Iliac Crest Harvest

Though not mandatory, a radiolucent table is recommended in the event intraoperative fluoroscopy is needed. The patient is positioned supine or lateral, depending on recipient site requirement. A linear incision is made starting approximately 3 cm posterior to the anterior superior iliac spine along the iliac crest to avoid injury to the lateral femoral cutaneous nerve and carried posteriorly as far as needed for the desired harvest, generally 3 to 5 cm. Be sure to next incise the external oblique fascia lateral and caudal to the palpable crest as the abdominal musculature inserts over the superior surface of the crest onto the lateral portion of the outer table. Sharply or with electrocautery elevate the external oblique fascia off of the bone and sweep away the iliacus muscle from the surface of the inner table as a single sleeve of tissue to protect the ilioinguinal and iliohypogastric nerves and facilitate closure. This exposes the iliac tubercle. The iliac tubercle and gluteal ridge provide a widened corridor of bone that is typically used for anterior iliac crest harvest. At this juncture, many techniques have been described[16,17,19-21] and are similar in the sense that cancellous bone within the inner and outer table is accessed through an osteotomy in the crest and harvested with a curet or similar instrument. When corticocancellous graft is desired, the authors' preferred technique is to split the crest and inner table with an oscillating saw to obtain only a unicortical segment of the inner table and crest with access to additional cancellous graft, as this maintains the shape of the outer table and pelvis facilitating an anatomic restoration of the abdominal musculature during closure. In a similar manner, a bicortical segment (the crest and inner table) or tricortical segment (the crest, inner, and outer table) can be obtained. The acetabular reaming technique can be used with this approach; the gluteal musculature is swept off of the outer table and an acetabular reamer, for total hip arthroplasty, is used to obtain graft by reaming the inner or outer table to obtain a morselized corticocancellous paste. This method yields as much as 90 cm^3 of graft and is reported to be faster than traditional methods decreasing operative time and cost (grade C).[16,17]

Posterior Iliac Crest Harvest

With the patient prone, an incision is made paralleling the posterior iliac crest centered over the posterior superior iliac spine with care to not injury the cluneal nerves. While maintaining the dorsal lumbar fascia and periosteum intact medially, expose the posterior superior iliac spine. With an osteotome or oscillating saw, create an osteotomy that hinges medially on the periosteal sleeve maintained to create a trapdoor opening, gaining access to cancellous graft. To decrease risk of penetrating the cortex of the greater sciatic notch or sacroiliac joint, limit the harvest to 4 cm deep and caudal to the posterior superior iliac spine.[2,19,22] The hinged cortical segment is then closed facilitating anatomic closure.

Complications

Although iliac crest is the most frequently used donor site for autogenous graft harvest, donor site morbidity is often stated as the decision to use allograft or other biologic treatment options. Complications are classified as either minor or major. Minor complications require no or minimal treatment and result in no long-term disability. Major complications require readmission, repeat surgery, prolonged hospital stay, or long-term disability. A review of the literature shows that minor complications occur in 7.1% to 39% and major complications in 1% to 10% depending on the series. Increased body mass index, medical comorbidities, and smokers have an increased risk of both major and minor complications (grade B recommendation).[16,23-26] Long-term pain at harvest site, superficial sensory nerve injury, superficial hematoma or seroma, and superficial infection are considered minor complications. Deep infection, hematoma or seroma that required operative drainage, permanent neurologic or vascular injury, incisional hernia, sacroiliac joint injury, ureteral injury, Trendelenburg gait, and donor site fracture are considered major complications. It is important to know and understand potential complications in order to minimize their occurrence.

GREATER TROCHANTER, PROXIMAL TIBIA, DISTAL TIBIA, DISTAL RADIUS

The greater trochanter, proximal tibia, distal tibia, and the distal radius all provide abundant cancellous, limited cortical and corticocancellous graft material and are generally selected when an ipsilateral limb is the recipient site due to ease of access and surgical positioning.

Greater Trochanter

Indications, Technique, and Complications

The greater trochanter is used as autograft during ipsilateral limb surgery, most commonly for acute femoral neck fractures with comminution. The authors' preferred method is to create a circular entry point within the lateral cortex of the greater trochanter with a trephine after a longitudinal incision has been made along the mid-axial line of the lateral thigh. Typically, about 5 to 10 cm of graft can readily be obtained, harvested in the direction of the femoral neck. Weight bearing is typically dictated by the fracture pattern but is usually restricted to a weight of leg, foot-flat protocol for the first few weeks in isolated scenarios. Persistent thigh pain has been reported in approximately 30% of patients but has been managed with conservative measures such as physical therapy and ice.[18,27]

Proximal Tibia

Indications, Technique, and Complications

The proximal tibia is an excellent source of autograft especially in the ipsilateral limb surgery as it is easily accessible and yields favorable volumes of not only cancellous graft but also corticocancellous and unicortical segments if desired. On average, this site produces about 25 cm^3 of cancellous graft but has reported volumes of up to 70 cm^3 (grade C).[21,28-32] Proximal tibia autograft harvest is contraindicated in patients with open physes. Medial and lateral condyle harvest site options have been described. The authors' preferred method is to use a 3-cm lateral approach centered over Gerdy tubercle. The incision is carried down to bone through the iliotibial band and anterior compartment fascia that are then reflected sharply anteriorly and posteriorly by elevating Sharpey fibers off of the bone, maintaining full thickness fascial layers for ease of closure. An oval osteotomy is then performed, as a rounded edge helps prevent propagation of fracture lines. The cancellous graft is then harvested using a curet or trephine, and the void is commonly filled with cancellous cadaveric allograft chips. The cortical segment is then replaced over the defect or morselized and inserted as autograft within the metaphyseal void. If metaphyseal bone is harvested beyond midline of the proximal tibia, the patient is restricted to non–weight bearing for 6 to 12 weeks (grade I). Complications have been reported as low as 1% to 2%, with persistent pain at harvest site being as high at 4% in some studies. Major complications are rare and include deep infection in less than 1%, joint perforation in 1.6%, and uncommonly nerve or vascular injury.[28,33,34]

Distal Tibia

Indications, Technique, and Complications

This site has traditionally been reserved to treat conditions of the foot and ankle due to its convenient location to the operative field, minimal blood loss, and short operative time (grade C).[35] The distal tibia metaphysis provides 2 to 3 cm of cancellous bone and even corticocancellous struts if desired (grade C).[36-38] A direct medial incision proximal to the medial malleolus above the level of the plafond is utilized with care to avoid the saphenous neurovascular bundle. A small cortical window is made with a trephine or osteotomes in an oval pattern to retrieve cancellous graft with a curet or similar instrument. A similar technique can be used from a direct anterior approach as well. The poor blood supply in this region makes this harvest site a poor choice to obtain larger quantities of graft, which has limited its use to surgery of the foot and ankle. Weight-bearing status is not influenced by this procedure and is usually dictated by the foot and ankle treatment. Rare complications of persistent donor site pain and hematoma can occur, but infection or fracture have not been reported (grade C).[36-38]

Distal Radius

Indications, Technique, and Complications

Similar to the distal tibia, the distal radius metaphyseal bone provides a readily accessible location for cancellous and corticocancellous graft harvest in the hand and upper extremity. This site can provide approximately 3 cm^3 of cancellous graft through a dorsal or volar approach (grade C).[35,39-44] The position of the limb, location of pathology needing treated, or areas of prior surgery will generally dictate the desired approach. The dorsal approach utilizes a longitudinal incision overlying Lister tubercle and dissection through the first and second extensor compartment with care to avoid injury to the superficial radial nerve. An alternative would be to use an incision and interval that is between the second and third extensor compartment to further protect the superficial radial nerve. A cortical window is then made with an osteotome, and cancellous graft is then harvested from the metaphyseal bone. The volar surface can be accessed with approaches used for fixing distal radius fractures and are familiar to most orthopedic surgeons. A longitudinal incision proximal to the wrist crease along the palpable tendon of the flexor carpi radialis or more radially centered over the radial styloid along the shaft of the radius is used for deep intervals between flexor carpi radialis and the radial artery or the radial artery and brachioradialis tendon, respectively. Pronator quadratus fascia is then incised along the radial border and swept ulnarly to gain access to the volar surface and obtain cancellous graft through a cortical window or corticocancellous segment as needed. The volar approach is perhaps more advantageous due to cosmetic concerns, familiarity of approach, avoiding insult to the extensor compartment tendons, painful adherence of scar tissue over the extensor surface, and less risk of injury to the superficial radial nerve.[43] Overall this site carries a low complication rate of less than 2% (grade C).[39]

Reamer-Irrigator-Aspirator

Indications

The reamer-irrigator-aspirator (RIA, RIA 2; Synthes) system is a single-use intramedullary reaming device that combines reaming with simultaneous intramedullary irrigation and aspiration. Its development was meant to decrease the risk of thermal injury to the bone from high-speed reaming of the canal and combat the pulmonary complications associated with standard reaming including fat embolism and acute respiratory distress syndrome secondary to high intramedullary pressures in polytraumatized patients. An unanticipated benefit was the harvest of large volumes autogenous intramedullary bone graft utilizing a minimally invasive technique.

The graft has been reported to effectively treat nonunion, segmental bone defects and for arthrodesis. Harvest volumes have been reported as high as 90 cm^3 in the femur and average about 30 cm^3 in the tibia and 40 cm^3 in the femur.[45-48] RIA autogenous graft harvest is indicated for patients at risk for infection at other harvest sites, who may have insufficient volumes of iliac crest bone stock, have previously had bone graft harvested from the iliac crest, or in patients in whom the volume of bone graft needed exceeds that which is available with traditional techniques (grade C).[46]

Studies show that graft material harvested in this manner maintain stem cell and osteocyte viability as well as the presence of biochemical proteins that are known to stimulate bone healing (grade B).[45,47,49,50] Studies comparing graft obtained from intramedullary reamings and iliac crest from the same patient and from different patients confirmed that angiogenic potential was lower in the RIA compared to IC-ABG samples but, via quantitative reverse transcription-polymerase chain reaction, showed that RIA had increased levels of growth factors including vascular endothelial growth factor, platelet-derived growth factor, and bone morphogenetic proteins (BMPs) among others.[47,49-51]

Specifically, from an *osteogenic* content perspective, RIA contains higher levels of mesenchymal stem cells, endothelial growth factors, and subsequently an increased calcium deposition.[52,53] A genome-wide transcriptional profiling of biochemical markers found in fracture healing demonstrated higher levels of vascular, skeletal, and hematopoietic transcription factors.[49] Histologic and transcription microscopy reviews demonstrate the *osteoconductive* macro- and micro-structure architecture of reamed intramedullary harvested bone is not disturbed.[54] Reamed debris and aspirate content showed higher levels of alpha fibroblast growth factor, platelet-derived growth factor, insulin-like growth factor 1, transforming growth factor-beta, and bone morphogenetic protein 2, all *osteoinductive* proteins. The total protein content was 2.1 times higher and only vascular endothelial growth factor and beta fibroblast growth factor were lower in the RIA versus the iliac crest samples.[50,55] Thus, intramedullary bone graft appears to be a viable alternative to the more traditional autogenous bone graft donor sites.

Technique

The reamed autograft is obtained by introducing the assembled RIA device over a guidewire within the intramedullary canal of either the femur or tibia using an inflow of normal saline and an outflow of suction that is collected in a filtered canister. The tibia is approached in an antegrade fashion similar to the approach used for intramedullary fixation of tibia fractures. The femur is approached through an antegrade or retrograde manner similar to that used for treating femoral fractures with an intramedullary device. The antegrade start point options for the femur are the greater trochanteric or piriformis fossa. Some authors suggest using the greater trochanteric start point, as the portal may theoretically decrease the risk of injury to the femoral neck compared to the piriformis start point (grade I)[45] though no difference in load to failure or mechanical behavior in biomechanical studies were found after cyclical loading of femora using greater trochanteric, piriformis, or retrograde intercondylar starting points (grade B).[56]

The reamer diameter is chosen by selecting a size 1 to 1.5 mm greater than the diameter of the isthmus of the femur or tibia being harvested. The RIA 2 system has a simplified unitized assembly and reamer diameters ranging from 10 to 18 mm. A 3.2-mm starting guidewire and fluoroscopy are used to find the desired start point. After insertion and confirmation of the position of the wire on the AP and lateral views, the wire is advanced, and the cortex is widened with an awl if necessary. This may not be required in scenarios with a patent canal from prior surgery. The starting wire is replaced with a ball tip guide wire, which may be slightly bent at the tip to manipulate the wire through the canal, ensure a centered wire within the canal, and prevent eccentric reaming. The guide wire advancement should stop at the level of the physeal scar of the distal femur and distal tibia and the area of the lesser trochanter of the proximal femur to prevent penetration of the adjacent joints and cortex.

If the greater trochanteric start point is chosen, ensure no greater than 10° of angulation of the guide wire from the canal is present as this may lead to eccentric reaming of the cortex and damage the reamer head connection. Prior to reaming, it is imperative to confirm the device and tubing are connected correctly and open, the desired filter is in the collection canister, and the irrigation and aspiration components are flowing appropriately. Continuously reaming while advancing is recommended as the initial torque and friction of the reamer head within a tight canal can cause iatrogenic fracture and fragmentation of the reamer head within the canal.[57] While reaming, the reamer should be advanced slowly, a few centimeters at a time, with frequent partial withdrawals to allow for emulsification of the canal material by the irrigation fluid and to avoid clogging of the aspiration portals. Once obtained, the intramedullary bone graft slurry can be mixed with cancellous allograft or demineralized bone matrix in a 3:1 ratio, three parts allograft or demineralized bone matrix to one part RIA, to increase graft volume.[58] After reaming procedure, fluoroscopy is performed to confirm no evidence of iatrogenic fractures or cortical breech. Reaming greater than 2 mm over the medullary canal diameter can decrease the torsional strength and lead to iatrogenic fracture (grade B).[45,48,59,60] Also, as a rule, the reamer should not be greater than 50% of the outer diaphyseal diameter.

Complications

Some advocate for reamed intramedullary autogenous bone graft versus IC-ABG due to donor site morbidity and limited volume of graft harvest reported with IC-ABG but RIA-ABG not without complication. The most notable complications are iatrogenic fracture and hemodynamic instability. Other issues regarding product malfunctions have been reported but eccentric reaming and aspiration of blood volume from the canal have been the most problematic. Due to the continuous suctioning of the canal during reaming, a large volume of blood has the potential to be aspirated. Average blood loss during RIA ranges from 200 to 500 mL, a mean hemoglobin drop of 4.4 mg/dL and in one study, 1 of 8 patients required blood transfusion.[46,60] Several case reports describe scenarios where up to 1,500 mL of blood have been aspirated, while reamer heads are incarcerated in the isthmus of the bone. In this event, the suction should be discontinued to prevent exsanguination. To reduce the risk of incarceration of the reamer head, reaming of no greater than 1.5 mm the diameter of the canal is recommended. Frequent fluoroscopic evaluation during reaming is important to ensure that eccentric reaming has not occurred and to reduce the risk of iatrogenic fracture. In the event significant eccentric reaming has occurred, the surgeon may advocate for a period of restricted weight bearing, usually non–weight bearing for approximately 6 weeks. The amount of restriction should be weighed by the goals of the surgeon and patient and the risk they are willing to allow with mobilization or restriction alike. In the event of an iatrogenic fracture, the fracture should be treated as the location and pattern dictates, which is usually an intramedullary implant.

Osteoporosis and osteopenia intuitively increase the risk of perforation and fracture; so, it is prudent to use additional caution and monitoring during reaming in this patient subset. In a series of 97 patients where RIA-ABG was harvested, 4.1% had iatrogenic fracture, and osteoporosis was noted as a risk factor.[48] Iliac crest has the aforementioned major complications in up to 18% and minor complications up to 39%. Qvick et al[61] noted a 1.96% major complication rate consisting of three donor site fractures and one femoral cortex penetration in a series of 204 RIA procedures. Belthur et al[45] reported a 4.8% complication rate in a comparison study of 41 patients with RIA-ABG harvest compared to an unmatched IC-ABG control group.

Outcomes and Clinical Applications

Reamed autogenous bone graft has been compared to other sources in the clinical settings of nonunion, segmental bone defects, and arthrodesis. Originally, Hammer et al[62] compared traditional reaming to RIA in tibia defects of sheep and found significant improvements in volume, stiffness, and strength of early callus signifying its utility in bone healing. Small series of studies demonstrate successful treatment of nonunions using RIA autograft.[46,47,63,64] Segmental bone loss has also been successfully treated using reamed autograft. McCall et al[47] reported that 85% of bone defects averaging 6.6 cm had healed by 11 months in their series of 21 patients. Similarly, Stafford and Norris demonstrated a union rate of 90% at 1 year in their series treating bone defects 5.8 cm on average with no RIA-related complications. A recent multicenter, prospective, randomized study of 133 patients comparing RIA and IC-ABG showed that reamed intramedullary autograft had comparable union rates, less donor site pain, and greater volume on average than IC-ABG (grade A).[65] This study noted that the RIA device is considerably more expensive than the bone graft harvest tray, but took significantly less time harvest, and after a comparison was found to be the cost conservative option.

RIA use in the setting of arthrodesis has primarily been studied for fusions in the foot and ankle as opposed to the spine likely due to the exposure required for surgery of the appendicular skeleton. Nodzo et al[66] reported a higher fusion rate with RIA compared to iliac crest in their matched cohort for arthrodesis of the tibiotalar joint. Though rare, reports of using RIA in spinal fusions have been successful when posterior iliac crest is contraindicated.[66,67] Overall, RIA is a viable, renewable, accessible, and cost-effective method to treat nonunion, segmental bone defects and arthrodesis procedures with the capacity to obtain large volumes of graft, quickly, with acceptable morbidity and complication rates.

CASE EXAMPLES

Case 1

A 66-year-old male presented to the authors' institution from an outside facility as a referral for hip pain, proximal femur nonunion, and implant failure (Figure 4.1). The patient sustained an isolated subtrochanteric femur fracture 4 months prior after falling from a height of about 4 ft and was treated acutely with a cephalomedullary implant. The patient had been gradually progressing but continued to have an antalgic gait and hip pain with new-onset thigh and knee pain and sought care. The injury was closed with no known history of infection. The patient is a nonsmoker, had no medical problems, no recent infections, and a remote history of a healed ipsilateral tibial shaft treated with open reduction internal fixation (ORIF) with no issues. On examination, the patient ambulated with an antalgic gait and proximal thigh and knee pain but otherwise neurovascularly intact with healed surgical wounds with no sign of infection.

- **Stage I**: Although a single stage procedure is often chosen, the authors elected a staged approach to ensure no occult infection was present. Removal of implant, tissue culture, and biopsy with implantation of antibiotic rod and closure. Plan to return to OR in 10 to 14 days after final cultures have resulted confirming no concomitant infection for revision fixation and autogenous grafting (Figure 4.2).
- **Stage II**: After confirmation of normal metabolic and inflammatory lab values and no organism growth from cultures, removal of the antibiotic rod and harvest of ipsilateral proximal tibia cancellous autograft was obtained for implantation. Reamed intramedullary graft harvest of the tibia is also a viable choice. Although RIA of ipsilateral femur is an option, we elected to

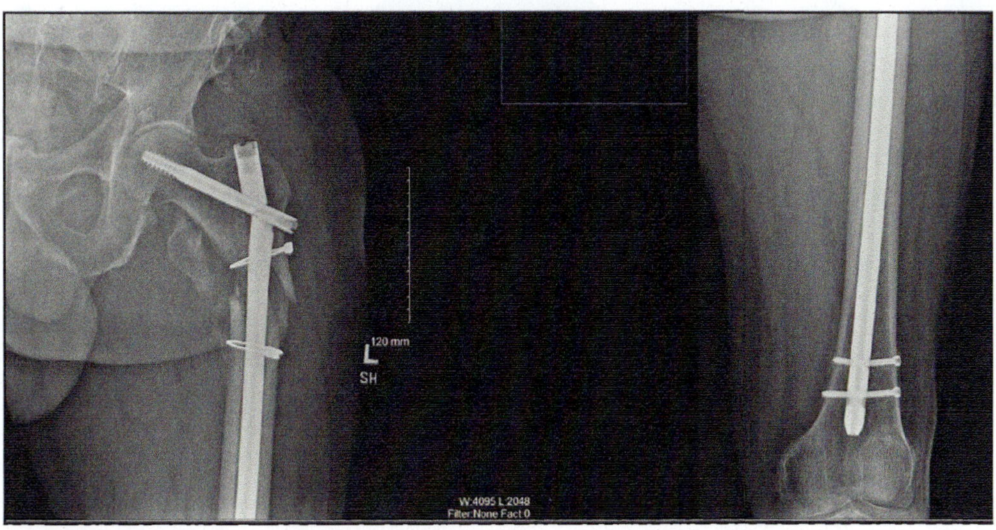

Figure 4.1. AP views of a left femur demonstrating a proximal femur nonunion and implant failure around a cephalomedullary implant.

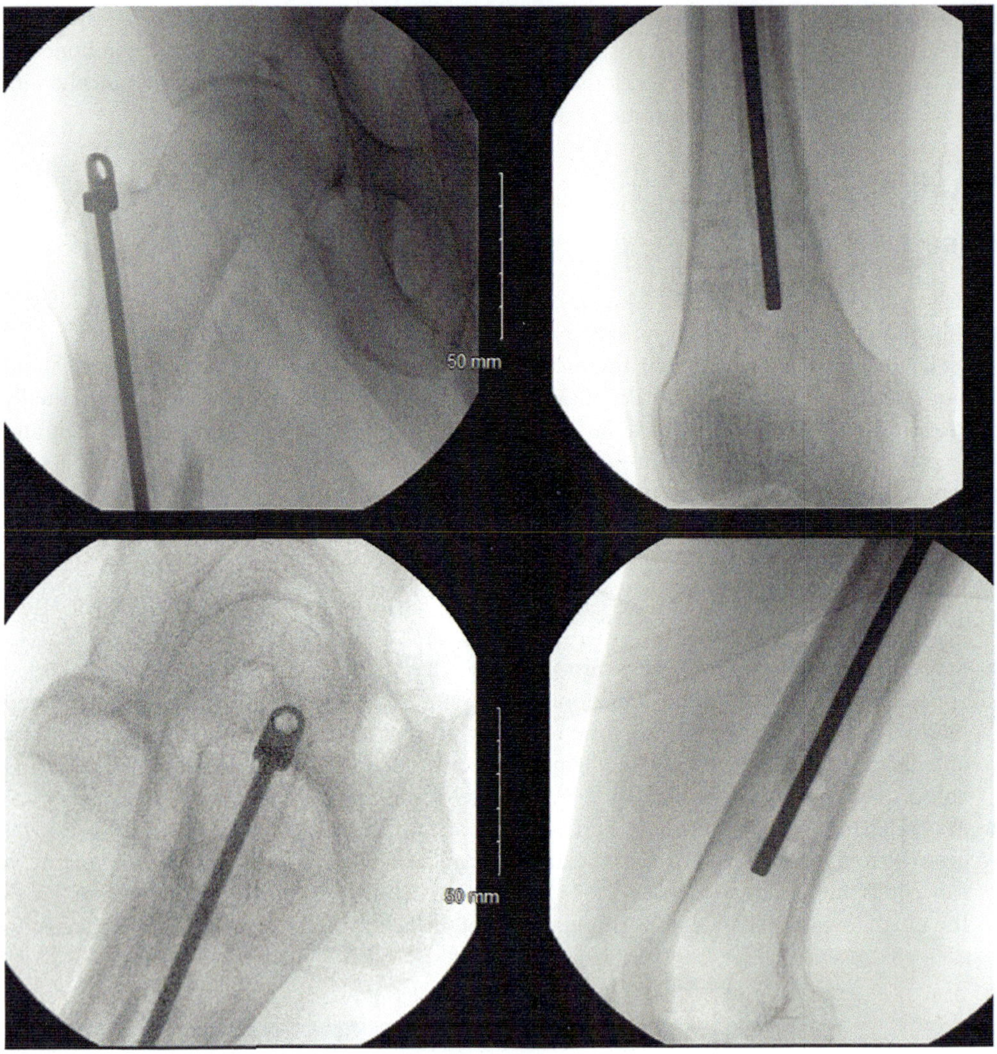

Figure 4.2. Fluoroscopic AP and lateral views of the proximal and distal femur demonstrating the implantation of the antibiotic rod in the location of the prior implant.

harvest graft from the proximal tibia to avoid an area with a prior implant placed, subclinical bacterial colonization, possibly fibrous scar tissue with fewer osteoinductive, osteoconductive, and osteogenic properties than the proximal tibia cancellous harvest, and avoid violating the knee joint. A 4-cm incision over Gerdy tubercle was carried through skin and subcutaneous tissue. The anterior compartment fascia and the iliotibial band were elevated in a subperiosteal manner exposing Gerdy tubercle, which was osteotomized with a Capener gouge. Twenty-five milliliters of cancellous autogenous bone graft was obtained from the proximal tibia. Fifty milliliters of cancellous allograft were packed into the wound and into the bone deficit in the proximal tibia. Layered closure and a sterile occlusive dressing were applied (Figure 4.3).

Revision cephalomedullary fixation was performed, and the autogenous graft was placed at the nonunion site (Figure 4.4).

The patient was followed with serial radiographs with 6-month follow-up images shown demonstrating abundant callus formation and healing of nonunion site (Figure 4.5).

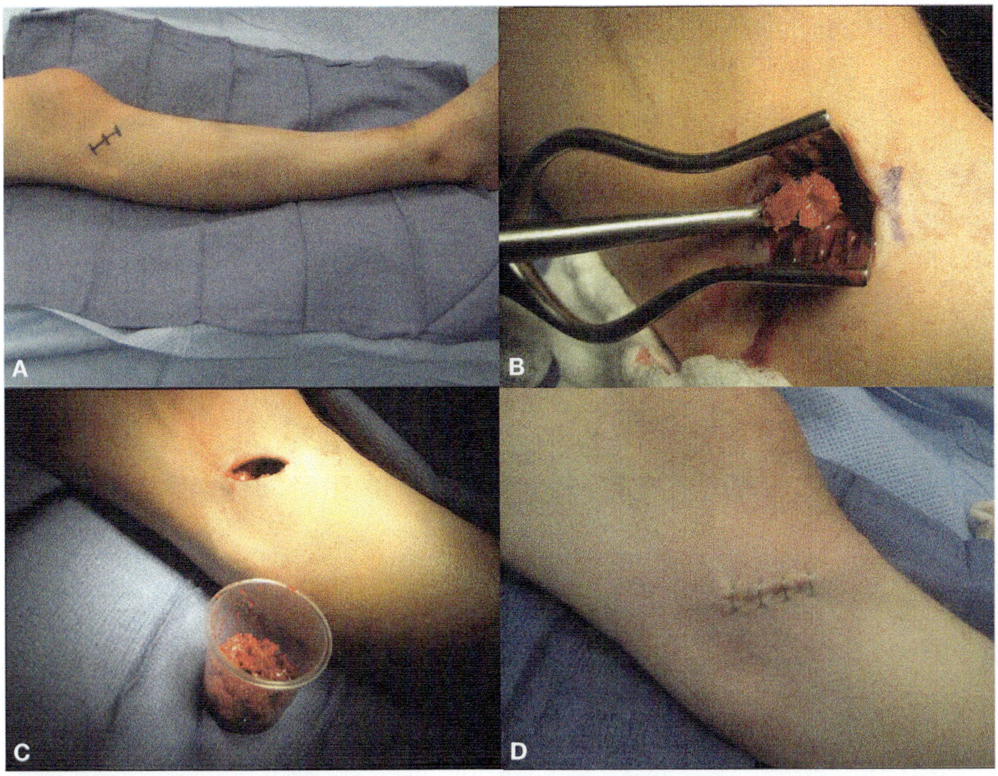

Figure 4.3. **A.** Marking for 3-cm incision over Gerdy tubercle. **B.** Cancellous autogenous bone graft from proximal tibia. **C.** Gross appearance of autogenous autograft and harvest site. **D.** Layered closure.

Case 2

A 26-year-old female, multiple injured trauma patient sustained operative upper and lower extremity injuries including a right open humeral shaft fracture that was treated with débridement, irrigation, and ORIF. At five months postoperative, the patient presented with an infected nonunion. Cultures were positive for methicillin-resistent Staphlococcus aureus consitent with a septic nonunion and osteomyelitis (Figure 4.6) that was treated with resection of nonviable bone, antibiotic spacer, and long-term intravenous antibiotics (Figure 4.7).

After inflammatory lab values normalized and another staged culture and débridement, a revision ORIF with bicortical iliac crest autograft was performed. A 10-cm direct approach to the iliac crest was carried through skin and subcutaneous tissue elevating the external oblique over the crest of the ilium. A bicortical graft from the iliac crest and the medial inner table preserving the outer table and proximal edge (Figure 4.8A) was obtained using a small saw. Multiple curettes were then used to obtain inner table cancellous bone graft. The wound was copiously irrigated, and the external oblique fascia was approximated in an anatomic manner to the tensor fascia lata and gluteus maximus fascia. The humerus was preliminarily fixated into place using a 2.7-mm plate to obtain length and alignment (Figure 4.8B). The bicortical iliac crest was then contoured with a rongeur to fit the defect and secured using 2.7-mm screws (see Figure 4.8B). Then a 3.5-mm dynamic compression plate was applied to the orthogonal surface (Figure 4.8C) and the remainder of the cancellous graft was packed around the defect and the wound closed in layers. Six-month follow-up demonstrates clinical and radiographic union of her humerus (Figure 4.9).

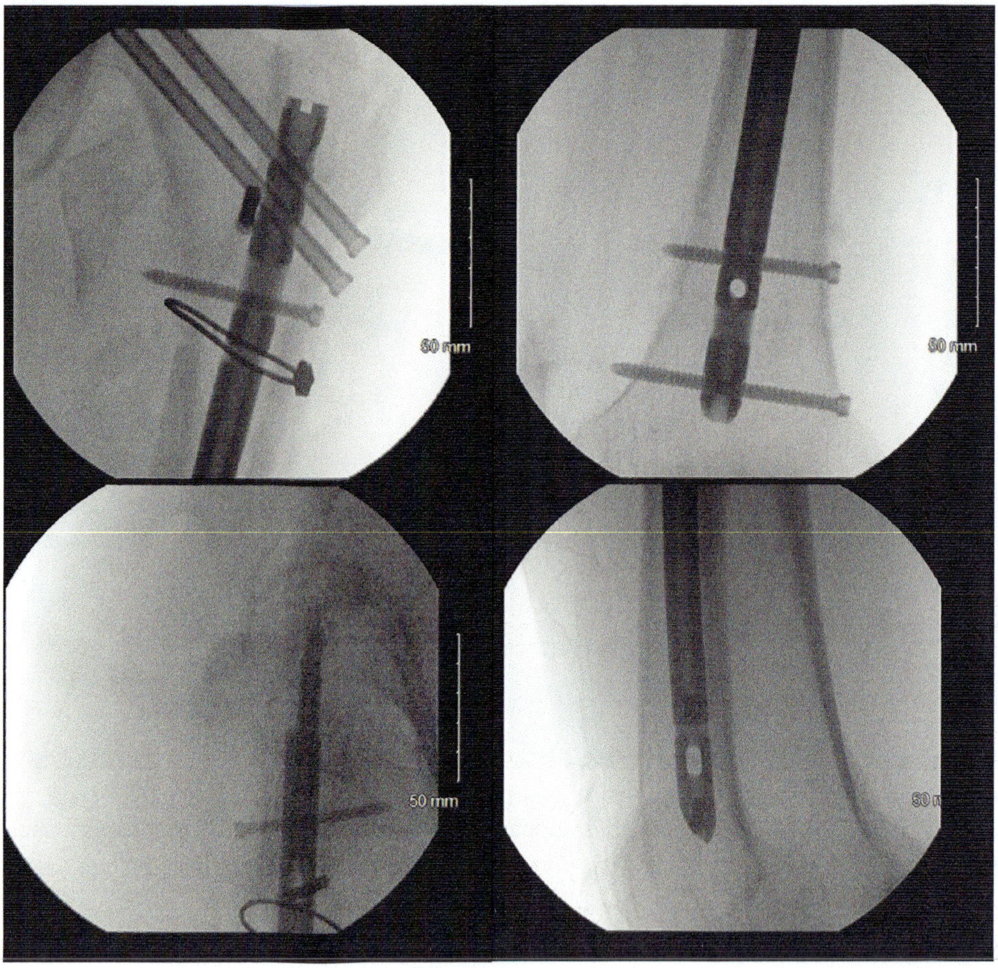

Figure 4.4. Intraoperative fluoroscopic images demonstrating the final revision construct with autogenous bone graft implantation of the left femur.

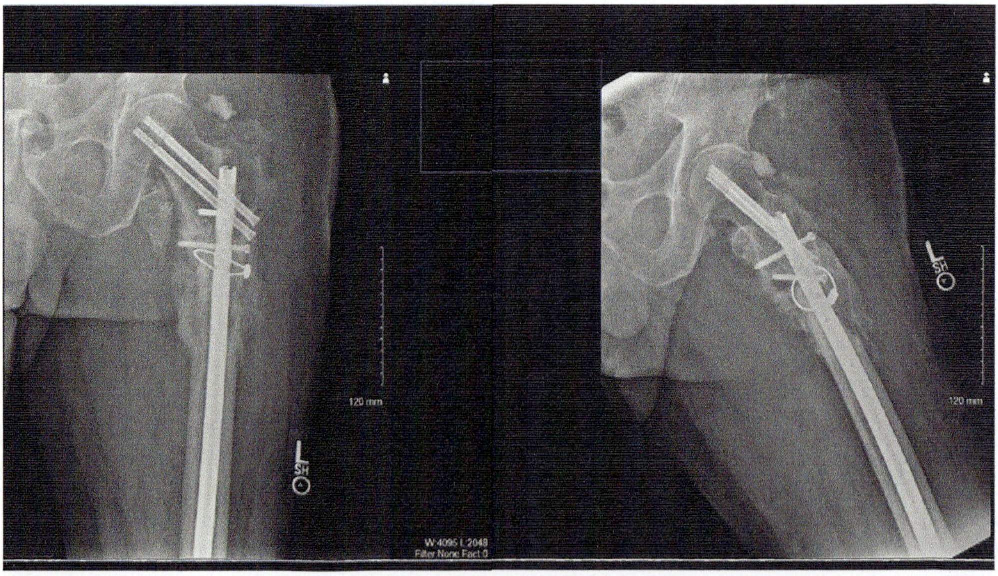

Figure 4.5. Six months postoperatively, radiograph demonstrating abundant callus and bone formation.

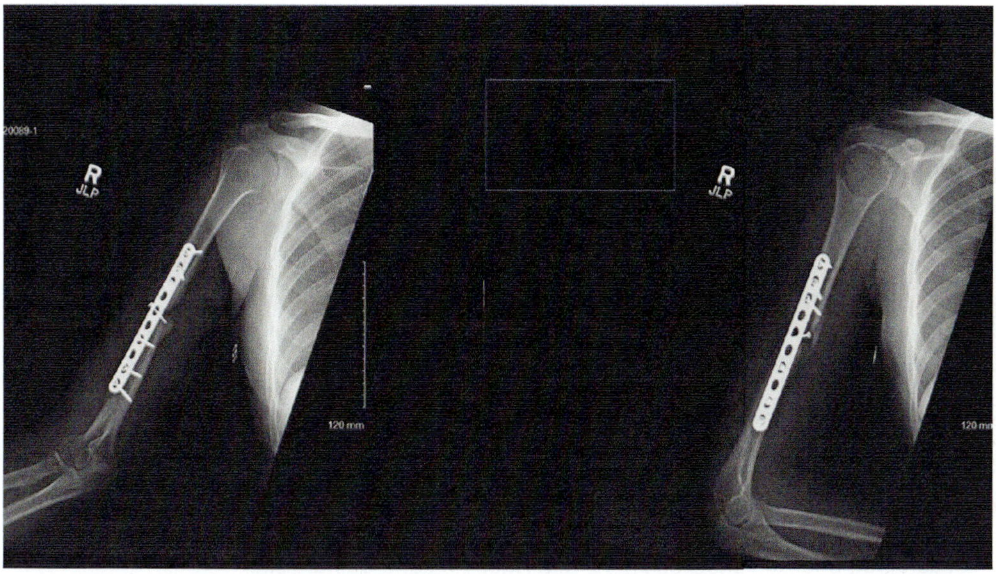

Figure 4.6. Right humeral shaft infected nonunion AP and lateral radiographs status post open reduction internal fixation.

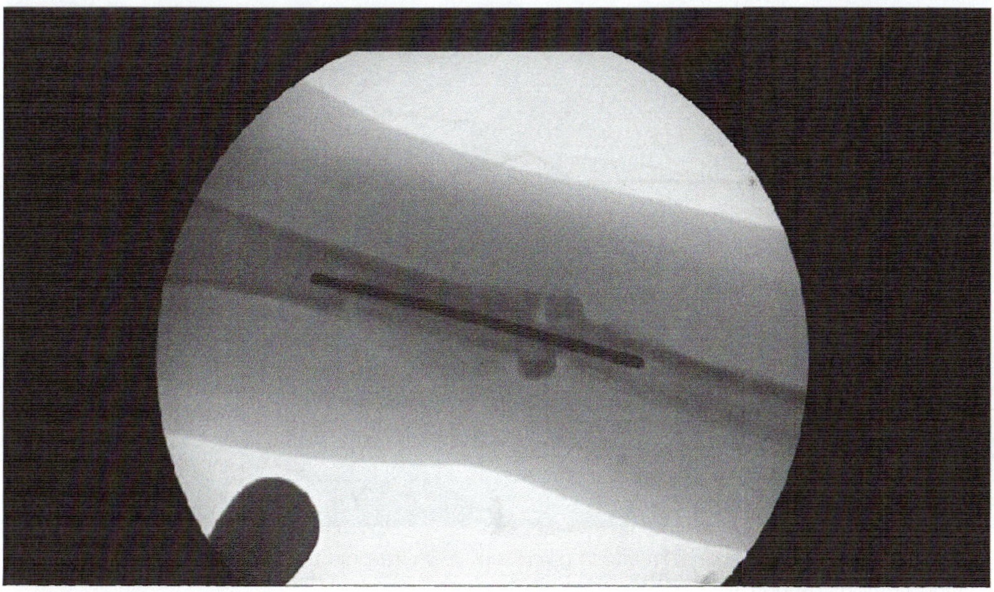

Figure 4.7. Fluoroscopic image of an antibiotic-coated Schanz pin and antibiotic spacer placement after resection of necrotic bone of right humeral shaft infected nonunion.

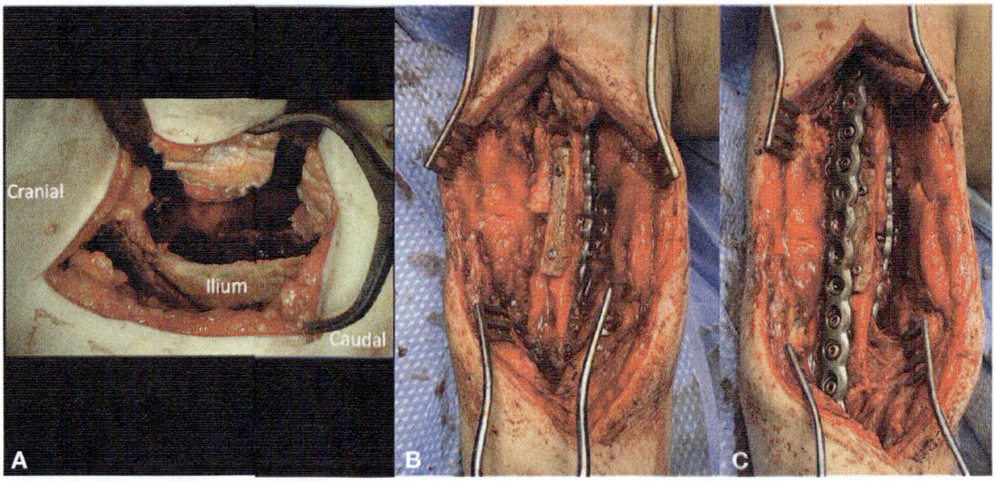

Figure 4.8. **A.** Right bicortical iliac crest donor site after harvest of graft. **B.** Right humerus demonstrating contoured bicortical graft fixated into place. **C.** Final fixation of bicortical iliac crest autograft prior to cancellous bone application around fracture site.

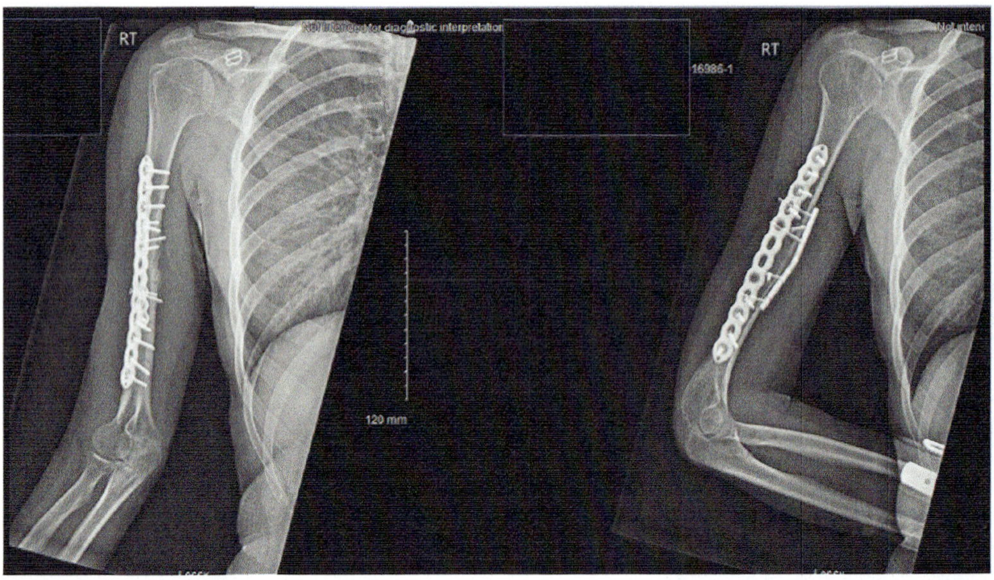

Figure 4.9. Right humeral shaft revision open reduction internal fixation and autogenous bone grafting demonstrating radiographic union at 6-month follow-up.

References

1. Finkemeier CG. Bone-grafting and bone-graft substitutes. *J Bone Joint Surg Am.* 2002;84(3):454-464.
2. Khan SN, Cammisa FPJ, Sandhu HS, Diwan AD, Girardi FP, Lane JM. The biology of bone grafting. *J Am Acad Orthop Surg.* 2005;13(1):77-86.
3. Wright JG, Swiontkowski MF, Heckman JD. Introducing levels of evidence to the journal. *J Bone Joint Surg Am.* 2003;85(1):1-3.
4. Wright JG, Einhorn TA, Heckman JD. Grades of recommendation. *J Bone Joint Surg Am.* 2005;87(9):1909-1910.
5. Gazdag AR, Lane JM, Glaser D, Forster RA. Alternatives to autogenous bone graft: efficacy and indications. *J Am Acad Orthop Surg.* 1995;3(1):1-8.

6. Dell PC, Burchardt H, Glowczewskie FPJ. A roentgenographic, biomechanical, and histological evaluation of vascularized and non-vascularized segmental fibular canine autografts. *J Bone Joint Surg Am.* 1985;67(1):105-112.
7. Sen MK, Miclau T. Autologous iliac crest bone graft: should it still be the gold standard for treating nonunions? *Injury.* 2007;38(Suppl 1):S75-S80.
8. Cypher TJ, Grossman JP. Biological principles of bone graft healing. *J Foot Ankle Surg.* 1996;35(5):413-417.
9. Easley ME, Trnka HJ, Schon LC, Myerson MS. Isolated subtalar arthrodesis. *J Bone Joint Surg Am.* 2000;82(5):613-624.
10. Sanders R. Displaced intra-articular fractures of the calcaneus. *J Bone Joint Surg Am.* 2000;82(2):225-250.
11. Bradbury N, Hutchinson J, Hahn D, Colton CL. Clavicular nonunion. 31/32 healed after plate fixation and bone grafting. *Acta Orthop Scand.* 1996;67(4):367-370.
12. Olsen BS, Vaesel MT, Søjbjerg JO. Treatment of midshaft clavicular nonunion with plate fixation and autologous bone grafting. *J Shoulder Elb Surg.* 1995;4(5):337-344.
13. Bauer TW, Muschler GF. Bone graft materials. An overview of the basic science. *Clin Orthop Relat Res.* 2000;(371):10-27.
14. Nusbickel FR, Dell PC, McAndrew MP, Moore MM. Vascularized autografts for reconstruction of skeletal defects following lower extremity trauma. A review. *Clin Orthop Relat Res.* 1989;243:65-70.
15. Ricci WM. In: Tornetta P III, Ricci WM, Ostrum RF, McQueen MM, McKee MD, Court-Brown CM, eds. *Rockwood and Green's Fractures in Adults 9th Edition.* Wolters Kluwer; Chapter 29: Principles of Nonunion and Bone Defect Treatment; 2020:865-869.
16. Westrich GH, Geller DS, O'Malley MJ, Deland JT, Helfet DL. Anterior iliac crest bone graft harvesting using the corticocancellous reamer system. *J Orthop Trauma.* 2001;15(7):500-506.
17. Brawley SC, Simpson RB. Results of an alternative autogenous iliac crest bone graft harvest method. *Orthopedics.* 2006;29(4):342-346.
18. Ahlmann E, Patzakis M, Roidis N, Shepherd L, Holtom P. Comparison of anterior and posterior iliac crest bone grafts in terms of harvest-site morbidity and functional outcomes. *J Bone Joint Surg Am.* 2002;84(5):716-720.
19. Ebraheim NA, Elgafy H, Xu R. Bone-graft harvesting from iliac and fibular donor sites: techniques and complications. *J Am Acad Orthop Surg.* 2001;9(3):210-218.
20. Behairy YM, Al-Sebai W. A modified technique for harvesting full-thickness iliac crest bone graft. *Spine (Phila Pa. 1976).* 2001;26(6):695-697.
21. Ilankovan V, Stronczek M, Telfer M, Peterson LJ, Stassen LF, Ward-Booth P. A prospective study of trephined bone grafts of the tibial shaft and iliac crest. *Br J Oral Maxillofac Surg.* 1998;36(6):434-439.
22. Meeder PJ, Eggers C. Techniques for obtaining autogenous bone graft. *Injury.* 1994;25(Suppl 1):A5-A16.
23. Arrington ED, Smith WJ, Chambers HG, Bucknell AL, Davino NA. Complications of iliac crest bone graft harvesting. *Clin Orthop Relat Res.* 1996;329:300-309.
24. Banwart JC, Asher MA, Hassanein RS. Iliac crest bone graft harvest donor site morbidity. A statistical evaluation. *Spine (Phila Pa 1976).* 1995;20(9):1055-1060.
25. Goulet JA, Senunas LE, DeSilva GL, Greenfield ML. Autogenous iliac crest bone graft. Complications and functional assessment. *Clin Orthop Relat Res.* 1997;(339):76-81.
26. Younger EM, Chapman MW. Morbidity at bone graft donor sites. *J Orthop Trauma.* 1989;3(3):192-195.
27. Hayes WRJ, Smith RW. Trochanteric bone grafts in foot and ankle surgery. *Foot ankle Int.* 1996;17(7):402-405.
28. Alt V, Nawab A, Seligson D. Bone grafting from the proximal tibia. *J Trauma.* 1999;47(3):555-557.
29. Herford AS, King BJ, Audia F, Becktor J. Medial approach for tibial bone graft: anatomic study and clinical technique. *J oral Maxillofac Surg.* 2003;61(3):358-363.
30. Judet H, Gilbert A, Mathoulin C, et al. Reconstruction of loss of bony substance in limbs by free vascularized fibula transplant. *Chirurgie.* 1991;117(5-6):469-476; discussion 477.
31. Wang K, Almeida LE, Olsson AB. Volume analysis of the proximal tibial metaphysis. *J Oral Maxillofac Surg.* 2007;65(12):2425-2429.
32. Catone GA, Reimer BL, McNeir D, Ray R. Tibial autogenous cancellous bone as an alternative donor site in maxillofacial surgery: a preliminary report. *J Oral Maxillofac Surg.* 1992;50(12):1258-1263.
33. O'Keeffe RMJ, Riemer BL, Butterfield SL. Harvesting of autogenous cancellous bone graft from the proximal tibial metaphysis. A review of 230 cases. *J Orthop Trauma.* 1991;5(4):469-474.
34. Frohberg U, Mazock JB. A review of morbidity associated with bone harvest from the proximal tibial metaphysis. *Mund Kiefer Gesichtschir.* 2005;9(2):63-65.
35. Biddulph SL. Bone donor site. Iliac crest or distal radius? *J Hand Surg Br.* 1999;24(6):645-646.
36. Saltrick KR, Caron M, Grossman J. Utilization of autogenous corticocancellous bone graft from the distal tibia for reconstructive surgery of the foot and ankle. *J Foot Ankle Surg.* 1996;35(5):406-412.
37. Mendicino RW, Leonheart E, Shromoff P. Techniques for harvesting autogenous bone graft of the lower extremity. *J Foot Ankle Surg.* 1996;35(5):428-435.
38. Weiss GA, Saxby TS. Distal tibial bone graft for foot and ankle surgery. *Foot Ankle Surg. [Internet].* 1998;4(2):93-97. https://www.sciencedirect.com/science/article/pii/S1268773198800088
39. Patel JC, Watson K, Joseph E, Garcia J, Wollstein R. Long-term complications of distal radius bone grafts. *J Hand Surg Am.* 2003;28(5):784-788.
40. Bruno RJ, Cohen MS, Berzins A, Sumner DR. Bone graft harvesting from the distal radius, olecranon, and iliac crest: a quantitative analysis. *J Hand Surg Am.* 2001;26(1):135-141.

41. Schuringa M, Fechner M. Cancellous bone grafting from the distal radius. *Eur J Plast Surg. [Internet].* 2002;25(6):319-322. https://doi.org/10.1007/s00238-002-0378-4
42. Horne LT, Murray PM, Saha S, Sidhar K. Effects of distal radius bone graft harvest on the axial compressive strength of the radius. *J Hand Surg Am.* 2010;35(2):262-266.
43. Mirly HL, Manske PR, Szerzinski JM. Distal anterior radius bone graft in surgery of the hand and wrist. *J Hand Surg Am.* 1995;20(4):623-627.
44. Jarrett P, Kinzel V, Stoffel K. A biomechanical comparison of scaphoid fixation with bone grafting using iliac bone or distal radius bone. *J Hand Surg Am.* 2007;32(9):1367-1373.
45. Belthur MV, Conway JD, Jindal G, Ranade A, Herzenberg JE. Bone graft harvest using a new intramedullary system. *Clin Orthop Relat Res.* 2008;466(12):2973-2980.
46. Quintero AJ, Tarkin IS, Pape H-C. Technical tricks when using the reamer irrigator aspirator technique for autologous bone graft harvesting. *J Orthop Trauma.* 2010;24(1):42-45.
47. McCall TA, Brokaw DS, Jelen BA, et al. Treatment of large segmental bone defects with reamer-irrigator-aspirator bone graft: technique and case series. *Orthop Clin North Am.* 2010;41(1):63-73; table of contents.
48. Lowe JA, Della Rocca GJ, Murtha Y, et al. Complications associated with negative pressure reaming for harvesting autologous bone graft: a case series. *J Orthop Trauma.* 2010;24(1):46-52.
49. Sagi HC, Young ML, Gerstenfeld L, Einhorn TA, Tornetta P. Qualitative and quantitative differences between bone graft obtained from the medullary canal (with a reamer/irrigator/aspirator) and the iliac crest of the same patient. *J Bone Joint Surg Am.* 2012;94(23):2128-2135.
50. Porter RM, Liu F, Pilapil C, et al. Osteogenic potential of reamer irrigator aspirator (RIA) aspirate collected from patients undergoing hip arthroplasty. *J Orthop Res.* 2009;27(1):42-49.
51. Higgins TF, Marchand LS. Basic science and clinical application of reamed sources for autogenous bone graft harvest. *J Am Acad Orthop Surg.* 2018;26(12):420-428.
52. Henrich D, Seebach C, Sterlepper E, Tauchmann C, Marzi I, Frank J. RIA reamings and hip aspirate: a comparative evaluation of osteoprogenitor and endothelial progenitor cells. *Injury.* 2010;41(Suppl 2):S62-S68.
53. Hak DJ, Pittman JL. Biological rationale for the intramedullary canal as a source of autograft material. *Orthop Clin North Am.* 2010;41(1):57-61; table of contents.
54. Wenisch S, Trinkaus K, Hild A, et al. Human reaming debris: a source of multipotent stem cells. *Bone.* 2005;36(1):74-83.
55. Schmidmaier G, Herrmann S, Green J, et al. Quantitative assessment of growth factors in reaming aspirate, iliac crest, and platelet preparation. *Bone.* 2006;39(5):1156-1163.
56. Finnan RP, Prayson MJ, Goswami T, Miller D. Use of the reamer-irrigator-aspirator for bone graft harvest: a mechanical comparison of three starting points in cadaveric femurs. *J Orthop Trauma.* 2010;24(1):36-41.
57. Yee MA, Hundal RS, Perdue AM, Hake ME. Autologous bone graft harvest using the reamer-irrigator-aspirator. *J Orthop Trauma.* 2018;32(Suppl 1):S20-S21.
58. Mauffrey C, Hake ME, Chadayammuri V, Masquelet A-C. Reconstruction of long bone infections using the induced membrane technique: tips and tricks. *J Orthop Trauma.* 2016;30(6):e188-e193.
59. Pratt DJ, Papagiannopoulos G, Rees PH, Quinnell R. The effects of medullary reaming on the torsional strength of the femur. *Injury.* 1987;18(3):177-179.
60. Conway JD. Autograft and nonunions: morbidity with intramedullary bone graft versus iliac crest bone graft. *Orthop Clin North Am. [Internet].* 2010;41(1):75-84; table of contents. http://europepmc.org/abstract/MED/19931055
61. Qvick LM, Ritter CA, Mutty CE, Rohrbacher BJ, Buyea CM, Anders MJ. Donor site morbidity with reamer-irrigator-aspirator (RIA) use for autogenous bone graft harvesting in a single centre 204 case series. *Injury.* 2013;44(10):1263-1269.
62. Hammer TO, Wieling R, Green JM, Südkamp NP, Schneider E, Müller CA. Effect of re-implanted particles from intramedullary reaming on mechanical properties and callus formation. A laboratory study. *J Bone Joint Surg Br.* 2007;89(11):1534-1538.
63. Newman JT, Stahel PF, Smith WR, Resende GV, Hak DJ, Morgan SJ. A new minimally invasive technique for large volume bone graft harvest for treatment of fracture nonunions. *Orthopedics.* 2008;31(3):257-261.
64. Kanakaris NK, Morell D, Gudipati S, Britten S, Giannoudis PV. Reaming irrigator aspirator system: early experience of its multipurpose use. *Injury.* 2011;42(Suppl 4):S28-S34.
65. Dawson J, Kiner D, Gardner W II, Swafford R, Nowotarski PJ. The reamer-irrigator-aspirator as a device for harvesting bone graft compared with iliac crest bone graft: union rates and complications. *J Orthop Trauma.* 2014;28(10):584-590.
66. Nodzo SR, Kaplan NB, Hohman DW, Ritter CA. A radiographic and clinical comparison of reamer-irrigator-aspirator versus iliac crest bone graft in ankle arthrodesis. *Int Orthop.* 2014;38(6):1199-1203.
67. Rankine JJ, Hodgson RJ, Tan HB, Cox G, Giannoudis PV. MRI appearances of the femur following bone graft harvesting using the reamer-irrigator-aspirator. *Injury.* 2015;46(Suppl 8):S65-S67.

5 Osteoconductive Graft Substitutes

David J. Hak

INTRODUCTION

Osteoconduction is defined as a three-dimensional process involving the ingrowth of capillaries, perivascular tissue, and osteoprogenitor cells from a bony bed into the three-dimensional structure of a porous scaffold, which serves as a guiding signal to fill a bone defect.[1] Bone graft substitutes that mimic the architecture of cancellous bone are known to provide the physical structure necessary for osteoconduction. The host substrate must also have very specific surface kinetics and biology to facilitate the migration, attachment, and proliferation of mesenchymal stem cells, which then differentiate into osteoprogenitor cells.

It is thought that there is an optimal range of pore sizes that encourage the ingrowth of blood vessels, mesenchymal tissues, and osteoprogenitor cells. Historically this optimal pore size has been considered to be between 0.3 and 0.5 mm (300-500 μm).

Newly developed additive ceramic manufacturing processes provide total control over pore size and distribution. Recent research suggests that the optimal pore size is in the range of 0.7 to 1.2 mm (700-1,200 μm), twofold to fourfold larger than previously thought.[2]

Osteoconductive bone graft substitutes are frequently used to fill metaphyseal voids following an injury with associated articular depression. They are typically used in conjunction with internal fixation implants. Their use is contraindicated in areas where there is known infection. Osteoconductive bone graft substitutes can also be used in conjunction with autogenous bone graft serving as an "extender" when the bone graft volume is insufficient.

There are several different osteoconductive bone graft substitutes available on the market. These products vary in their chemical composition, structural strength, and resorption/remodeling rates (Table 5.1). To select a bone graft substitute that provides the properties desired for a specific clinical situation, the surgeon should understand the differences between these products. Unfortunately, there are a limited number of clinical studies and a lack of direct comparison studies between these products. Although bone graft substitutes are subject to some degree of regulatory scrutiny, specific proof of their efficacy is not usually required.[3] In the United States, most bone graft substitutes are approved by the Food and Drug Administration through the 510k process, which only requires that the product be substantially equivalent (at least as safe and effective) to a product that had been marketed prior to May 28, 1976. Most bone graft substitutes only provide animal study data in their submission. In a review of 59 bone graft substitutes marketed in the United Kingdom, researchers found that only 37% of the products had published clinical data evaluating their human use.[4]

CALCIUM PHOSPHATE

Calcium phosphate is a synthetic resorbable bone graft substitute with a very high mechanical strength, and therefore, it is often referred to as a cement. It has a compressive strength that is 4 to 10 times greater than the average compressive strength of cancellous bone. The high compressive strength has led some surgeons to advocate immediate weightbearing with its use in circumstances where weightbearing would typically be restricted.[5]

TABLE 5.1 Characteristics of Osteoconductive Bone Graft Substitutes

Bone Graft Substitute	Compressive Strength	Resorption Rate	Advantages/Unique Features
Calcium phosphate	Highest of all products, 4-10 times greater than cancellous bone	Slow, 30%-60% resorbed at 1 year	Strength may permit earlier weightbearing
Calcium sulfate	Similar to cancellous bone	Fast, 4-12 wk	May be combined with antibiotics to provide gradual local delivery
Bioglass	Slightly less than to slightly greater than cancellous bone depending on structure	Fast, 6-12 wk	
Hydroxyapatite	Much greater than cancellous bone	Precipitated low temperature form: 6-12 mo Sintered high temperature form: 10 y plus	
Coralline hydroxyapatite	Slightly greater than cancellous bone	Depends on specific variety, ranges from 1 to 10 y	
Tricalcium phosphate	Equal to or slightly less than cancellous bone	Alpha: slow, 6-18 mo Beta: fast 6-12 wk	

Calcium phosphate is an injectable paste of inorganic calcium and phosphate that hardens in situ and cures by a crystallization reaction to form dahllite, a carbonated apatite which is similar to that found in the mineral phase of bone. The gradual resorption of calcium phosphate bone graft substitutes mimics the normal bone remodeling process.[6] Over time the calcium phosphate undergoes osteoclastic resorption followed by the invasion of small blood vessels that become surrounded by circumferential lamellae of new bone.[7]

The clinical use of calcium phosphate was initially studied in fractures of the distal radius. In one prospective study of 110 patients greater than age 50 with distal radius fractures, patients were randomized to receive either closed reduction and cast immobilization for 6 weeks or closed reduction and percutaneous injection of calcium phosphate. Because of the stability provided by the calcium phosphate, the latter group was only immobilized for 2 weeks and then allowed to begin early wrist range of motion. The patients treated with calcium phosphate had less pain and earlier restoration of their motion. There was a higher incidence of malunions in the control group compared to the calcium phosphate group (42% vs 18%).[8]

In another study, 323 patients with displaced distal radius fractures were randomized to receive conventional treatment or conventional treatment plus calcium phosphate.[9] As in the previous study patients that received the calcium phosphate were permitted to begin wrist range of motion at 2 weeks, while the other patients were maintained either in a cast or external fixator for 6 to 8 weeks. Patients that were treated with calcium phosphate and permitted early wrist motion had significantly better function when evaluated 6 to 8 weeks postoperatively. This included better grip strength, wrist range of motion, and digital motion. However, by 3 months postoperatively, only digital motion remained significantly better in the calcium phosphate–treated patients, and at 1 year, no clinical differences were detected. The authors concluded that the use of calcium phosphate may allow for accelerated rehabilitation following operatively managed distal radius fractures.

The use of calcium phosphate bone graft substitute has also been studied in depressed intra-articular tibial plateau fractures. In a study of 26 patients undergoing open reduction and internal fixation of displaced tibial plateau fractures, calcium phosphate was found to produce good outcomes. Because of the high mechanical strength of the cement, the authors allowed early weightbearing after a mean postoperative period of 4.5 weeks, with a range from 1 to 6 weeks. Despite early weightbearing, only two patients in this series suffered from a partial loss of reduction.[10] Calcium phosphate was compared to autogenous bone graft in a larger study of 120 tibial plateau fractures. All patients underwent open reduction with standard plate-and-screw or screw-only fixation and then either the calcium phosphate or autogenous bone graft was placed in the defect cavity for subarticular support. There was a statistically higher rate of articular subsidence during the 3 to 12-month follow-up period in the bone graft group. The investigators concluded that calcium phosphate bone graft substitute appears to be a better choice, at least in terms of the prevention of subsidence, than autogenous iliac bone graft for the treatment of subarticular defects associated with unstable tibial plateau fractures.[11]

Newer formulations of calcium phosphate products include a moldable putty, which has been shown to prevent articular subsidence when used as a metaphyseal void filler with fixation of a variety of periarticular fracture.[12] An additional benefit of this formulation is there was no soft tissue or intra-articular extravasation as can occur with the injectable formulation.

The strength of calcium phosphate bone graft substitute leads surgeons in one clinical study to begin full weightbearing at 3 weeks following open reduction and internal fixation and reported no subsequent radiographic evidence of reduction loss.[5] Investigators compared injected calcium phosphate to no graft in a prospective randomized study of 47 patients with 52 closed displaced intra-articular calcaneus fractures undergoing open reduction and internal fixation. While there was no difference in the degree of collapse of Böhler angle compared to the initial postoperative values at 6 weeks and 3 months, there was a statistically greater mean loss of Böhler angle at 6 months in the group not treated with calcium phosphate cement.[13] The investigators concluded that their results support the use of calcium phosphate to fill the bone void in displaced intra-articular calcaneal fractures undergoing open reduction and internal fixation.

CALCIUM SULFATE

The hemihydrate form of calcium sulfate is known more commonly as Plaster of Paris. When the hemihydrate form of calcium sulfate ($CaSO_4$-½H_2O) is mixed with water, a dihydrate form ($CaSO_4$-2H_2O) known as gypsum is formed. Reports as early as 1892 described successful healing in 6 of 9 cavitary bone defects treated with plaster of Paris.[14] Peltier documented his use of calcium sulfate for cavitary bone defects in reports published beginning in the 1950s.[15-18]

Calcium sulfate is available as either individual pellets or as a powder that can be mixed in solution to form an injectable paste or molded to form desired shapes. The setting solution used with the powder form may be proprietary and differ between companies. Antibiotics can also be added to the powder variety as described below.

While most authors classify calcium sulfate as an osteoconductive bone graft substitute, some authors feel that the material is resorbed too rapidly to provide a long-term three-dimensional framework to support osteoconduction.[19] Calcium sulfate resorbs in a period of 4 to 12 weeks, depending on defect size. Walsh et al hypothesized that the mechanism of calcium sulfates bone regenerative action was related to the local acidity produced during its resorption. They postulated that in a confined cancellous defect, this local acidity results in demineralization of the adjacent bone with a release of matrix bound bone morphogenetic proteins (BMPs) that have a stimulatory effect on bone formation.[20] It has been shown that osteoblasts attach to the calcium sulfate, and this may represent another possible in vivo mechanism of action for the resorption and rapid regeneration of bone defects.[21,22]

Since calcium sulfate has compressive strength that is equal to or slightly greater than cancellous bone, it is indicated for the filling of bone defects that are not intrinsic to the stability of the bone structure.[23] Its use in filling benign bone defects has been described.[24,25] Other uses include expansion of autogenous or allogeneic bone grafts in spinal fusion, backfilling of bone graft harvest sites, and periprosthetic bone loss.[26,27]

Prolonged postoperative wound drainage can be seen following the use of calcium sulfate. It has been theorized that this serous drainage is due to the osmotic effect of the calcium sulfate, and the serous drainage subsides with calcium sulfate eventual resorption. Serous drainage has been reported in different series to occur in 4% to 51% of cases. Wound drainage occurs more frequently when large volumes of calcium sulfate are used or when they are placed in a subcutaneous location such as might occur in the tibia or ulna.[28]

The use of calcium sulfate has been reported in small series of tibial plateau and acetabular fractures.[29,30] However, it may not be the optimal bone graft substitute for these conditions due to its rapid resorption and incomplete bone regeneration.

The relatively rapid resorption of calcium sulfate makes it a useful carrier for the gradual release of antibiotics. Antibiotics may be added to the powder varieties of calcium sulfate prior to mixing with the solution. Bead molds are available to allow the surgeon to create resorbable antibiotic beads. Several basic science studies have examined the elution characteristics of cephalexin and tobramycin from calcium sulfate.[31,32] Calcium sulfate impregnated with tobramycin was found to be more effective at eradication of infection than either debridement alone or treatment with intramuscular antibiotics in a rabbit osteomyelitis model.[33] In a preliminary published report of its use in patients with infected long bone defects and nonunions, successful eradication of infection was achieved in 23 of 25 patients.[34] A meta-analysis including 16 studies with 917 patients with chronic osteomyelitis found that debridement with the use of antibiotic-loaded calcium sulfate showed an overall eradication rate of 92%. The overall reoperation rate was 9%, overall refracture rate was 2%, overall delayed wound healing rate was 20%, and the rate of aseptic wound leakage was 12%.[35]

BIOGLASS

The original investigation of bioglass as a bone graft substitute dates back to the late 1960s.[36] Bioactive glass products have been used as a bone graft substitute in dentistry since 1993 and approved for orthopedic use in 2002. It is a silica-based melt-derived glass characterized by a SiO_2 content of less than 60%, which is a critical feature for its rate of bioactivity.[37] In vivo, the material is highly osteoconductive, and it also promotes the growth of new bone on its surface.[38] Currently available bioactive glass beads are composed of silica (45%), calcium oxide (24.5%), disodium oxide (24.5%), and pyrophosphate (6%). The beads range in size from 90 to 170 μm. After implantation, the silica breaks down rapidly as local hydrogen ions replace sodium, and the surface layer of silica repolymerizes to form a layer rich in $Si(OH)_4$. At the same time, calcium and phosphate that is released combines to form an amorphous surface layer that binds to collagen, growth factors, and fibrin. Bioactive glass undergoes resorption by a combination of cellular mechanisms and chemical dissolution. Upon implantation, the surface area of bioactive glass increases multifold. This provides greater exposure to interstitial fluid and blood resulting in faster resorption. The bioglass particles are gradually consumed as they are constantly reexposed during bone remodeling. Unlike hydroxyapatite, the majority of bioglass material is fully resorbed within 6 to 12 weeks after implantation.

There are two published randomized clinical studies of the use of bioglass in orthopedic trauma. Bioactive glass was compared with a control in a prospective randomized study of 78 patients with a high-energy open or closed tibial shaft fracture treated with a reamed interlocked nail. All fractures were treated with bioglass healed, while there were 4 cases (10.5%) in the control group that failed to heal by 7 to 8 months postoperatively. At 12 weeks, 88% of the bioglass treated fractures were rated as excellent or good compared to 50% of the controls, and at 26 weeks, 100% of the bioglass treated fractures were rated as excellent or good compared to 89% of the controls ($P < .05$). The authors concluded that the use of bioglass accelerated fracture healing.[39]

Bioglass was compared with autogenous bone graft in a small prospective randomized study of depressed lateral tibial plateau fractures. There were no differences in the subjective evaluation, functional tests, and clinical examination between the two groups during 1-year follow-up. The authors concluded that bioactive glass granules can be clinically used as filler material instead of autogenous bone in depressed lateral tibial plateau fractures.[40]

HYDROXYAPATITE AND SUBSTITUTED HYDROXYAPATITES

Calcium hydroxyapatite is formed by the precipitation of calcium nitrate and ammonium-dihydrogen phosphate with a chemical formula $Ca_{10}(PO_4)_6(OH)_2$. Nearly 70% of the mineral component of teeth and bone is hydroxyapatite. Hydroxyapatite is slowly resorbed but has relatively high mechanical strength. Calcium hydroxyapatite is often combined with tricalcium phosphate to yield a more physiological balance between mechanical support and bone resorption.[41]

Hydroxyapatite can be prepared using a number of different methods including dry methods, wet methods, high temperature processes, and method based on biogenic sources or bioinspired approaches.[42]

Recently, substituted hydroxyapatites have been developed in which silicon, magnesium, or carbonate replace the hydroxyl or phosphate groups of the apatite structure. Silicon is thought to play an important role in bone metabolism, and its deficiency can result in abnormal bone formation due to decreased collagen and hydroxyapatite deposition. Magnesium ions have been shown to activate the hydroxyapatite crystal cell structure promoting rapid cell-mediated resorption, new bone formation, and remodeling.

CORALLINE HYDROXYAPATITE

Coralline hydroxyapatite was one of the first widely marketed osteoconductive bone graft substitutes and initially studied in orthopedic trauma. It is now most commonly used for various dental, maxillofacial, and spinal indications. It is produced from marine coral exoskeletons that have a very regular pore structure that resembles that of cancellous bone. The genus *Goniopora* has a microstructure with parallel longitudinal pores of 600 μm, with interconnecting channels ranging from 220 to 260 μm. Optimal pore size and interconnectivity are important for vascular ingrowth. The coral is subjected to high pressure and heated in an aqueous phosphate solution, converting the calcium carbonate coral skeleton into hydroxyapatite $[C_{10}(PO_4)_6(OH)_2]$.[43] Coralline hydroxyapatite acts as an osteoconductive bone graft substitute. Animal and human studies have shown that the pore structure allows invasion of vascular and fibrous tissue, which is later converted to mature lamellar bone. This process is similar to the healing process seen with autogenous bone grafts.[44-46]

Coralline hydroxyapatite has only slightly greater compressive strength than cancellous bone, and it is indicated to be used with internal fixation. In addition to filling metaphyseal defects, it has also been reported useful as a bone graft expander in spinal surgery.[47] It is brittle and weak in tension. With tissue ingrowth, the strength of the implant increases proportionally to the amount of tissue ingrowth.[48] Coralline hydroxyapatite is available as various sized blocks, wedges, and granules. It is also available in different porosities. Resorption of the original material is extremely slow with most material remaining present for several years. A faster resorbing material that has only a very thin layer of hydroxyapatite was developed in order to provide resorption at a predictable rate that corresponds to the rate of anticipated bone ingrowth.

Coralline hydroxyapatite was compared with autogenous bone graft in a randomized study of 40 patients undergoing open reduction and internal fixation of tibial plateau fractures. Radiographic and clinical assessment at follow-up showed no significant differences between the two groups. Seven patients that received coralline hydroxyapatite subsequently underwent elective hardware removal, and biopsy of the bone graft substitute showed bone ingrowth in all specimens, with the fractional percentage of bone ingrowth ranging from 25% to 47%.[49] Coralline hydroxyapatite was used in a series of 21 comminuted and displaced distal radius fractures that were treated with open reduction, external fixation, and k-wires. The coralline hydroxyapatite was effective in maintaining the articular surface reduction and had a favorable safety profile compared to other forms of treatment.[50]

TRICALCIUM PHOSPHATE

Tricalcium phosphate [$Ca_3(PO_4)_2$] bone graft substitutes are composed of 39% calcium and 20% phosphorus by weight in a molar concentration of 1.5, a composition that is similar to human bone. The material has a range of multidirectional interconnected pores. Tricalcium phosphate was one of the earliest materials used as a bone graft substitute, with Albee and Morrison reporting its successful use in bone defects in 1920.[51]

Tricalcium phosphate can assume one of two crystalline structures. α-Tricalcium phosphate has a polygonal shape, while β-tricalcium phosphate is spherical, has a higher porosity, and can be packed more densely in a bone defect. β-Tricalcium phosphate has a finer microarchitecture, which results in a faster resorption rate.[52] Most commercially available tricalcium phosphate bone graft substitutes are of the β variety. It is available as granules, wedges, cubes, and cylinders. The compressive and tensile strength of β-tricalcium phosphate is similar to cancellous bone.[53] It is brittle and weak under tension and shear forces.

Tricalcium phosphates may be produced by a conventional high temperature ceramic processing or by a low-temperature aqueous chemical method. Various proprietary processes have been developed to optimize the properties of the tricalcium phosphate bone graft substitute. Tricalcium phosphate undergoes resorption via dissolution and fragmentation over 6 to 18 months.[54] Resorption of tricalcium phosphate occurs by osteoclasts without an inflammatory or giant cell response. The bone volume produced is always less than the volume of the tricalcium phosphate that is resorbed.[54] Tricalcium phosphate is hydrophilic permitting the wicking and absorption of blood and marrow, which may assist the migration of osteogenic cells into the scaffold.

Bucholz et al[55] reported on the use of tricalcium phosphate as a bone graft substitute in 24 patients with a posttraumatic bone defect and 8 patients with a benign tumor or cyst. They reported excellent results in the 14 tibia fractures, 6 radius fractures, 3 ulna fractures, and 1 humerus fractures.

McAndrew et al reported on the use of tricalcium phosphate to fill defects in 30 patients with fractures and 13 patients with nonunions. With a minimum follow-up of 6 months and an average follow-up of 1 year, they reported that 90% of the fractures and 85% of the nonunions were successfully healed. They estimated a resorption rate of the tricalcium phosphate of approximately 10% per month, with complete resorption occurring in 6 to 24 months.[56]

The use of β-tricalcium phosphate has been described to fill the defect created during opening wedge proximal tibial osteotomies.[57] A potential role as a graft extender in impaction grafting during revision arthroplasty surgery has also been suggested.[58] Several potential roles for β-tricalcium phosphate have also been explored in spine surgery, including as a carrier for growth factors and as a bone graft extender.[59-62]

COMBINATION PRODUCTS AND ADDITIVE MANUFACTURING

Increasingly, commercial entities interested in new bone graft substitutes are developing combination products. As previously discussed, calcium hydroxyapatite is often combined with tricalcium phosphate to yield a more physiological balance between mechanical support and bone resorption.[41]

Another commercially available combination product consists of 40% hydroxyapatite and 60% calcium sulfate and the radiocontrast agent iohexol. It is an injectable, moldable, and drillable osteoconductive bone void filler, which is designed to resorb at the same rate that bone forms. This bone graft substitute was compared to iliac crest bone graft in a randomized, controlled, multicenter study of 135 patients with an acute tibial plateau fracture that underwent open reduction and internal fixation. Investigators found no significant differences between the two groups in the short form-12 physical component score, rates of fracture healing, defect remodeling, or articular subsidence at 26 weeks postoperatively. They concluded that the bone graft substitute was noninferior to autologous bone graft with regard to both patient-reported and radiographic outcomes.[63]

Additive manufacturing with three-dimensional printing is another area of increasing interest. Additive manufacturing is a broad term encompassing three-dimensional printing and several other varieties of material manufacturing, which involve computer-directed layer-by-layer synthesis of a material such as a bone graft substitute.[64] Current technology allows the development of custom-designed three-dimensional scaffolds with a specific microarchitecture that can match specific patient needs.[1] One of the many benefits of additive manufacturing is that it offers precise control over porosity, pore interconnectivity, filament size, and filament alignment. Extrusion-based additive manufacturing is a technique that is particularly well suited to the creation of osteoconductive bone graft substitutes. Inkjet and extrusion-based additive manufacturing systems such as three-dimensional bioplotting can be used for simultaneous scaffold formation, cell and growth factor delivery when used under sterile conditions.[64]

The potential clinical translation of additive manufacturing has been established in an animal long bone defect model.[65] Investigators used fused deposition molding of medical-grade polycaprolactone-tricalcium phosphate to produce cylindrical scaffolds. The scaffolds were implanted in a sheep tibial critical-sized bone defect model. Scaffolds were implanted alone and in combination with BMP-7 or bone marrow cells. Comparison was made to empty defects and to defects filled with an autologous bone graft. Histological, biomechanical, and micro-computed tomography analysis was performed at 3 and 12 months. They found that scaffolds combined with BMP-7 produced a bone regenerate equivalent to autologous bone graft, while the scaffolds combined with bone marrow cells did not seem to augment bone formation.

COMMON INDICATIONS AND CASE EXAMPLES

Osteoconductive bone graft substitutes can be used to support any reduced articular surface, filling the subchondral or metaphyseal void created by the injury. One of the most common uses is in the tibial plateau (Figures 5.1 and 5.2) where articular impaction is frequently seen. Osteoconductive bone graft substitutes are indicated to be used in conjunction with internal fixation. While some can be placed prior to insertion of the fixation, sometimes described as drillable products, most are paced after completion of the internal fixation. Other common indication for the use of osteoconductive bone graft substitutes include the tibial pilon and distal radius. Several injectable bone graft substitutes where originally studied in the distal radius.[8,9] This location was primarily selected because of the frequency of the injury. Since then, the introduction and widespread adoption of locked plate fixation has decreased the need for metaphyseal void filling in these injuries.

As previously described, calcium sulfate is commonly combined with antibiotics and used as a drug delivery vehicle to provide local release of antibiotics in an area of deep infection. Other frequent uses of osteoconductive bone graft substitutes are as a bone graft extender when the defect or fusion area is larger than the available autogenous bone graft.

The market for osteoconductive bone graft substitutes is very large and profitable leading to an ever-increasing number of available products. Most of these products have not undergone clinical evaluation and most available literature consists of low-level studies and case series. Further comparative clinical evaluations, ideally in randomized controlled trials including an arm without any graft substitute, would be helpful in determining which osteoconductive bone graft substitute best optimizes patient outcomes for a specific indication.

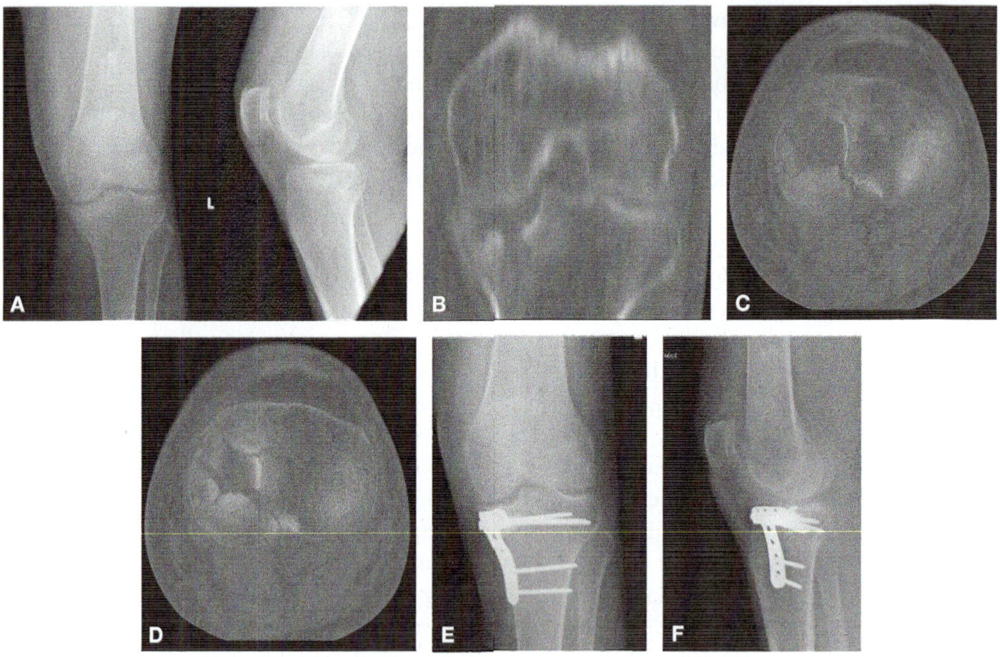

Figure 5.1. **A.** Anteroposterior and lateral radiographs of an 81-year-old female community ambulator who sustained a lateral tibial plateau fracture with 11 mm of central depression as the result of a ground-level fall. **B-D.** Computerized tomography scan with coronal reconstruction demonstrating the location and size of the articular depression. **E, F.** The patient underwent open reduction and internal fixation. Injectable calcium phosphate bone graft substitute was inserted beneath the reduced articular depression. Anteroposterior and lateral radiographs at 4-month follow-up show maintenance of the articular reduction without subsidence.

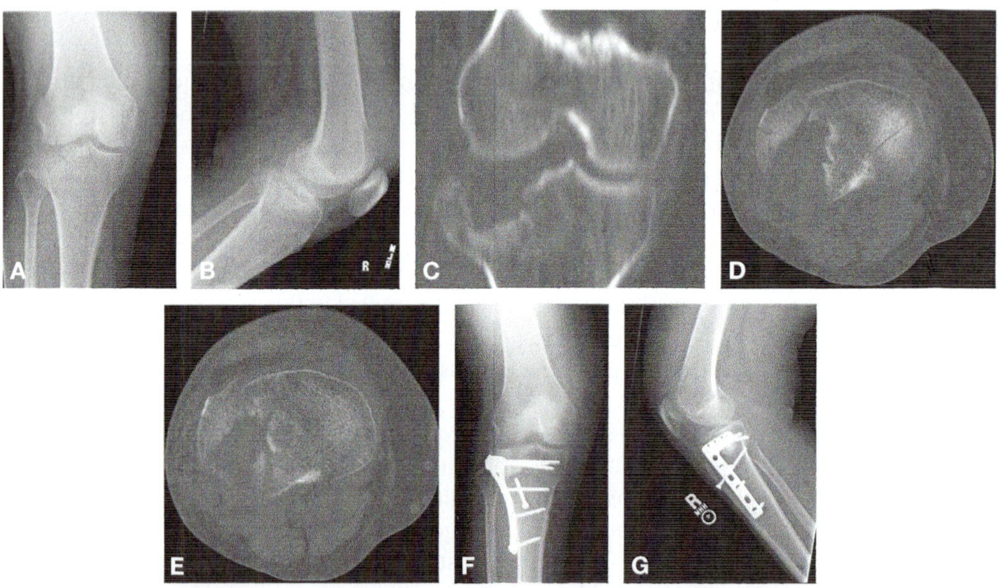

Figure 5.2. **A, B.** Anteroposterior and lateral radiographs of a 52-year-old female who sustained a lateral tibial plateau fracture with 16 mm of articular depression as the result of a 3-foot fall from a ladder. **C-E.** Computerized tomography scan with coronal reconstruction demonstrating the location and size of the articular depression. **F, G.** The patient underwent open reduction and internal fixation. A block of hydroxyapatite bone graft substitute was inserted beneath the reduced articular depression. Postoperative anteroposterior and lateral radiographs at 3 months show maintenance of the articular reduction without subsidence.

References

1. Weber FE. Reconsidering osteoconduction in the era of additive manufacturing. *Tissue Eng Part B Rev.* 2019;25(5):375-386.
2. Ghayor C, Weber FE. Osteoconductive microarchitecture of bone substitutes for bone regeneration revisited. *Front Physiol.* 2018;9:960. eCollection 2018. doi:10.3389/fphys.2018.00960
3. Bauer TW, Smith ST. Bioactive materials in orthopaedic surgery: overview and regulatory considerations. *Clin Orthop Relat Res.* 2002;395:11-22.
4. Kurien T, Pearson RG, Scammell BE. Bone graft substitutes currently available in orthopaedic practice: the evidence for their use. *Bone Joint J.* 2013;95-B:583-597.
5. Schildhauer TA, Bauer TW, Josten C, Muhr H. Open reduction and internal fixation with an injectable skeletal cement for the treatment of complex calcaneal fractures. *J Orthop Trauma.* 2000;14:309-317.
6. Constanz BR, Ison IC, Fulmer MT, et al. Skeletal repair by in situ formation of the mineral phase of bone. *Science.* 1995;267:1796-1799.
7. Frankenburg EP, Goldstein SA, Bauer TW, et al. Biomechanical and histologic evaluation of calcium phosphate cement. *J Bone Joint Surg.* 1998;80A:1112-1124.
8. Sanchez-Sotelo J, Munuera L, Madero R. Treatment of Fractures of the distal radius with a remodellable bone cement: a prospective, randomized study using Norian SRS. *J Bone Joint Surg Br.* 2000;82B:856-863.
9. Cassidy C, Jupiter JB, Cohen M, et al. Norian SRS cement compared with conventional fixation in distal radius fractures: a randomized study. *J Bone Joint Surg.* 2003;85A:2127-2137.
10. Lobenhoffer P, Gerich T, Witte F, Tscherne H. Use of injectable calcium phosphate cement in the treatment of tibial plateau fractures: a prospective study of twenty-six cases with twenty-month mean follow-up. *J Orthop Trauma.* 2002;16:143-149.
11. Russell TA, Leighton RK; Alpha-BSM Tibial Plateau Fracture Study Group. Comparison of autogenous bone graft and endothermic calcium phosphate cement for defect augmentation in tibial plateau fractures. A multicenter, prospective, randomized study. *J Bone Joint Surg Am.* 2008;90(10):2057-2061.
12. Atassi OH, Busel G, De La Fuente G, et al. The use of a novel moldable calcium phosphate putty (montage) for periarticular fractures: early clinical results. *Tech Orthop.* 2021;36(4):505-508.
13. Johal HS, Buckley RE, Le IL, Leighton RK. A prospective randomized controlled trial of a bioresorbable calcium phosphate paste (alpha-BSM) in treatment of displaced intra-articular calcaneal fractures. *J Trauma.* 2009;67(4):875-882.
14. Dressmann H. Ueber Knochenplombierung. *Bietr Klin Chir.* 1892;9:804-810.
15. Peltier LF, Lillo R. The substitution of plaster of Paris rods for portions of the diaphysis of the radius in dogs. *Surg Forum.* 1955;6:556-558.
16. Peltier LF. The use of plaster of Paris to fill large defects in bone. *Am J Surg.* 1959;97:311-315.
17. Peltier LF. The use of plaster of Paris to fill defects in bone. *Clin Orthop.* 1961;21:1-29.
18. Peltier LF, Jones RH. Treatment of unicameral bone cysts by curettage and packing with plaster of Paris pellets. *J Bone Joint Surg Am.* 1978;60:820-822.
19. Stubbs D, Deakin M, Chapman-Sheath P, et al. In vivo evaluation of resorbable bone graft substitutes in a rabbit tibial defect model. *Biomaterials.* 2004;25:5037-5044.
20. Walsh WR, Morberg P, Yu Y, et al. Response of a calcium sulfate bone graft substitute in a confined cancellous defect. *Clin Orthop.* 2003;406:228-236.
21. Sidqui M, Collin P, Vitte C, Forest N. Osteoblast adherence and resorption activity of isolated osteoclasts on calcium sulphate hemihydrate. *Biomaterials.* 1995;16:1327-1332.
22. Bucholz RW. Nonallograft osteoconductive bone graft substitutes. *Clin Orthop.* 2002;395:44-52.
23. Pietrzak WS, Ronk R. Calcium sulfate bone void filler: a review and look ahead. *J Craniofac Surg.* 2000;11:327-333.
24. Gitelis S, Pinsecki P. Use of a calcium sulfate-based bone graft substitute for benign bone lesions. *Orthopaedics.* 2001;24:162-166.
25. Mirzayan R, Panossian V, Avedian R, Forrester DM, Menendez LR. The use of calcium sulfate in the treatment of benign bone lesions. *J Bone Joint Surg.* 2001;83A:355-358.
26. Blaha JD. Calcium sulfate bone-void filler. *Orthopedics.* 1998;21:1017-1019.
27. Turner RM, Urban RM, Gitelis S, Kuo KN, Andersson GB. Radiographic and histologic assessment of calcium sulfate in experimental animal models and clinical use as a resorbable, bone-graft substitute, bone-graft expander, and a method for local antibiotic delivery: one institution's experience. *J Bone Joint Surg.* 2001;83A(Suppl 2, part 1):8-18.
28. Beuerlein MJ, McKee MD. Calcium sulfates: what is the evidence? *J Orthop Trauma.* 2010;24(suppl 1):S46-S51.
29. Watson JT. The use of an injectable bone graft substitute in tibial metaphyseal fractures. *Orthopedics.* 2004;27(1 Suppl):s103-s107.
30. Moed BR, Carr SEW, Craid JG, Watson JT. Calcium sulfate used as bone graft substitute in acetabular fracture fixation. *Clin Orthop.* 2003;410:303-309.
31. Doadrio JC, Arcos D, Cabañas MV, Vallet-Regi M. Calcium sulphate-based cements containing cephalexin. *Biomaterials.* 2004;25:2629-2635.

32. Pietrzak WS, Eppley BL. In vitro analysis of the elution of tobramycin from a calcium sulfate bone void filler. *J Craniofacial Surg.* 2004;15:752-757.
33. Nelson CL, McLaren SG, Skinner RA, et al. The treatment of experimental osteomyelitis by surgical debridement and the implantation of calcium sulfate tobramycin pellets. *J Orthop Res.* 2002;20:643-647.
34. McKee MD, Wild LM, Schemitsch EH, Waddell JP. The use of an antibiotic-impregnated, osteoconductive bioabsorbable bone substitute in the treatment of long bone defects: Early results in a prospective trial. *J Orthop Trauma.* 2002;16:622-627.
35. Shi X, Wu Y, Ni H, et al. Antibiotic-loaded calcium sulfate in clinical treatment of chronic osteomyelitis: a systematic review and meta-analysis. *J Orthop Surg Res.* 2022;17(1):104. doi:10.1186/s13018-022-02980-2
36. Hench LL. The story of Bioglass. *J Mater Sci Mater Med.* 2006;17:967-978.
37. Thomas MV, Puleo DA, Al-Sabbagh M. Bioactive glass three decades on. *J Long Term Eff Med Implants.* 2005;15:585-597.
38. Valmaki VV, Aro HT. Molecular basis for the action of bioactive glasses as bone graft substitute. *Scand J Surg.* 2006;95:95-102.
39. Sun JY, Hao SC, Sun RB, Yang YS. Treatment of high-energy tibial shaft fractures with internal fixation and early prophylactic NovaBone grafting. *Orthop Surg.* 2009;1(1):17-21.
40. Heikkilä JT, Kukkonen J, Aho AJ, Moisander S, Kyyrönen T, Mattila K. Bioactive glass granules: a suitable bone substitute material in the operative treatment of depressed lateral tibial plateau fractures: a prospective, randomized 1 year follow-up study. *J Mater Sci Mater Med.* 2011;22(4):1073-1080.
41. Boyan BD, McMillan J, Lohmann CH, Ranly DM, Schwartz Z. Basic information for successful clinical use with special focus on synthetic graft substitutes. In: Laurencin CT, ed. *Bone Graft Substitutes.* ASTM Int; 2002:231-259.
42. Fiume E, Magnaterra G, Rahdar A, Verné E, Baino F. Hydroxyapatite for biomedical applications: a short overview. *Ceramics.* 2021;4:542-563.
43. Roy DM, Linnehan SK. Hydroxyapatite formed from coral skeletal carbonate by hydrothermal exchange. *Nature.* 1974;247:220-222.
44. Cornell CN, Lane JM. Current understanding of osteoconduction in bone regeneration. *Clin Orthop.* 1998;355:S267-S273.
45. Holmes RE, Bucholz RW, Mooney V. Porous hydroxyapatite as a bone-graft substitute in metaphyseal defects: a histometric study. *J Bone Joint Surg.* 1986;68:904-911.
46. Holmes R, Mooney V, Bucholz R, Tender A. A coralline hydroxyapatite bone graft substitute: preliminary report. *Clin Orthop.* 1984;188:252-262.
47. Boden SD, Martin GJ Jr, Morone M, Ugbo JL, Titus L, Hutton WC. The use of coralline hydroxyapatite with bone marrow, autogenous bone graft, or osteoinductive bone protein extract for posterolateral lumbar spine fusion. *Spine.* 1999;24:320-327.
48. Martin RB, Chapman MW, Sharkey NA, Zissimos SL, Bay B, Shors EC. Bone ingrowth and mechanical properties of coralline hydroxyapatite 1 yr after implantation. *Biomaterials.* 1993;14:341-348.
49. Bucholz RW, Carlton A, Holmes R. Interporous hydroxyapatite as a bone graft substitute in tibial plateau fractures. *Clin Orthop.* 1989;240:53-62.
50. Wolfe SW, Pike L, Slade JF III, Katz LD. Augmentation of distal radius fracture fixation with coralline hydroxyapatite bone graft substitute. *J Hand Surg (Am).* 1999;24:816-827.
51. Albee FH, Morrison HF. Studies in bone growth, triple calcium phosphate as a stimulus to osteogenesis. *Ann Surg.* 1920;71:32-39.
52. Wiltfang F, Merten MA, Schlegel KA, et al. Degradation characteristics of α and β tri-calcium phosphate (TCP) in minipigs. *J Biomed Mater Res.* 2002;63:115-121.
53. Jarcho M. Calcium phosphate ceramics as hard tissue prosthetics. *Clin Orthop.* 1981;157:259-278.
54. Moore WR, Graves SE, Bain GI. Synthetic bone graft substitutes. *ANZ J Surg.* 2001;71:354-361.
55. Bucholz RW, Carlton A, Holmes RE. Hydroxyapatite and tricalcium phosphate bone graft substitutes. *Orthop Clinic North Am.* 1987;18:323-334.
56. McAndrew MP, Gorman PW, Lange TA. Tricalcium phosphate as a bone graft substitute in trauma: preliminary report. *J Orthop Trauma.* 1988;2:333-339.
57. van Hemert WL, Willems K, Anderson PG, van Heerwaarden RJ, Wymenga AB. Tricalcium phosphate granules or rigid wedge performs in open wedge high tibial osteotomy: a radiological study with a new evaluation system. *Knee.* 2004;11:451-456.
58. van Haaren EH, Smit TH, Phipps K, Wuisman PIJM, Blunn G, Heyligers IC. Tricalcium phosphate and hydroxyapatite bone-graft extender for use in impaction grafting revision surgery: An in vitro study on human femora. *J Bone Join Surg Br.* 2005;87:267-271.
59. Erbe EM, Marx JG, Clineff TD, Bellincampi LD. Potential of an ultraporous β-tricalcium phosphate synthetic bone void filler and bone marrow aspirate composite graft. *Eur Spine J.* 2001;10:S141-S146.
60. Gunzburg R, Szpalski M. The use of a novel beta-tricalcium phosphate-based bone void filler as a graft extender in spinal fusion surgeries. *Orthopedics.* 2002;25(5 Suppl):S591-S595.
61. Meadows DR. Adjunctive use of intraporous beta-tricalcium phosphate bone void filler in spinal arthrodesis. *Orthopedics.* 2002;25(5 Suppl):S579-S584.

62. Ohyama T, Kubo Y, Iwata H, Taki W. Beta-tricalcium phosphate combined with recombinant human bone morphogenetic protein-2: a substitute for autograft, used for packing interbody fusion cages in the canine lumbar spine. *Neurol Med Chir (Tokyo).* 2004;44:234-240.
63. Hofmann A, Gorbulev S, Guehring T, et al; CERTiFy Study Group. Autologous iliac bone graft compared with biphasic hydroxyapatite and calcium sulfate cement for the treatment of bone defects in tibial plateau fractures: a prospective, randomized, open-label, multicenter study. *J Bone Joint Surg Am.* 2020;102(3):179-193.
64. Gibbs DMR, Vaezi M, Yang S, Oreffo ROC. Hope versus hype: what can additive manufacturing realistically offer trauma and orthopedic surgery? *Regen Med.* 2014;9:535-549.
65. Reichert JC, Cipitria A, Epari DR, et al. A tissue engineering solution for segmental defect regeneration in load-bearing long bones. *Sci Transl Med.* 2012;4:141ra93.

6 Demineralized Bone Matrix and Clinical Uses

Jack Zhong, Benjamin C. Schaffler, and Philipp Leucht

INTRODUCTION

A variety of orthobiologics are at the disposal of the orthopedic surgeon to enhance fracture healing, fusion, and reconstruction of bone defects. Understanding the capabilities and shortcomings of each biologic will help the orthopedic surgeon select the correct one for application. This review will focus on one such orthobiologic: demineralized bone matrix (DBM). The molecular mechanism and clinical applications of DBM will be unpacked, and clinical cases of its use will be described.

Orthobiologics are grouped into osteoconductive (matrix substitutes), osteoinductive (growth factors), and osteogenic (stem/progenitor cells). DBM falls under the osteoinductive and osteoconductive categories.[1] DBM is thought to have osteoinductive properties by mobilizing growth factors left in the extracellular matrix during the demineralization process.[2] Depending on its form, DBM may have an osteoconductive effect while its scaffolding is present.[3] DBM is used as a bridging material, providing a wide surface area to serve as cellular attachment sites. It functions similar to alloplastic void fillers, although its strength in compression is relatively weak.[1] Therefore, it is not an appropriate option when structural support is needed for the particular bone defect to be reconstructed.

DBM has been described as early as 1965 when Urist[4] described decalcified bone causing formation of new bone by autoinduction on histological study. DBM processing involves pulverizing allograft bone and decalcification with hydrochloric acid solution.[4] The mineral components are removed and the collagen matrix, growth factors, proteins remain.[3] Modern processing of DBM has introduced variability in the protocol, but the theory behind the graft remains the same.

BIOLOGY AND MECHANISM OF ACTION

Early studies of DBM compared mineralized bone particles to demineralized bone particles (DBPs) in rat cranial defect models.[5] It was found DBP elicited migration of connective tissue cells, conversion of those cells to chondroblasts and extracellular cartilage matrix, and replacement of matrix with bone.[5] This process is similar to endochondral ossification. Meanwhile, mineralized bone particles elicited osteoclast differentiation and resorption, mediated by the presence of minerals and osteocalcin.[6]

From in vitro studies, DBM is thought to contain inductive growth factors such as bone morphogenetic protein (BMP)-2 and BMP-7 and transforming growth factor-β (TGF-β).[7] Culturing human dermal fibroblasts with DBPs modulated TGF-β and Hedgehog signaling pathways.[8] Zhou et al[9] demonstrated summative effects of BMP-2 and TGF-β1 modulation of the Wnt signaling, which are implicated in the regulation of chondrocyte, osteoblast, and osteoclast differentiation. Glowacki et al[6] investigated the effects of DBM compared with BMP-2 and/or TGF-β. BMP and TGF-β mixture stimulated chondroitin production that was similar in composition but to a lesser amount than that stimulated by DBP.

In vivo, DBM has been shown to induce cartilage formation in various rat tissues, with the most effect in muscle, followed by subcutaneous tissue, and then bone.[10] DBM is understood to mainly elicit bone formation through endochondral ossification.[11] In a mouse cortical bone defects model, DBM has also been reported to induce bone formation through intramembranous ossification.[12] DBM has been shown to have osteoinductive properties. Tavakol et al[13] demonstrated that albumin instead of carboxymethyl cellulose used as carrier for DBM demonstrated improved bone regeneration in rats in vivo at 8 weeks.

CLINICAL APPLICATIONS

DBM can be used as a graft in isolation or as a graft expander in combination with allograft or autologous cell populations. Although it lacks a structural benefit, DBM alone can be used as a bone void filler or isolated graft choice in different realms of orthopedic surgery. DBM alone has been demonstrated in the literature to have similar rates of fusion following instrumented procedures to allograft.[3] In fracture care, DBM can be utilized in areas of bone loss as well as in nonunion repair. While there are no studies directly comparing the rates of union in fractures treated with DBM alone and other types of allograft, Brink[3] did note that the efficacy of DBM in promoting healing is dependent on proper graft processing and it has a relatively higher cost than other graft alternatives.

Although isolated use of DBM is rare, there have been several case series that describe its use alone. Haß et al.[14] described a case series where juvenile bone cysts were curettaged and packed with DBM. Radiographic changes were reported to start at 3 to 4 months, followed by cortical remodeling at 6 months, and total radiopaque filling of the defect at 8 months.[14] There was one distal tibia pathologic fracture at 5 months postoperatively. Wilkins and Kelley[15] reported the use of DBM for the treatment of 35 fracture nonunions and 41 benign bone tumor excision. DBM alone was used in 97% of patients, bone marrow aspirate (BMA) was added in two tibial nonunion, and strut allograft was added in three humeral nonunion. The bone healing rate was 85.1% for fracture nonunion and 93% for benign tumor excision.[15]

DBM is often combined with other autologous compounds in hopes of improving its successes in orthopedics. Researchers have experimented with combining DBM with platelet-rich plasma (PRP) as well as mesenchymal stromal cells (MSCs). Autogenous PRP contains endogenous growth factors found in platelets, and its precise role in orthopedics has not been fully elucidated. MSCs are a heterogeneous population of mesenchymal and hematogenous cells, which are not well-defined but likely contain a small fraction of progenitor cells that possess a secretory profile that contributes to bone regeneration.[16] In a canine study, Brodke et al[17] noted that the combination of DBM with retained progenitor cells and PRP may contribute to more mature bone formation, although the results were not significant. Conversely, Boyan et al[18] noted decreased osteoinduction in DBM combined with activated PRP. This point was echoed by Ranly et al[19] who also noted in a mouse model that DBM infused with PRP actually had less osteoinductive capacity. In fracture healing and trauma surgery, there is not yet a clear indication for PRP enhanced with MSCs or PRP.

BMA concentrate is often combined with DBM with the intention of adding an osteogenic cell population to the DBM allograft (Figure 6.1). DBM in combination with BMA concentrate has demonstrated good clinical results in achieving fusion and promoting bony union. Lindsey et al[20] compared DBM augmented with BMA to iliac crest autograft in augmenting long bone fractures and noted improved rates of union in the composite DBM group. Tricot et al[21] reported in patients undergoing hindfoot fusion that DBM + BMA had equivalent clinical outcomes to DBM used in combination with autograft, with no significant increase in nonunion or reoperation. In posterior spinal fusion, DBM + BMA is equally as effective, promoting high fusion rates without the complications of seroma associated with BMP.[22]

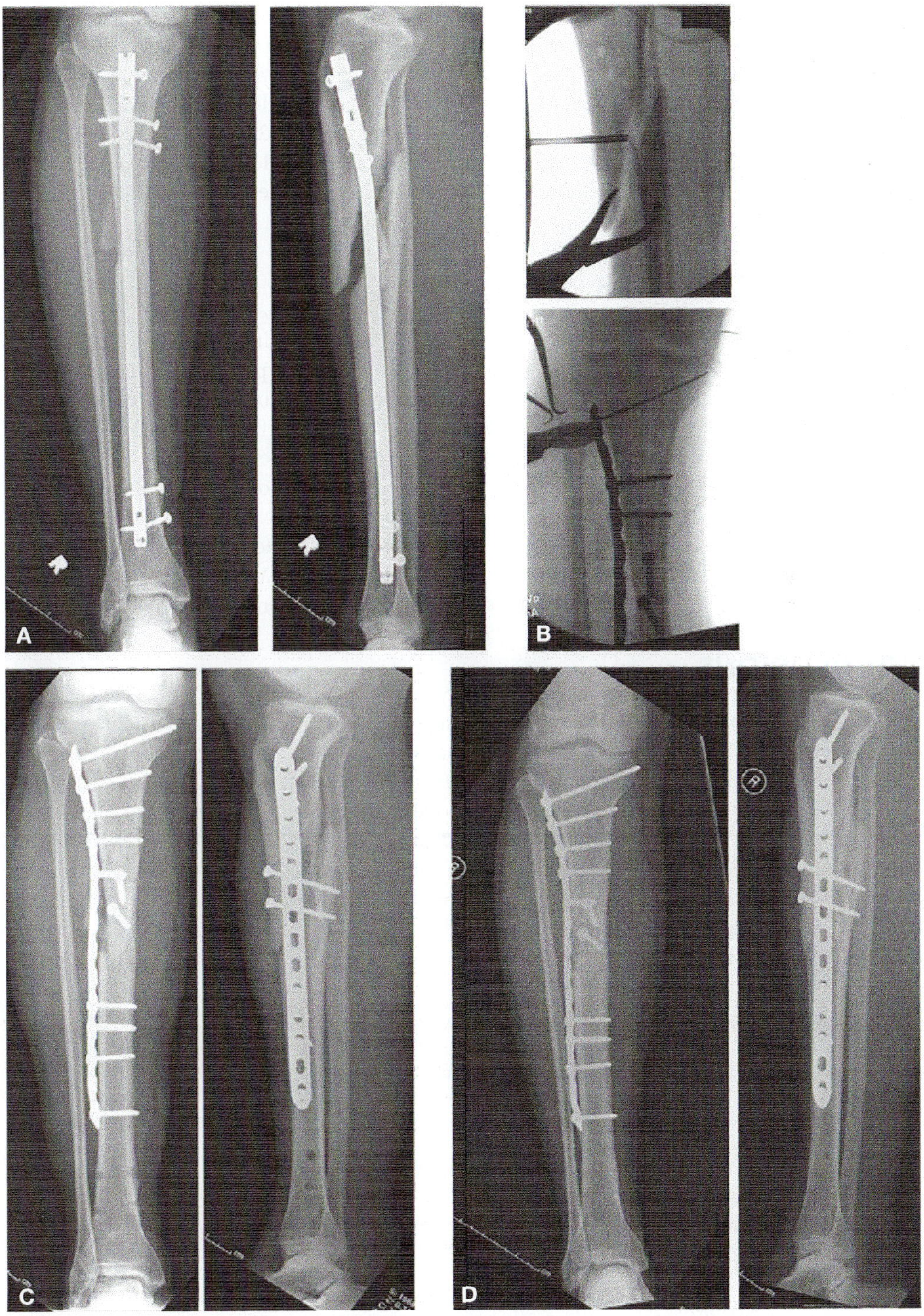

Figure 6.1. **A.** Atrophic nonunion at 5 months tibial nailing with large fracture gap. **B.** Intraoperative images demonstrating intramedullary application of demineralized bone matrix + bone marrow aspirate concentrate composite graft with revision plating. **C.** Initial postoperative x-ray. **D.** Final x-ray at 6 months demonstrating vigorous callous with complete bridging of the nonunion.

Differences exist in DBM type and effectiveness, attributed to nonstandardization in processing techniques and donor bone quality. DBM can be manufactured as freeze-dried powder, granules, gel putty, or strips. The formulation can be changed based on manufacturing and combining with other materials such as allogenic bone chips or calcium sulfate granules. Interestingly, there seems to be significant lot-to-lot variability in terms of BMP-2/7 concentrations in DBM purchased commercially. BMP-2/7 concentration had a dose-dependent effect on fusion in a rat model.[23] Comparison of different brands of DBM showed brand-related differences in fusion rates ranging from 0% to 100% in a mouse model of spinal fusion.[24]

FUTURE DIRECTIONS

Although an abundance of studies have analyzed DBM in vitro and in animal models, there has been no level I evidence analyzing its use and effectiveness in human patients. DBM is often used in conjunction with other allograft and autograft materials, which confounds its true effects on patients. More high-level studies are needed to analyze the clinical effects of DBM compared to other grafts. New technology is being leveraged to make improvements to DBM. Presently, 3D printing technology has been described to coat porous polycaprolactone/β-tricalcium phosphate scaffolds with nano-DBM and demonstrated this material to enhance cell proliferation in vitro.[25] DBM with hydrogel has also been investigated as a delivery system for bone-derived stem cells, and it has been shown to have higher osteogenicity than standard DBM in vivo rat model.[26] It will be interesting to see the clinical effects of these improvements on bone healing.

CONCLUSIONS

DBM is a versatile, processed allograft product that contains osteoinductive and osteoconductive properties but lacks osteogenic potential. DBM has many reported uses in orthopedic surgery, both in isolation and in combination with other orthobiologic factors. Due to its weak structure, DBM is most appropriate to promote fusion and bone healing in sites not exposed to high forces. DBM can have wide variability in its structure and content based on how it is processed and between commercial retailers. Research efforts have been focused on combining DBM with other osteogenic factors to improve its osteogenic potential, although no large clinical studies exist in this realm. DBM is available as a commercial product and thus cost considerations should come into play when considering its use.

REFERENCES

1. Leucht P, Watson JT. Orthobiologics for fracture healing: opportunities and risks. *AAOS Now*. 2015;42.
2. Kinney RC, Ziran BH, Hirshorn K, Schlatterer D, Ganey T. Demineralized bone matrix for fracture healing: fact or fiction? *J Orthop Trauma*. 2010;24. https://journals.lww.com/jorthotrauma/fulltext/2010/03001/demineralized_bone_matrix_for_fracture_healing_.11.aspx
3. Brink O. The choice between allograft or demineralized bone matrix is not unambiguous in trauma surgery. *Injury*. 2021;52:S23-S28. doi:10.1016/j.injury.2020.11.013
4. Urist MR. Bone: formation by autoinduction. *Science*. 1965;150(3698):893-899. doi:10.1126/science.150.3698.893
5. Glowacki J, Altobelli D, Mulliken JB. Fate of mineralized and demineralized osseous implants in cranial defects. *Calcif Tissue Int*. 1981;33(1):71-76. doi:10.1007/BF02409414
6. Glowacki J, Zhou S, Mizuno S. Mechanisms of osteoinduction/chondroinduction by demineralized bone. *J Craniofac Surg*. 2009;20:634-638. https://journals.lww.com/jcraniofacialsurgery/fulltext/2009/03001/mechanisms_of_osteoinduction_chondroinduction_by.17.aspx
7. Mohan S, Baylink DJ. Bone growth factors. *Clin Orthop*. 1991;263:30-48.
8. Yates KE, Mizuno S, Glowacki J. Early shifts in gene expression during chondroinduction of human dermal fibroblasts. *Exp Cell Res*. 2001;265(2):203-211. doi:10.1006/excr.2001.5192
9. Zhou S, Mizuno S, Glowacki J. Wnt pathway regulation by demineralized bone is approximated by both BMP-2 and TGF-β1 signaling. *J Orthop Res Off Publ Orthop Res Soc*. 2013;31(4):554-560. doi:10.1002/jor.22244

10. Inoue T, Deporter DA, Melcher AH. Induction of chondrogenesis in muscle, skin, bone marrow, and periodontal ligament by demineralized dentin and bone matrix in vivo and in vitro. *J Dent Res*. 1986;65(1):12-22. doi:10.1177/00220345860650010101
11. Yasko AW, Lane JM, Fellinger EJ, Rosen V, Wozney JM, Wang EA. The healing of segmental bone defects, induced by recombinant human bone morphogenetic protein (rhBMP-2). A radiographic, histological, and biomechanical study in rats. *J Bone Joint Surg Am*. 1992;74(5):659-670.
12. Colnot C, Romero DM, Huang S, Helms JA. Mechanisms of action of demineralized bone matrix in the repair of cortical bone defects. *Clin Orthop Relat Res*. 2005;435. https://journals.lww.com/clinorthop/fulltext/2005/06000/mechanisms_of_action_of_demineralized_bone_matrix.12.aspx
13. Tavakol S, Khoshzaban A, Azami M, et al. The effect of carrier type on bone regeneration of demineralized bone matrix in vivo. *J Craniofac Surg*. 2013;24(6):2135-2140. https://journals.lww.com/jcraniofacialsurgery/fulltext/2013/11000/the_effect_of_carrier_type_on_bone_regeneration_of.60.aspx
14. Haß HJ, Krause H, Kroker S, Wagemann W. Implantation humaner demineralisierter Knochenmatrix (DBM) zur Behandlung juveniler Knochenzysten. *Oper Orthop Traumatol*. 2006;18(1):19-33. doi:10.1007/s00064-006-1160-8
15. Wilkins Ross M, Kelly CM. The effect of allomatrix injectable putty on the outcome of long bone applications. *Orthopedics*. 2003;26(5):S567-S570. doi:10.3928/0147-7447-20030502-08
16. Keating A. Mesenchymal stromal cells. *Curr Opin Hematol*. 2006;13(6):419-425. doi:10.1097/01.moh.0000245697.54887.6f
17. Brodke D, Pedrozo HA, Kapur TA, et al. Bone grafts prepared with selective cell retention technology heal canine segmental defects as effectively as autograft. *J Orthop Res Off Publ Orthop Res Soc*. 2006;24(5):857-866. doi:10.1002/jor.20094
18. Boyan BD, Ranly DM, Schwartz Z. Use of growth factors to modify osteoinductivity of demineralized bone allografts: lessons for tissue engineering of bone. *Dent Clin North Am*. 2006;50(2):217-228, viii. doi:10.1016/j.cden.2005.11.007
19. Ranly DM, Lohmann CH, Andreacchio D, Boyan BD, Schwartz Z. Platelet-rich plasma inhibits demineralized bone matrix-induced bone formation in nude mice. *J Bone Joint Surg Am*. 2007;89(1):139-147. doi:10.2106/JBJS.F.00388
20. Lindsey RW, Wood GW, Sadasivian KK, Stubbs HA, Block JE. Grafting long bone fractures with demineralized bone matrix putty enriched with bone marrow: pilot findings. *Orthopedics*. 2006;29(10):939-941. doi:10.3928/01477447-20061001-07
21. Tricot M, Deleu PA, Detrembleur C, Leemrijse T. Clinical assessment of 115 cases of hindfoot fusion with two different types of graft: allograft+DBM+bone marrow aspirate versus autograft+DBM. *Orthop Traumatol Surg Res OTSR*. 2017;103(5):697-702. doi:10.1016/j.otsr.2017.03.014
22. Rodgers WB, Gerber EJ. A DBM, BMA, local bone graft composite in multi-level PLIF: fusion rates. *Spine J*. 2010;10(9):S26. doi:10.1016/j.spinee.2010.07.076
23. Bae H, Zhao L, Zhu D, Kanim LE, Wang JC, Delamarter RB. Variability across ten production lots of a single demineralized bone matrix product. *JBJS*. 2010;92(2):427-435. https://journals.lww.com/jbjsjournal/fulltext/2010/02000/variability_across_ten_production_lots_of_a_single.20.aspx
24. Russell N, Walsh WR, Lovric V, et al. In-vivo performance of seven commercially available demineralized bone matrix fiber and putty products in a rat posterolateral fusion model. *Front Surg*. 2020;7:10. https://www.frontiersin.org/articles/10.3389/fsurg.2020.00010
25. Yuan B, Wang Z, Zhao Y, et al. In vitro and in vivo study of a novel nanoscale demineralized bone matrix coated PCL/β-TCP scaffold for bone regeneration. *Macromol Biosci*. 2021;21(3):2000336. doi:10.1002/mabi.202000336
26. Vurat MT, Parmaksiz M, Elçin AE, Elçin YM. Bioactive composite hydrogels as 3D mesenchymal stem cell encapsulation environment for bone tissue engineering: in vitro and in vivo studies. *J Biomed Mater Res A*. 2023;111(2):261-277. doi:10.1002/jbm.a.37457

7 Basic Science

Michael J. Beltran

INTRODUCTION

Bone marrow is a dynamic tissue found within trabecular portions of both the axial and appendicular skeleton, most notably from the pelvis.[1] Composed of hematopoietic, adipose, and stromal support cells (which includes the important nonhematopoietic mesenchymal stem cells [MSCs]), its makeup changes over time; aging leads to a decrease in hematopoietic cells ("red marrow") and an increase in adipose tissue ("yellow marrow").[2] In addition to macroscopic changes to bone marrow with aging, the cellular function of MSCs found in bone marrow also appears to be affected by age, perhaps due to increased cellular senescence.[2] Diabetes and metabolic conditions have also been shown to affect MSC function in vivo.[2-4] Nonhematopoietic MSCs were first identified in bone marrow in 1968, and since then have been studied intensely due to their obvious utility in the field of regenerative medicine.[5] MSCs can assume an osteoprogenitor cell lineage based on local chemotactic and other growth factors, making their use advantageous when the goal is bony union; while other tissues have been shown to yield MSCs in varying quantities and concentrations, bone marrow represents the most readily available source of MSCs for clinical use in orthopedic surgery—particularly for trauma and nonunion applications.

Compared to autogenous corticocancellous bone graft material, bone marrow aspirate (BMA) does not have osteoconductive properties but does exhibit both osteoinductive and osteogenic potential due to the presence of MSCs and harvested growth factors; osteoconductivity can be obtained by mixing with allograft, a graft substitute such as demineralized bone matrix, or by augmenting already obtained autogenous graft (composite bone grafting). Centrifugation increases the concentration of MSCs that can be injected or mixed with allograft or a graft substitute but will not increase the absolute number of MSCs present in the aspirated sample. Both MSC concentration and absolute number of MSCs implanted at the site of a nonunion have been correlated with the likelihood of obtaining union. Concentrating BMA with a centrifuge does not compensate for poor harvest techniques.[6] In the author's opinion, its major benefit is the ability to handle a lower volume of material while maintaining a persistently high concentration and absolute number of MSCs, making percutaneous injection simpler or giving the surgeon more control over graft saturation during open grafting procedures.

Centrifuging BMA separates a sample into three distinct layers based on nuclear weight. The platelet poor plasma layer and the hematopoietic layer containing red blood cells are both discarded, leaving a "buffy coat" rich in MSCs, growth factors, and other cellular proteins.[7] This buffy coat layer often makes up approximately 10% to 15% of the harvested volume, meaning if 120 mL of BMA are harvested from the iliac crest, only 10 to 12 mL is available to be mixed with graft material or percutaneously injected. Centrifuging BMA does not guarantee that all MSCs harvested will be collected in the desired layer, however, and does not account for possible cell loss on filters within the system. Clinical series studying the use of BMA in the treatment of nonunions have demonstrated comparable efficacy regardless of whether concentration is performed.[6,8-10]

HARVEST TECHNIQUE

Hernigou's initial clinical and basic science research into bone marrow aspiration has been refined through subsequent study by his group and many others, most notably by Muschler and colleagues, and this body of scientific evidence provides surgeons with a technical blueprint for maximizing the harvest of MSCs, minimizing hemodilution, and obtaining predictable union with BMA or bone marrow aspirate concentrate (BMAC). It is important to understand the specific technical steps that should be taken to maximize MSC number and concentration—as mentioned previously, merely placing a needle into a random bony location and aspirating may not lead to sufficient stem cell harvest. The overarching goal when harvesting from bone marrow is to maximize the yield of MSCs while minimizing hemodilution. Unfortunately, there are peer-reviewed publications related to clinical harvest techniques that are fraught with common mistakes and pitfalls. Improper harvest technique may jeopardize the likelihood of obtaining a sufficient concentration of MSCs.[11]

Technical Considerations

While the use of a larger syringe and/or higher volume aliquots are both easier and faster intraoperatively for the surgeon, they are each associated with hemodilution and a lower harvest of MSCs; this appears to be the most common mistake cautioned by both centrifuge and BMA system manufacturers as well as authors describing their own technique for BMA harvest. A smaller syringe (10 mL) has demonstrable superiority over larger syringe sizes; this is postulated to be due to the generation of higher negative pressures within the syringe—a higher pressure gradient at the tip of the needle preferentially aspirates bone marrow adjacent to the needle tip before hemodilution occurs. In one study comparing 10 and 50 mL syringes, the concentration and number of MSCs harvested, independent of each aliquot volume drawn, was superior with the use of a 10 mL syringe.[12] Furthermore, the force with which the 10 mL syringe plunger is drawn back has also been shown to affect MSC harvest by creating a similar mechanical environment—demonstrating that higher negative pressures within the syringe are associated with a greater harvest of MSCs.[13] This rapid "jerk" technique requires that the plunger be drawn back as quickly as possible and immediately released once a small volume (2-4 mL) is acquired. The use of multiple small aliquot draws from multiple sites within the bone is recommended to maximize harvest and decrease hemodilution. At the histologic level within spongy cancellous bone such as the pelvis, only a small amount of cellular marrow is present immediately adjacent to the needle port(s). After the first 2 to 4 mL of BMA is aspirated, any additional volume consists mainly of hemodilution.[14]

Location of harvest must also be considered when deciding how to maximize MSC yields with BMA. Multiple sites of harvest have been described in orthopedic surgery, including the iliac crest, distal femur, proximal tibia, and calcaneus. However, only the iliac crest has shown promise in maximizing harvest of MSCs; sites outside the iliac crest should be avoided if possible for trauma and nonunion applications, especially if centrifugation is not planned.[15,16] Pierini et al[17,18] have demonstrated that harvest from the posterior iliac crest yields superior concentrations and absolute numbers of MSCs compared to more anterior locations on the iliac crest; violation of the inner or outer table of the crest is also less likely to occur posteriorly. However, both anterior and posterior iliac crest harvest sites have been shown to generate sufficiently high MSC concentrations to allow for predictable healing in numerous clinical series. Practically speaking, the site of harvest is likely to be chosen based on other intraoperative factors, such as patient positioning for a given clinical scenario, body habitus, and whether prior surgery to the pelvis has taken place. Whether the patient is supine or prone, the pelvis should always be prepped into the operative field to avoid settling for harvest from an inferior location.

Because factors such as syringe size and bony location affect cell harvest, it is not surprising that debate exists regarding which type of needle design is best used to maximize yield of MSCs. A simple needle with a single 45° beveled end port has been shown to be highly effective at harvesting BMA by Hernigou and others (Figure 7.1). Because the tip is facing a different area of marrow after the needle is rotated, it is possible to aspirate small aliquots of BMA from eight distinct areas (by rotating 45° prior to each syringe draw) before having to advance or pull back the needle tip to a new area of bone. This needle design has been extensively studied by Hernigou et al[6,19,20] for BMA applications in orthopedics, including nonunion applications. Needle length and diameter (gauge) should also be considered. While a small needle would in theory also contribute to generating a larger pressure gradient, in clinical practice, needles smaller than 11 gauge are difficult to work with and more prone to breakage as the needle is passed between the narrow inner and outer tables of the pelvis. Muschler et al[14] have previously demonstrated no difference in MSC harvest using either an 8- or 11-gauge needle and both are commonly available. The aspiration needle should be as long as necessary to maximize a given surgical technique; most needles available are up to 12 cm long, which is sufficient if the needle is entering the pelvis anywhere along the crest even in obese individuals. The authors prefer to use a longer needle, 15 cm in length, for technical reasons discussed later in this chapter.

Manufacturers of BMA harvest and centrifuge systems also provide their own aspiration needles in disposable kits and packs, meaning other needle designs are available and the surgeon should recognize if a given needle is worthy of use in BMA harvest. A commonly available needle

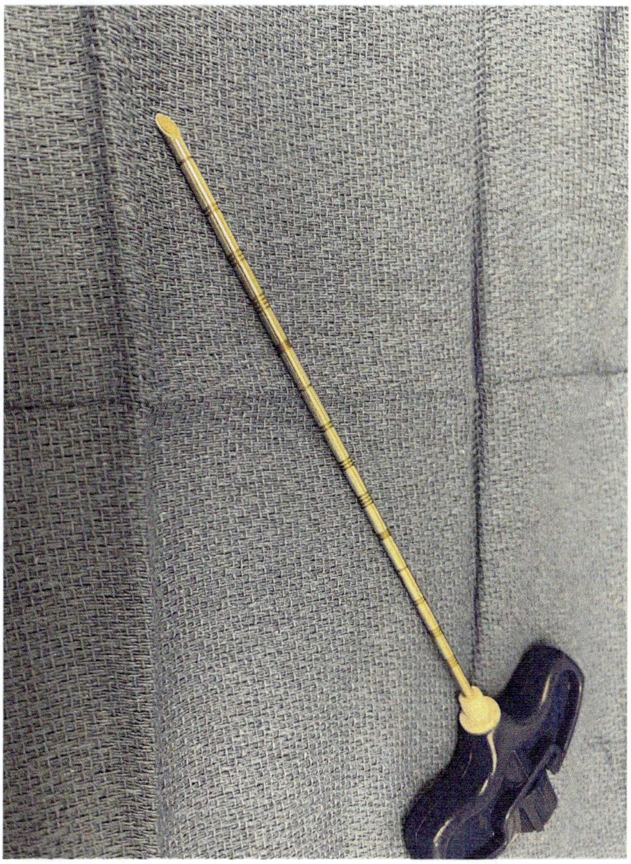

Figure 7.1. A beveled 45° end port needle permits multiple low volume aliquots at a given needle depth.

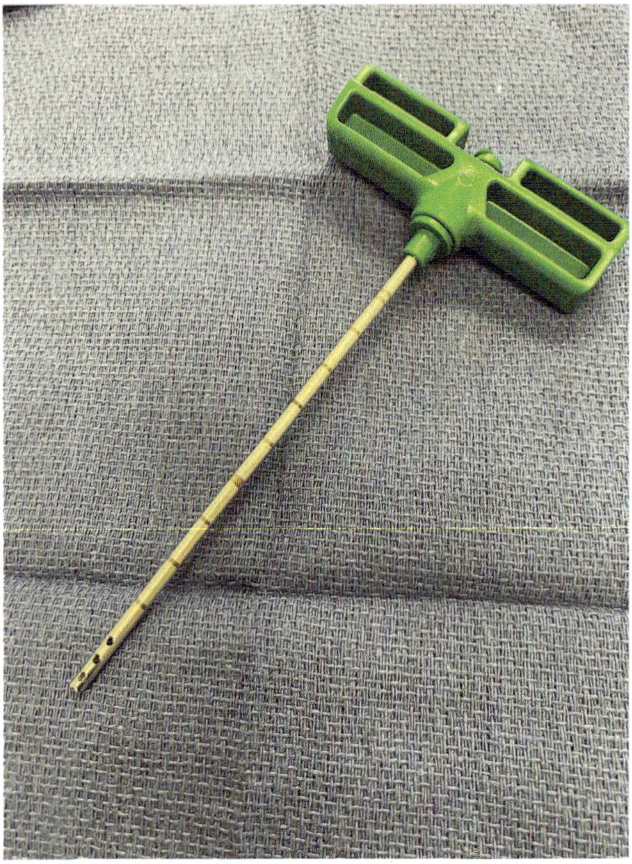

Figure 7.2. Multiple side port needle. Note the side port needle includes a straight open end port after trocar removal for aspiration, which increases hemodilution if the needle is pulled back versus advanced during aspiration.

design incorporates multiple side ports (usually four or six), which in theory allows for aspiration of cells from multiple areas simultaneously (Figure 7.2). Because side ports are present on either side of the needle, it should be rotated only four times before advancing or drawing back for repeat aspiration. The needle should be moved 2 cm to ensure that fresh areas of marrow are sampled. In clinical practice, this needle design requires more frequent redirection to new areas of the pelvis for aspiration if small aliquot sampling (as should be the goal) is utilized prior to centrifugation. Surgeons should avoid a single end port design, like the commonly available Jamshidi needle. This needle is prone to hemodilution, especially if the needle is pulled back prior to each aspiration; as the needle is pulled back, blood predictably fills the needle track, and no new MSC cells should be expected to be harvested. While in theory multiport designs make sense, to date no published data are available which suggest they are superior to a simple single port design to maximize harvest of MSCs. In clinical practice, the decision to utilize a specific needle may be dictated by hospital inventory and whether concentration is anticipated. BMAC disposable packs with syringes and aspiration trochars come standard with most centrifuge vendors.

Bone Marrow Aspirate Concentrate Preparation

The decision to proceed with producing concentrated BMA should be made prior to beginning the aspiration since appropriate measures must be taken to prevent premature clotting of the aspirated sample. The surgeon should have knowledge of their own hospital system regarding availability of a centrifuge, which will often be tied to using disposables for a specific vendor. Availability of the centrifuge and disposables should be coordinated ahead of time to ensure accessibility and avoid untimely delays in patient care.

Preventing premature clotting of the aspirated sample typically requires the use of heparinized saline and/or an anticoagulant citrate dextrose solution A (ACD-A). At least 1,000 units/mL of heparin is recommended to prevent clotting; the use of ACD-A is system dependent and typically is included with BMAC disposables. In addition, the aspiration needle and syringe should be flushed with ACD-A or heparin prior to beginning collection, adding another layer of protection to maximize the cellular yield from the concentrated specimen. Most systems require no less than 15 minutes of centrifugation before the aspirated sample has been separated out into its defined layers; some systems allow for "superconcentration" via an additional spin, adding time to the procedure. Based on the type of procedure being performed, the surgeon should time the aspiration portion of a case to coincide with additional surgical work that must be done (eg, a posterolateral approach to the tibia for nonunion) so that the increased surgical time associated with BMAC does not have an adverse effect on clinical outcomes.

Common Pitfalls and Mistakes

Numerous pitfalls and technical errors are possible during the harvesting of bone marrow. Understanding these issues helps to minimize adverse events while ensuring that a sufficient concentration of MSCs have been harvested to maximize the likelihood of obtaining bony union. Adverse events are commonly related to poor needle insertion technique and/or a poor understanding of pelvic anatomy, whereas technical errors leading to insufficient MSC harvest are easily remedied via appropriate harvest techniques.

Hernigou et al[21] have previously shown that compared to iliac crest bone graft (ICBG) harvest, bone marrow aspiration of MSCs has a predictably lower incidence of adverse events, including need for transfusion, donor site pain, and hematoma formation. However, adverse events are still possible with BMA, and compared to open ICBG, errant needle positioning has the potential to damage the bowel, pelvic vessels, or nerves (ie, sciatic nerve). Hernigou et al[22,23] have described safe zones for needle placement into the iliac crest, with six zones based on iliac crest landmarks. Furthermore, surgeons should recognize that because the pelvis thins out substantially between the iliac crest and supraacetabular bone, needles should not be inserted more than 3 to 4 cm deep to avoid cortical perforation. One technique that provides for deeper needle placement is to insert the needle from anterior to posterior along the iliac crest, where the bone remains wider. Furthermore, especially in outpatient situations where fluoroscopy may not be available, ultrasound has been described in multiple papers as an effective means of safe needle placement into the pelvis for harvesting of bone marrow.[24,25]

Technical errors related to poor MSC harvest usually start with attempts to harvest as quickly as possible. The details that have been shown to maximize MSC harvest extend surgical time. Furthermore, many surgeons are not well-informed on the myriad ways to maximize MSC harvest and yield. Experienced surgeons are more likely to spend the additional time necessary to obtain sufficient MSCs, and the additional operative time can be minimized by timing centrifugation with other aspects of the surgical procedure (ie, nonunion exposure).

The use of large volume syringes is perhaps the most common technical error encountered. The reasons for this are both obvious and less intuitive. First, large syringes allow the surgeon to quickly aspirate volume, either all at once (nearly all hemodilution and fewer cells) or if they are somewhat facile with BMA, by using smaller aspiration aliquots. As previously described, the use of a smaller syringe leads to a greater pressure gradient and harvest of more MSCs compared to a larger syringe. Despite published research demonstrating superiority of smaller syringes, commonly available BMA kits and disposable packs routinely come with larger diameter syringes provided (60 mL). Unless a surgeon is aware of the benefits of smaller syringes, they will instinctively use what is available intraoperatively in a given system. In addition, it is a common mistake to fill the entire syringe before exchange. Syringes should be exchanged after they are 50% full because of the benefits of a more rapid pull of the stopper.

A more subtle technical consideration that may have a major impact on harvest and unwanted hemodilution is whether the needle is advanced to full depth then slowly pulled back as sites are aspirated or if the needle is aspirated then advanced forward. In the case of the former technique, surgeons must recognize that the needle track will predictably fill with blood. For needle designs that may have an open-end port, this technique should be avoided, as hemodilution is much more of a problem. With the use of the author's recommended needle with a single beveled side port, this issue is mitigated; however, numerous commercially available needles including multiple side port designs all include an end port (because the sharp cutting trocar must exit the needle somewhere). At least one manufacturer has addressed this by including an aspiration cannula that goes through the needle. There are two main drawbacks to advancing the needle forward as they aspirate. First, each time they advance they should replace the stylet or trocar to prevent the cannula from becoming plugged by cancellous bone, which adds considerable time to the procedure if harvest is occurring from multiple sites in the pelvis. Second, additional ultrasound or other confirmatory measures may be necessary as the needle is advanced more deeply to ensure that adverse events do not occur from penetration of the inner or outer table of the pelvis.

The last major technical error surgeons encounter routinely with BMA is related to poor preoperative planning. Failing to prep out the entire pelvis limits the surgeon's ability to harvest from the best source of MSCs, as well as potentially forcing the surgeon to aspirate larger aliquots than might be necessary. One example of this is the management of large segmental bone defects. If BMA with or without centrifugation is to be used as a standalone source of osteoprogenitors alongside allograft and/or other bone graft extenders, a surgeon might need to aspirate up to or beyond 240 mL of marrow to get a sufficient quantity of MSCs, and access to both sides of the pelvis allows for multiple fresh harvest sites. In another scenario, BMA may be used to augment ICBG in tandem with a graft extender. If only one side of the pelvis is prepped, the surgeon may find themselves harvesting ICBG from the pelvis and BMA from the calcaneus or knee, both of which are inferior locations for MSCs. In short, prepping out both sides of the pelvis on a routine basis during ICBG and BMA harvest affords the surgeon more options of ensuring that the graft and BMA quality obtained is sufficient to obtain union.

AUTHOR'S PREFERRED SURGICAL TECHNIQUE

Maximizing the harvest of MSCs should be the primary goal, and to that end, the author's recommended surgical technique is standardized to achieve this goal. The decision to centrifuge a harvested sample should be weighed against the increased cost associated with use of a system, the potential increased surgical time (although mitigated by harvesting first and spinning during subsequent portions of the procedure), and the individual requirements of a specific case; in the author's experience, uncentrifuged aspirates are best utilized as part of open surgical procedures, where a greater volume of aspirate may be required to hydrate a large amount of graft material. Because concentrated samples involve less volume, they are ideal for smaller defects and are much easier to inject percutaneously.

1. The needle selected should be a large-gauge needle—preferably 8 or 11 gauge, with an inner diameter of no greater than 1.5 mm. When available, a single beveled end port needle is preferable, as the best available scientific evidence has demonstrated efficacy with this needle design. The author prefers a longer needle when available, ideally 15 cm in length, as this allows the surgeon to aspirate a greater area of bone before needle redirection is required, especially in morbidly obese patients.

2. Multiple 10 mL syringes (3-4) should be opened on the back table and preloaded with 0.5 mL of heparin (1,000 units/mL). The use of multiple syringes allows the surgeon to rapidly aspirate bone marrow without sacrificing on technique.
3. A "jerk" technique should be utilized—if rapid pulls of the syringe lead to aspiration volumes of greater than 4 mL, a slower pull may be advised to reduce hemodilution. In the author's experience, young patients with rich, well-vascularized bone tend to be difficult to maintain small aliquot volumes (<4 mL) with a jerk technique.
4. Aspiration volumes at each position should be as small as possible, ideally 2 mL and not greater than 4 mL. The syringe is exchanged for an empty syringe after becoming half full.
5. For surgeons familiar with pelvic anatomy and fluoroscopic imaging, the author recommends the use of the sciatic corridor technique (description below). Using a long (15 cm) single beveled side port needle placed along the sciatic corridor, more than 200 mL of high-quality BMA can be obtained without the need to redirect the needle to a new area of the pelvis. This accelerates the process of obtaining high quality marrow with a large concentration and absolute yield of MSCs. Furthermore, because most surgeons managing long bone and other nonunions have additional expertise in trauma, the bony landmarks and fluoroscopic images necessary to ensure safe placement are well known and commonly utilized. Last, this technique allows harvesting from both the posterior and anterior portions of the pelvis regardless of positioning (supine or prone).

The sciatic corridor technique for needle placement mirrors the placement of external fixator pins into the anterior inferior iliac spine (AIIS) and directed along the sciatic buttress from anterior to posterior. The placement of these pins is now routine in pelvic external fixation because of improved construct stability. For that reason, this is a technique that many surgeons managing nonunions should be comfortable with. After a 2-mm stab incision is made 1 cm inferior and medial to the palpable anterior superior iliac spine (ASIS), blunt dissection is carefully down until the AIIS is felt with the needle tip. Blunt dissection is necessary to avoid injury to the lateral femoral cutaneous nerve. After the trocar and needle are advanced through the cortex, alternating obturator inlet and iliac oblique views are used to ensure the needle stays directed above the sciatic notch (to protect the sciatic nerve and arteries) and between the inner and outer table of the pelvis. A long needle (15 cm) can safely be passed all the way into the posterior pelvis unless redundant soft tissue limits depth (ie, morbid obesity). Because of the needle depth, a greater volume of high-quality aspirate can be obtained using this technique before redirection is necessary—and in most circumstances, sufficient quantity is obtained with just a single pass. Surgeons should not use a needle possessing an end port with this technique unless advancement is taking place given the length of the needle track. Furthermore, surgeons must recognize the need to utilize a radiolucent flat top table in order to ensure reliable fluoroscopic views can be obtained. Blind passage of a needle along the sciatic corridor should never be attempted. When prone positioning is utilized, the posterior superior iliac spine (PSIS) represents the insertion point for the needle, but the trajectory remains the same.

CLINICAL APPLICATIONS AND OUTCOMES

The current body of literature regarding BMA and BMAC in the field of orthopedic trauma is centered on the treatment of presumed aseptic, atrophic nonunions. With multiple studies demonstrating union in up to 90% of patients, it would seem that the use of BMA or BMAC would be an obvious first-line choice in the management of nonunions.[6,8-10,26-28] However, while nonunion studies reporting on the use of BMA or BMAC are generally positive, many of these studies are adversely affected by small sample size, selection bias, and treatment heterogeneity.

Series Utilizing Bone Marrow Aspirate Without Concentration

Connolly et al[26] reported the first known use of bone marrow aspiration in an attempt to treat delayed union or nonunion of the tibia. They demonstrated union in 18 of 20 nonunions, many of which were the result of open fractures. However, their patient cohort was not uniform in initial treatment or in the timing until nonunion surgery was performed. Patients were initially treated with external fixators, casting, or intramedullary nailing, and upon return to the operating room for nonunion surgery, half of the patients had a new intramedullary nail placed. It is difficult to determine if union was the result of using BMA or was related to other factors such as reaming of the endosteal canal. They did however utilize a standardized technique. Bone marrow was aspirated from the posterior iliac crest using small aliquots and was not concentrated, and they injected the posterolateral tibia in most cases.[26]

Smaller series of patients treated with BMA also demonstrate similar results. Braly et al studied atrophic metadiaphyseal distal tibial nonunions treated with BMA percutaneously at a mean time from injury to surgery of 8 months. In their series, they obtained union in 9 of 11 patients (82%).[27] In another small series by Garg et al addressing nonunion of the femur, humerus, or ulna, they obtained union in 17 of 20 patients (85%). The PSIS was used for harvest in all cases, and 15 to 20 mL of BMA was injected percutaneously.[28]

Series Utilizing Bone Marrow Aspirate Concentrate

While efficacy appears to be present when centrifugation is not utilized, a few larger series of patients utilizing BMAC appear to be of higher quality and yield comparable results to BMA alone. Hernigou et al[6] previously reported on a series of 60 tibial nonunions treated with BMAC using a standardized technique. Eighty-eight percent of patients obtained union without further surgical interventions and were percutaneously injected at an average of 8 months from injury. No patients were initially managed with intramedullary nailing, with 48 of the 60 patients having open fractures definitively managed in an external fixator and the remaining 12 patients being closed injuries managed in a cast. And while most fractures were isthmal injuries (31 of 60), the remainder were proximal or distal metaphyseal/metadiaphyseal injuries, indicating significant patient heterogeneity. Hernigou's surgical technique for aspiration and centrifugation was standardized across all patients, and samples were also studied in the laboratory, providing a framework for understanding the relationship between concentration of MSC, the absolute number of MSCs, and the likelihood of obtaining union. In another series of femoral nonunions managed with BMAC, Guimaraes et al[29] demonstrated a 50% union rate, obtaining healing in 8 of 16 patients at an average time of 41 months after the index surgery. While not approaching the success rate found in nonunions of the tibia, their 50% success rate nearly 4 years out from a femur fracture is encouraging, especially when compared with exchange nailing of femur nonunion, which has published success rates as low as 53%.[30]

More recently, a larger comparative study was presented in which 51 long bone nonunions were managed with either BMAC and cancellous allograft or autogenous ICBG. Lin et al demonstrated that the union rate in both groups was similar: 78% of nonunions treated with ICBG successfully united, while 75% of nonunions treated with BMAC healed. However, in their series, the successful BMAC cases healed at an average of 3.5 versus 5.7 months for ICBG cases.[8] Furthermore, these results compare favorably with those from another study randomizing patients with aseptic tibial nonunions to the use of allograft with bone morphogenic protein-7 or autograft.[31] Additionally, they reported that 20% of patients randomized to autograft had chronic pain related to their donor site.[31]

Other Clinical Series Using Bone Marrow Aspirate Concentrate for Other Trauma Applications

While most literature describes the use of BMAC for nonunion repair, a few series have studied the use of BMAC in the setting of limb salvage with distraction osteogenesis. In these scenarios, BMA with or without concentration has been studied as a means of increasing healing at the docking site, as well as for improving maturation and healing of the regenerate bone. In one small series, Gessman et al augmented regenerate bone at the completion of the distraction phase. The average bone defect was 82.4 mm, and all eight patients in the series went on to heal without secondary surgery or delays in regenerate maturation with a mean healing index of 36.9 d/cm.[32] In another series by Lee et al,[33] BMAC was used to augment healing at the site of fresh osteotomies performed as part of limb lengthening procedures. Compared to the control group, the group treated with BMAC demonstrated a lower healing index at all four cortices (ie, more rapid consolidation). In another study, Hatzokos et al studied the use of BMAC with demineralized bone matrix as a carrier in the management of bone transport docking sites. They found BMAC + DBM (composite grafting) to be equivalent to the use of autogenous ICBG in reducing the time to union after docking, and it was superior to simple docking site compression alone.[34]

Use of Bone Marrow Aspirate for Acute Fractures and Future Direction

At present, no data currently exists to support the use of BMA or BMAC for the management of acute fractures, including those at higher risk for nonunion. While the idea is appealing, acute trauma presents unique challenges when compared to nonunion situations. First, high-energy fractures commonly involve significant associated soft tissue injury within the zone of injury, especially for tibia fractures. The distorted soft tissue planes adjacent to a fracture would suggest that locally applied aspirate is unlikely to remain in place at the fracture location and may leak away from the location where it is most needed to encourage bone formation, regardless of whether the MSCs are applied locally or percutaneously. One remedy for this issue would be to apply the BMA on a local carrier adjacent to the fracture. Concerns arise with this technique, however, because most fractures at a greater risk of nonunion, like open tibia fractures, are associated with a greater risk of deep infection when necrotic bone or other foreign bodies are acutely left at the site of a fracture.[35] It seems the ideal carrier for acute use of BMA would also be capable of being loaded with antibiotics to protect the carrier from acting as a nidus for infection. Unfortunately, at this time, no carrier has been identified that can provide the benefits of both controlling for infection with local antibiotics and acting as a carrier for MSCs. In the future as bone graft substitutes continue to evolve, a tailorable drug delivery device that can provided controlled release of both antibiotics and MSCs at the site of a high-risk fracture may serve as a useful adjuvant to increase the rate of union and decrease time to union after open fracture, especially of the tibia.

Complication Rates Between Bone Autograft Harvest and Bone Marrow Aspirate

While complications related to open bone graft harvest are well published, much less has been written regarding the drawbacks and limitations of harvesting BMA. In general, the major concerns with BMA pertain to injury to local neurovascular structures, hematoma formation, and the need for blood transfusion.

Hernigou et al[22,23] previously studied computed tomography angiograms of the pelvis to better delineate theoretical risks to neurovascular structures in the pelvis. As expected, large deviations of up to 20° in needle trajectory had the potential to place important structures, including the external iliac artery and superior gluteal vessels. Risk to the external iliac artery and vein was greatest with anterior harvest sites, whereas violation of the sciatic notch was possible with posterior harvest locations. Despite these theoretical risks, Hernigou et al[6] demonstrated no adverse neurovascular injuries in his large series of BMAC cases for tibial nonunion. In a separate review of more than 500 BMA cases, an overall complication rate of 7.6% was identified, with the most common event as anemia which did not require transfusion.[21] This compared quite favorably to a complication rate of over 80% in a comparison cohort of patients undergoing open ICBG harvest. In the author's experience, major complications related to BMA harvest are easily mitigated with the use of intraoperative fluoroscopy, which can and should be used to confirm correct needle placement into the desired area of the pelvis and which is typically already in the operating room during long bone nonunion surgery.

CASE EXAMPLES

Case 1

A 58-year-old male was referred from outside facility for nonunion surgery 8 months after an 8-ft fall in which he injured his knee. Initially placed into a knee immobilizer and treated nonoperatively, with initiation of weightbearing 3 months after injury and knee range of motion permitted in hinged brace 6 weeks after injury. Plain radiographs and computed tomography scan of the knee demonstrated a unicondylar medial tibial plateau nonunion with metaphyseal bone resorption (Figure 7.3A-E).

The patient was taken for a formal nonunion repair in the prone position via a posteromedial approach. After débridement of all fibrous nonunion tissue, the wound was packed to allow for hemostasis. A 15-cm single beveled end port needle was used to obtain BMA using the sciatic corridor technique. A 5-mm stab incision was made over the PSIS, and the needle was introduced and carefully advanced down the corridor into the anterior pelvis using alternating iliac oblique (to confirm needle advancement above the sciatic notch) and obturator inlet views (to confirm needle remains between inner and outer table of pelvis) (Figure 7.4A and B). Two to four milliliter aliquots were then aspirated at each needle location eight times by rotating the needle 45°, before pulling back 1 cm and repeating. In this manner, 240 mL of high-quality BMA was obtained without having to redirect the needle to a new location. The nonunion was then packed with a combination of 15 mL of allograft bone and 10 mL demineralized bone matrix mixed with 15 mL of concentrated BMAC prepared using the SmartPrep2 system (Terumo BCT, Lakewood, CO). An additional centrifuge spin ensures that a higher concentration will be present in a smaller volume of aspirate fluid, allowing for better control of graft saturation at the time of implantation. Lag screws at the articular surface and a buttress plate stabilize the partial articular nonunion and allow for predictable healing.

Case 2

A 28-year-old female s/p motor vehicle collision versus pedestrian sustaining type 1 open comminuted fracture of tibia at distal metadiaphysis (Figure 7.5A and B). Patient with history of long-term tobacco usage (2+ packs per day for >10 years). Taken urgently to operating room for wound débridement, intramedullary nailing, and primary wound closure. Given the fracture location, comminution, and patient history, it was felt that acute fracture augmentation would facilitate more predictable healing and avoid the need for reoperation or other secondary surgery.

After placement of the statically locked intramedullary nail, a 5-mm stab incision 1 cm inferior and medial to the palpable anterior superior iliac spine is made. Blunt dissection is carried down to the AIIS to avoid injury to the lateral femoral cutaneous nerve, which is at risk in the

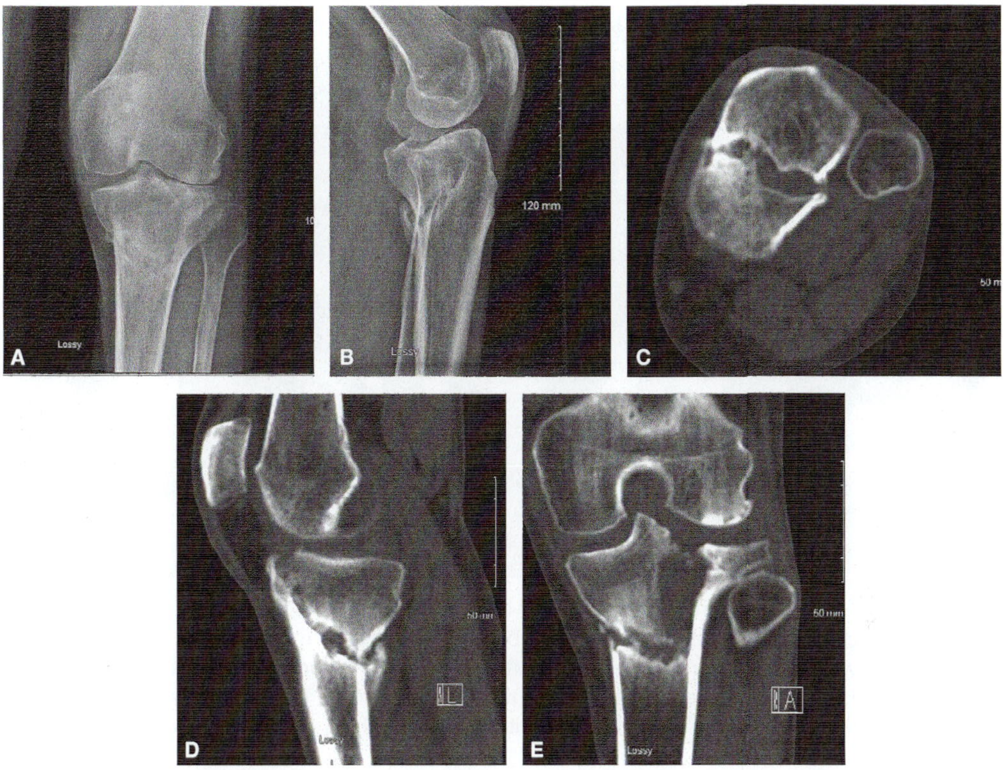

Figure 7.3. **A-E.** Radiographs and computed tomography scan from a 58-year-old male with medial tibial plateau nonunion after failed conservative treatment. After nonunion repair with buttress plate fixation, biology is augmented using concentrated bone marrow aspirate mixed with allograft and demineralized bone matrix. Healing reliably occurs in setting of rigid fixation of nonunion augmented with appropriate biology.

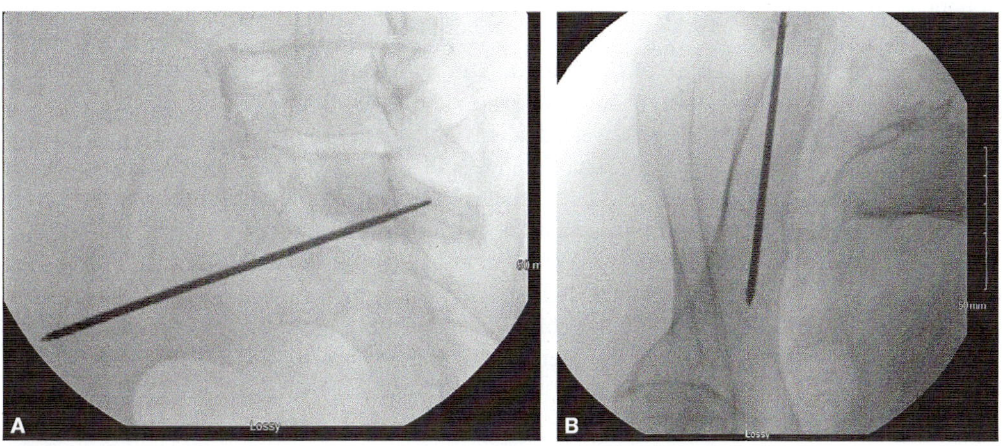

Figure 7.4. **A, B.** The sciatic corridor can safely be utilized to obtain multiple 2 to 4 mL aliquots of high-quality bone marrow aspirate without the need to redirect the needle. The imaging is identical to the views utilized to place an external fixator pin from the AIIS. An iliac oblique view safely allows the needle to be placed deep into the pelvis and above the sciatic notch, while the obturator inlet view ensures the needle remains between the inner and outer table of the pelvis.

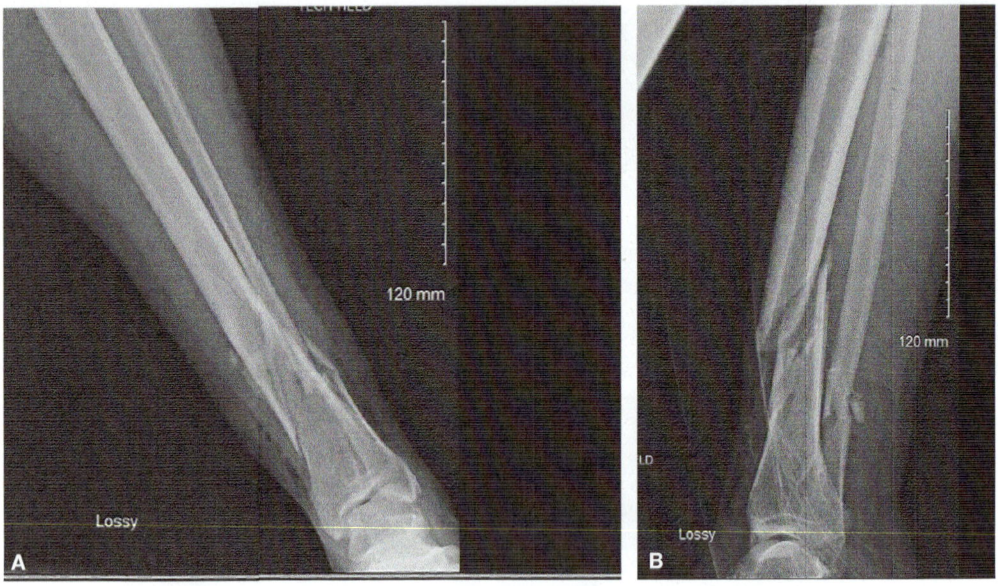

Figure 7.5. A, B. Radiographs from a 28-year-old female with type 1 open tibial shaft fracture. Heavy two pack per day smoker. To augment biology and ensure more reliable bone healing, bone marrow was aspirated from the pelvis. After closure of the wound and placement of an intramedullary nail, the entire bone marrow aspirate amount (120 mL) was injected percutaneously at the fracture site without centrifugation—which comes with added health care costs.

field. Using alternating iliac oblique and obturator inlet views, a 15-cm, 11-gauge single beveled end port aspiration needle is carefully advanced deep into the posterior pelvis, and high-quality BMA aliquots were collected until 120 mL of BMA is harvested. Because the wound is closed primarily prior to aspiration, the BMA sample must be injected percutaneously, and heparinization of the sample during collection is paramount to ensure the syringe does not become plugged or prevent percutaneous injection. Because the fracture was open, a carrier for the BMA in the form of bone graft or substitute is not advised, as foreign material at the site of an open tibia fracture serves as a nidus for infection.

Because of the acute nature of the fracture and additional costs associated with use of a centrifuge system, concentration of the BMA sample was not performed. Under fluoroscopic guidance, an 18-gauge spinal needle was advanced adjacent to the fracture, and all 120 mL of BMA was slowly injected. The author's preference is to inject along the posterior cortex, under the deep posterior compartment musculature, as well as anterolaterally along the crest under the anterior compartment. Injecting subcutaneous along the anteromedial face of the tibia, where host biology and vascularity is minimal, is not felt to substantially aid in healing, as the stem cells may not be supported by local chemotactic and angiogenic factors. The patient was allowed to bear immediate weight on the tibia after surgery and was followed at regular intervals to ensure fracture healing. At 3 months, her fracture demonstrated bridging callous on all four cortices (Figure 7.6A and B).

Case 3

A 19-year-old female s/p type 1 open, low-energy tibial shaft fracture while playing soccer. Initially the fracture was stabilized by another surgeon with an intramedullary nail placed via a suprapatellar approach after débridement of the open fracture. The patient subsequently developed an acute surgical site infection at 3 weeks postop, which was treated with incision and drainage,

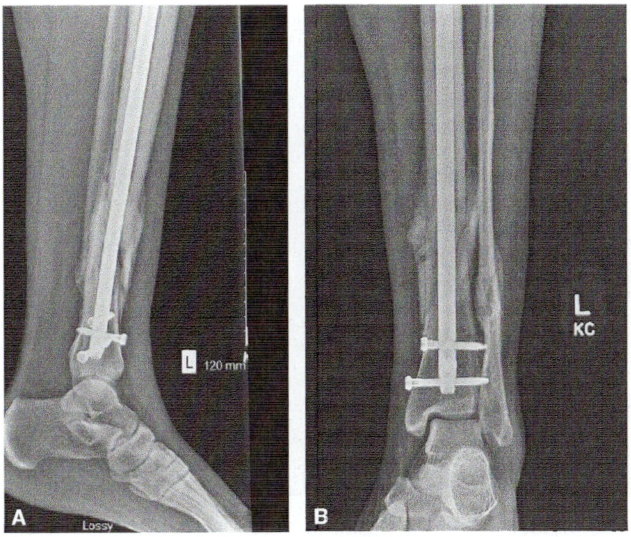

Figure 7.6. **A, B.** At 3 months, the fracture is reliably healing, with bridging callous seen on all four cortices.

primary closure, and culture-specific antibiotics for methicillin-sensitive *Staphylococcus aureus* for 6 weeks followed by oral suppressive antibiotics for 6 additional weeks. At 9 months after an exchange nail failed, she was referred for treatment of her tibial nonunion (Figure 7.7A and B).

On presentation to clinic, her leg showed a well-healed soft tissue envelope, with no swelling but with pain on palpation of the fracture site. Repeat inflammatory indices were negative (erythrocyte sedimentation rate, C-reactive protein). The patient then underwent a scheduled two-stage treatment of presumed aseptic nonunion with the known possibility of an occult infected

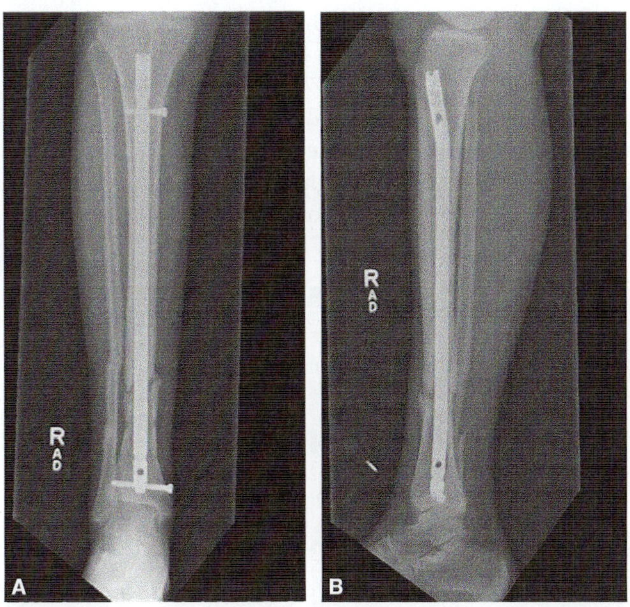

Figure 7.7. **A, B.** Radiographs from a 19-year-old female with recalcitrant tibial nonunion after previous open tibia fracture complicated by acute surgical site infection and then treated later with exchange nail. Nine months after the exchange nail, she continues to have pain and an obvious ununited fracture.

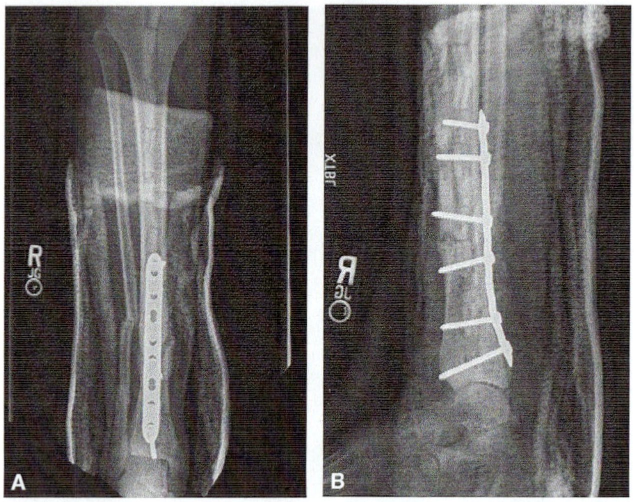

Figure 7.8. **A, B.** After staged nonunion repair (due to history of prior infection) with removal of hardware and placement of resorbable antibiotic carrier, the nonunion was débrided through a posterolateral approach and compression plating performed. To augment her biology, bone marrow was aspirated and then centrifuged, again using the sciatic corridor but in the prone position. The bone marrow aspirate concentrate was mixed with demineralized bone matrix and packed along the nonunion to aid in healing.

nonunion given her prior history. During the first stage, the intramedullary rod was removed and calcium sulfate "bullets" were placed down the intramedullary canal to act as a resorbable, high-dose local antibiotic delivery device. Reamings and nonunion aspirate samples were also sent for culture. One week later, with cultures showing no growth, she returned to the operating room for open nonunion repair via a posterolateral approach in the prone position. After débridement of fibrous nonunion tissue and osteotomy of the fibula, compression plating of the tibial nonunion was performed (Figure 7.8A and B). BMA was harvested from the posterior iliac crest using a multiple fenestrated side port aspiration needle 11 cm in length. Multiple passes were made to harvest 180 mL of high-quality BMA using 2 to 4 mL aliquot aspirations with a 10-mL syringe. After centrifugation, 18 mL of BMAC was mixed with 20 mL of demineralized bone matrix and 2 g of vancomycin powder and packed along the nonunion medially and posterolaterally to aid in repair. The patient was permitted to bear weight 4 weeks after surgery and demonstrated complete healing of her nonunion by 5 months postoperatively (Figure 7.9A and B).

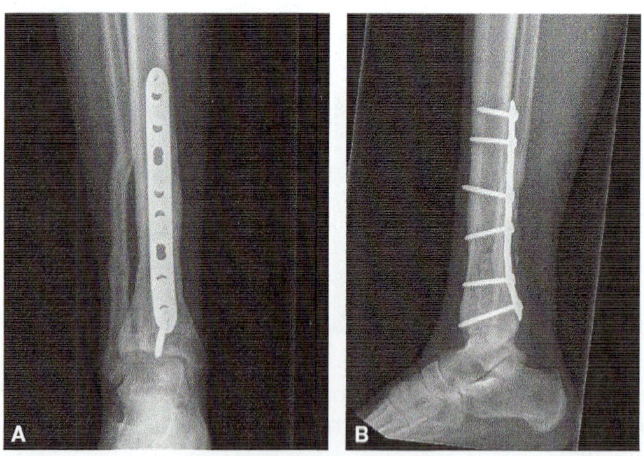

Figure 7.9. **A, B.** After 5 months, the nonunion has healed.

FUTURE SCIENTIFIC DIRECTION AND EMERGING THERAPIES

Human Amniotic Membrane and Cord Blood Derivatives in Fracture Care

The use of human amniotic membrane (HAM) or cord blood derivatives as an adjunct to obtain union is an emerging area of research with clear clinical applications. Its potential for use has been explored in surgical fields outside of orthopedics with mixed results. Within the field of orthopedics, the use of HAM has been most widely adopted in the sports medicine literature as a potential alternative to host derived tissue, with the potential to accelerate and enhance healing of soft tissue in the setting of poor tissue quality and/or host biology. There is a paucity of evidence, especially as it relates to human trials, supporting its use in fracture care. However, the use of HAM in the treatment of rat models of diaphyseal tibia fractures has shown promise in promoting callous formation at 6 weeks postoperatively.[36] The authors suggest that HAM may prove useful at the time of initial fixation in fractures that are expected to have delayed union or those at risk for nonunion. One small clinical series investigated the use of amniotic cord-derived membrane to minimize wound complications following extensile lateral approach for open reduction internal fixation of calcaneus fractures. While the series was small, it suggested an ability to reduce wound complications as well as the risk of progressing to nonunion.[37]

Amniotic cord blood derivatives present another attractive alternative for the treatment of fractures and nonunion. They theoretically have a high concentration of mesenchymal or pluripotent stem cells, which could accelerate fracture healing, perhaps more effectively than host-derived graft sources. Cord blood derivative use has been most widely studied for cartilaginous regenerative potential and as an adjunct for rotator cuff repair.[38] Unfortunately, there is little documented use in the setting of either acute fracture surgery or nonunion repair. Arguably the most limiting factor in the study and use of these products is the proprietary process described by each individual manufacturer. By removing transparency with regard to the various products available, surgeons are left to guess at whether the science can or should support clinical use in fracture care; as a result, their use remains poorly described in the literature. Their current use in the treatment of fractures or nonunions is purely experimental at this time.

Use of Bone Marrow Aspirate Concentrate on Composite Grafts

The use of biomaterials to serve as carriers for autogenous MSCs is another emerging field of preclinical research with potential for translation into the clinical setting. While demineralized bone matrix and other processed allograft bone products have been used for years as effective carriers and bone graft extenders, the biomaterials of greatest interest and potential for future clinical direction include ceramics, biodegradable polymers, and composite biomaterials. Regardless of the makeup of these materials, they each serve as a three-dimensional framework for the incorporation of MSCs into bony or soft tissue defects. They must be relatively biologically inert to avoid eliciting an immune response (which could lead to resorption), provide structure and stability as bony incorporation occurs, and ideally create an osteoinductive and osteoconductive environment where MSCs can differentiate into bone precursors and facilitate healing. Marcacci et al[39] report on a four patient clinical series where a hydroxyapatite scaffold impregnated with culture-expanded MSCs was used in the treatment of large diaphyseal defects of the tibia. They demonstrated complete healing of the graft to the host bone and no late fractures through the implant site. While a very small series, these results are encouraging that future larger studies evaluating hydroxyappetite scaffolds may show promise for the management of bone defects. One major limitation of ceramics like hydroxyapatite is that their application is limited to clinical scenarios where little to no loading of the scaffold occurs due to the low toughness of ceramics (ie, they are brittle).

Polymers also demonstrate several qualities that may prove useful in orthopedic applications, namely their ability to support tissue growth prior to gradual degradation and integration into host tissue. Polylactic acid, polyglycolide, and poly(ε-caprolactone) are the most widely studied polymers and have shown some promise in preclinical research in providing favorable tissue environments for the delivery of MSCs in fracture models. However, they also demonstrate several limitations. Most notably, the biomechanical properties of these polymers differ significantly from both cortical and cancellous bone. Furthermore, their degradation products are typically acids and can lead to a less favorable tissue environment for MSCs to differentiate into bone-producing cells.

Finally, composite materials have shown early promise due to their ability to provide the optimal qualities of both ceramics and polymers. They have been employed in oral and maxillofacial surgery, where a resorbable composite "fleece" loaded with periosteum-derived stem cells has shown promise in the ability to form lamellar bone within 3 months after implantation.[40] The ideal composite would present mixed properties that support osteoconduction and osteoinduction while protecting the biologic properties of the BMAC/MSC, during a controlled, steady degradation while bony ingrowth occurs.

References

1. Bianco P. Stem cells and bone: a historical perspective. *Bone.* 2015;70:2-9.
2. Baker N, Boyette LB, Tuan RS. Characterization of bone marrow-derived mesenchymal stem cells. *Bone.* 2015;70:37-47.
3. Mansilla E, Diaz Aquino V, Zambon D, et al. Could metabolic syndrome, lipodystrophy, and aging be mesenchymal stem cell exhaustion syndromes? *Stem Cell Int.* 2011;2011:943216.
4. Leslie WD, Rubin MR, Schwartz AV, Kanis JA. Type 2 diabetes and bone. *J Bone Miner Res.* 2012;27:2231-2237.
5. Friedenstein AJ, Petrakova KV, Kurolesova AI, Frolova GP. Heterotopic of bone marrow. Analysis of precursor cells or osteogenic and hematopoietic tissues. *Transplantation.* 1968;6:230-247.
6. Hernigou P, Poignard A, Beaujean F, Rouard H. Percutaneous autologous bone-marrow grafting for nonunions. Influence of the number and concentration of progenitor cells. *J Bone Joint Surg Am.* 2005;87:1430-1437.
7. Connolly JF. Clinical use of marrow osteoprogenitor cells to stimulate osteogenesis. *Clin Orthop Relat Res.* 1998;355(Suppl):S257-S266.
8. Lin K, Vandenberg J, Putnam S, et al. Bone marrow aspirate concentrate with cancellous allograft versus iliac crest bone graft in the treatment of long bone nonunions. *OTA Int.* 2019;2:e012.
9. Sugaya H, Mishima H, Aoto K, et al. Percutaneous autologous concentrated bone marrow grafting in the treatment for nonunion. *Eur J Orthop Surg Traumatol.* 2014;24:671-678.
10. Connolly JF. Injectable bone marrow preparations to stimulate osteogenic repair. *Clin Orthop Relat Res.* 1995;313:8-18.
11. Chahla J, Mannava S, Cinque ME, Geeslin AG, Codina D, LaPrade RF. Bone marrow aspirate concentrate harvesting and processing technique. *Arthrosc Tech.* 2017;6:e441-e445.
12. Hernigou P, Homma Y, Flouzat Lachaniette CH, et al. Benefits of small volume and small syringe for bone marrow aspirations of mesenchymal stem cells. *Int Orthop.* 2013;37:2279-2287.
13. Gronkjaer M, Hasselgren CF, Osteergaard AS, et al. Bone marrow aspiration: a randomized controlled trial assessing the quality of bone marrow specimens using slow and rapid aspiration techniques and evaluating pain intensity. *Acta Haematol.* 2016;135:81-87.
14. Muschler GF, Boehm C, Easley K. Aspiration to obtain osteoblast progenitor cells from the human bone marrow: the influence of aspiration volume. *J Bone Joint Surg Am.* 1997;79:1699-1709.
15. Hyer CF, Berlet GC, Bussewitz BW, Hankins T, Ziegler HL, Philbin TM. Quantitative assessment of the yield of osteoblastic connective tissue progenitors in bone marrow aspirate from the iliac crest, tibia, and calcaneus. *J Bone Joint Surg Am.* 2013;95:1312-1316.
16. Narbona-Carceles J, Vaquero J, Suarez-Sancho S, Suárez-Sancho SBS, Forriol F, Fernández-Santos ME. Bone marrow mesenchymal stem cell aspirates from alternative sources: is the knee as good as the iliac crest? *Injury.* 2014;45(Suppl 4):S42-S47.
17. Pierini M, Di Bella C, Dozza B, et al. The posterior iliac crest outperforms the anterior iliac crest when obtaining mesenchymal stem cells from bone marrow. *J Bone Joint Surg Am.* 2013;95:1101-1107.
18. Hernigou P. The history of bone marrow in orthopaedic surgery (part I trauma): trepanning, bone marrow injection in damage control resuscitation, and bone marrow aspiration to heal fractures. *Int Orthop.* 2020;44:795-808.
19. Hernigou P, Mathieu G, Poignard A, Manicom O, Beaujean F, Rouard H. Percutaneous autologous bone-marrow grafting for nonunions. Surgical technique. *J Bone Joint Surg Am.* 2006;88(Suppl 1):322-327.

20. Hernigou P, Beaujean F. Treatment of osteonecrosis with autologous bone marrow grafting. *Clin Orthop Relat Res.* 2002;405:14-23.
21. Hernigou P, Desroches A, Queinnec S, et al. Morbidity of graft harvesting versus bone marrow aspiration in cell regeneration therapy. *Int Orthop.* 2014;38:1855-1860.
22. Hernigou J, Picard L, Alves A, Silvera J, Homma Y, Hernigou P. Understanding bone safety zones during bone marrow aspiration from the iliac crest: the sector rule. *Int Orthop.* 2014;38:77-2384.
23. Hernigou J, Alves A, Homma Y, Guissou I, Hernigou P. Anatomy of the ilium for bone marrow aspiration: map of sectors and implication for safe trocar placement. *Int Orthop.* 2014;38:2585-2590.
24. Shapiro SA, Arthurs JR. Bone marrow aspiration for regenerative orthopedic intervention: technique with ultrasound guidance for needle placement. *Regen Med.* 2017;12:917-928.
25. Long JR, Stensby JD, Wiesner EL, Bryson WN, Hillen TJ, Jennings JW. Efficacy and safety of bone marrow aspiration and biopsy using fluoroscopic guidance and a drill-powered needle: clinical experience from 775 cases. *Eur Radiol.* 2020;30:5964-5970.
26. Connolly JF, Guse R, Tiedeman J, Dehne R. Autologous marrow injection as a substitute for operative grafting of tibial nonunions. *Clin Orthop Relat Res.* 1991;266:259-270.
27. Braly HL, O'Connor DP, Brinker MR. Percutaneous autologous bone marrow injection in the treatment of distal meta-diaphyseal tibial nonunions and delayed unions. *J Orthop Trauma.* 2013;27:527-533.
28. Garg NK, Gaur S, Sharma S. Percutaneous autogenous bone marrow grafting in 20 cases of ununited fracture. *Acta Orthop Scand.* 1993;64:671-672.
29. Guimaraes JA, Duarte ME, Fernandes MB, et al. The effect of autologous concentrated bone-marrow grafting on the healing of femoral shaft non-unions after locked intramedullary nailing. *Injury.* 2014;45:S7-S13.
30. Weresh MJ, Hakanson R, Stover MD, Sims SH, Kellam JF, Bosse MJ. Failure of exchange reamed intramedullary nails for ununited femoral shaft fractures. *J Orthop Trauma.* 2000;14:335-338.
31. Friedlaender GE, Perry CR, Cole JD, et al. Osteogenic protein-1 (bone morphogenetic protein-7) in the treatment of tibial nonunions. *J Bone Joint Surg Am.* 2001;83(Suppl 1):S151-S158.
32. Gessman J, Koller M, Godry H, Schildhauer TA, Seybold D. Regenerate augmentation with bone marrow concentrate after traumatic bone loss. *Orthop Rev (Pavia).* 2012;4:e14.
33. Lee DH, Ryu KJ, Kim JW, Kang KC, Choi YR. Bone marrow aspirate concentrate and platelet-rich plasma enhanced bone healing in distraction osteogenesis of the tibia. *Clin Orthop Relat Res.* 2014;472:3789-3797.
34. Hatzokos I, Stavridis SI, Iosifidou E, Karataglis D, Christodoulou A. Autologous bone marrow grafting combined with demineralized bone matrix improves consolidation of docking site after distraction osteogenesis. *J Bone Joint Surg Am.* 2011;93:671-678.
35. Edwards CC, Simmons SC, Browner BD, Weigel MC. Severe open tibial fractures. Results treating 202 injuries with external fixation. *Clin Orthop Relat Res.* 1988;230:98-115.
36. Sarı E, Yalçınozan M, Polat B, Özkayalar H. The effects of cryopreserved human amniotic membrane on fracture healing: animal study. *Acta Orthop Traumatol Turc.* 2019;53:485-489.
37. Stewart CM. Theg use of cryopreserved umbilical cord in open reduction and internal fixation of calcaneus fractures. *J Trauma Emerg Med Acute Care.* 2019;1(1001):1-6.
38. Song J, Hong K, Kim N, et al. Cartilage regeneration in osteoarthritic knees treated with distal femoral osteotomy and intra-lesional implantation of allogenic human umbilical cord blood-derived mesenchymal stem cells: a report of two cases. *Knee.* 2019;26:1445-1450.
39. Marcacci M, Kon E, Moukhachev V, et al. Stem cells associated with macroporous bioceramics for long bone repair: 6-to 7-year outcome of a pilot clinical study. *Tissue Eng.* 2007;13:947-955.
40. Schimming R, Schmelzeisen R. Tissue-engineered bone for maxillary sinus augmentation. *J Oral Maxillofac Surg.* 2004;62:724-729.

8 Platelet-Rich Plasma

Tristan McMillan, Luke Farrow, Iain Stevenson, and Emil Schemitsch

WHAT IS PLATELET-RICH PLASMA?

Platelets are small anucleate blood cells that are generated from megakaryocytes in bone marrow and play a functional role in inflammation, hemostasis, angiogenesis, wound healing, growth and development, and innate immunity.[1] This is largely due to the release of the contents of intracellular platelet granules that remain stored in circulating platelets until activation, adhesion, or aggregation. There are three types of granules: lysosome, dense, and alpha granules. The lysosome granules contain a variety of digestive enzymes. The dense granules contain serotonin, histamine, dopamine, and adenosine that are all essential in the initial inflammatory response to tissue injury through promotion of platelet aggregation, an increase in capillary permeability, and attracting and activating macrophages.[2] The alpha granules represent the major granule population in size and number, containing over 30 bioactive proteins that include adhesive glycoproteins, clotting factors and cofactors, protease inhibitors as well as a multitude of important mitogenic growth factors: platelet-derived growth factor (PDGF), transforming growth factor-beta (TGF-β), vascular endothelial growth factor (VEGF), epidemic growth factor, fibroblast growth factor (FGF) endothelial cell growth factor, insulin-like growth factor (IGF), and interleukin-β.[3] This content, together with their supply of cytokines and chemokines, plays a significant role in healing through cellular chemotaxis, proliferation, and differentiation, and laying down of extracellular matrix.[4]

Platelet-rich plasma (PRP) is generated through the processing of blood to produce plasma which contains a more concentrated platelet content than whole blood. With an estimated platelet concentration of up to 1,407,640 platelets/μL, it is typically more than five times that of whole blood (266,040 ± 60,530 platelets/μL).[5] The resultant platelet concentrate is rich in platelet granules. Once in the presence of a blood clot, degranulation of these granules begins to occur with active secretion of their content. Specifically, a concentrated secretion of growth factors occurs within 10 minutes and 95% of the presynthesized growth factors is secreted within 60 minutes.[6] The ability to deliver these bioactive molecules in a concentrated and focused manner offers the potential to augment and improve the body's ability to heal. PRP has therefore increased in popularity over the last three decades with increasing clinical applications within a variety of medical specialties including orthopedics, maxillofacial surgery, dentistry, plastic surgery, and ophthalmic surgery.

In orthopedics, soft tissue and cartilaginous applications are growing in popularity with evidence in support. Though not the specific focus of this book chapter, it is important to note that the potential benefits of PRP have been explored in a wide range of soft tissue and degenerative conditions. This includes tendinopathy (rotator cuff,[7] elbow extensors,[8] Achilles,[9] hip abductors,[10] and patellar tendons[11]), osteoarthritis,[12] chronic wounds,[13] and meniscal repair.[14] Scientific rationale focuses on the identification of significant abnormal local histopathology in these degenerative conditions—such as abnormal vascularity, atypical collagen content, and dysregulation of cytokine production.[15-17] As previously described, PRP provides several bioactive proteins that may help to restore normal tissue structure, function, and local homeostasis.[18]

The overall evidence for benefit of PRP in soft tissue and degenerative conditions remains uncertain, with contrasting views seen across the breadth of literature, and between different anatomical sites. This is likely to relate to the known heterogeneity in the production, formulation, and use of PRP in different studies. It may, however, also be associated with the different pathological mechanisms occurring at various anatomical locations, for example, mid-portion versus insertional Achilles tendinopathy. Further high-level evidence with homogeneity in the design and reporting of randomized controlled trials (RCTs) for each anatomical site of degenerative injury would be of significant benefit to determine the potential for widespread PRP use in this area.

THE ROLE OF PLATELET-RICH PLASMA IN BONE HEALING

The healing of human tissue, including bone, is achieved by a series of complex cellular events under the control of signaling proteins. Following an acute fracture or an operative intervention, platelets are normally activated by thrombin and subendothelial collagen leading to fusion of the platelet granules with the plasma membrane and secretion of their contents. The addition of human platelet concentrate has been shown to promote the proliferative and functional activity of human fetal osteoblastlike cells in both short-term and long-term culture.[19] Furthermore, outside of orthopedics, PRP has been shown to improve bone formation and osseointegration around dental implants.[20] In order to understand the scientific potential of PRP to enhance osteoinduction and bone healing, it is important to look at how the individual bioactive molecules secreted by platelets influence bone. This includes the effects of the following growth factors: PDGF, TGF-β, IGF, FGF, and VEGF, although these materials by themselves are not directly osteoinductive. These factors serve to augment the normal bone healing pathways and have been called "osteopromotive" in nature.

The influence of PDGFs on bone healing are the most frequently investigated, particularly with their availability in a recombinant form. PDGFs are dimeric glycoproteins with three PDGF dimer forms (PDGF-AA, PDGF-AB, and PDGF-BB) existing within human platelets.[21] PDGFs are proinflammatory and promote mesenchymal stem cell (MSC) proliferation along with osteoblast differentiation, increasing bone matrix apposition and stimulation of bone formation.[22] The alpha granules also secrete the serum proteins fibronectin and vitronectin that promote osteogenic cell adhesion and proliferation.[23]

TGF-β is involved in fibroblast activation and proliferation, as well as MSC proliferation and osteogenic/chondrogenic differentiation.[24] A subgroup of the TGF-β superfamily are the bone morphogenic proteins (BMPs). BMPs are growth and differentiation factors that are important in bone formation and fracture healing. Their role includes bone matrix production, neovascularization, and MSC recruitment and augment the direct conversion of undifferentiated cells to an osteoblastic lineage. BMPs 2 and 7 are most commonly associated with fracture healing. BMPs 2, 4, 6, and 7 have all been identified within platelet concentrates; however, there are large variations in BMP content between platelet donors with some donors having no detectable amounts of any BMP.[25]

The IGF regulatory system plays an important role in skeletal growth and maintenance. IGF-I is a single-chain protein that is secreted by platelets when activated, binding to a specific cell surface receptor (IGF-IR) and directly increasing bone formation by regulation of the differentiated function of the osteoblast.[26] Wildemann et al[27] has shown the local application of IGF-I and TGF-β1 leads to faster fracture healing. Osteoclasts also express IGF-IR, and in vitro IGF-I induces RANK-L leading to osteoclastogenesis and a subsequent increase in bone resorption, placing IGF-I as a "coupler," assisting in bone remodelling.[28]

FGF promotes the growth and differentiation of a variety of cells including osteoblasts and chondrocytes. This is in addition to their role in angiogenesis and mesenchymal cell mitogenesis.[29] VEGF also contributes to angiogenesis, in addition to its role in extracellular matrix remodeling and endochondral ossification.[30] These two growth factors are present within PRP, and when bFGF and VEGF were added in the early proliferating stage, osteogenic differentiation of MSCs could be enhanced effectively.[31]

PRP also contains pro-inflammatory cytokines such as interleukins and tissue necrosis factor. While the inflammatory response is important in fracture healing, the influence of this potential upregulation of the inflammatory response on acute fracture healing is not fully understood.

CLASSIFICATION OF PLATELET-RICH PLASMA

There continues to be significant variation in the nomenclature and classification of platelet-rich plasma preparations with biological differences in PRP preparations potentially influencing the quantity of platelets and bioactive proteins at the site of application, which may account for the large variability in the clinical benefits of PRP reported in the literature. One of the first classifications proposed was in 2009 by Ehrenfest et al[32] who classified the different platelet concentrates into four categories, depending on the presence of leucocytes and the fibrin structure:

- P-PRP: pure or leucocyte-poor platelet-rich plasma. No or low leucocyte levels and a low-density fibrin network after activation.
- L-PRP: leucocyte and platelet-rich plasma. Elevated leucocyte content and a low-density fibrin network after activation.
- P-PRF: pure or leucocyte-poor platelet-rich fibrin. No or low leucocyte levels and a high-density fibrin network.
- L-PRF: leucocyte and platelet-rich fibrin. Elevated leucocyte content and a high-density fibrin network.

In 2016, Magalon et al[33] proposed the DEPA (Dose of injected platelets, Efficiency of production, Purity of PRP, Activation of PRP) classification that takes into consideration the dose of injected platelets, the efficiency of the production, the purity of the PRP obtained, and the activation process. The classification is summarized in Table 8.1, and the tool can help institutions to assess the quality of the PRP being produced.

In addition to these two systems, a multitude of other classification systems have been proposed including those by Mishra et al,[34] DeLong et al,[35] Mautner et al,[36] and Lana et al.[37] With this many variations in classification, there remains no clear consensus of opinion; nonetheless, it is important for clinicians to consider the type and quality of PRP prior to clinical application.

TABLE 8.1 Summary of the DEPA Classification Proposed by Magalon et al

	Dose of Injected Platelets (Billions)	Efficiency of the Process (Platelet Recovery Rate %)	Purity of the Platelet-Rich Plasma (PRP) (Relative Composition in Platelets %)
A	>5, very high dose	>90, high	>90, very pure PRP
B	3-5, high dose	70-90, medium	70-90, pure PRP
C	1-3, medium dose	30-70, low	30-70, heterogeneous PRP
D	<1, low dose	<30, poor	<30, whole blood PRP

Reproduced from Magalon J, Chateau AL, Bertrand B, et al. DEPA classification: a proposal for standardising PRP use and a retrospective application of available devices. *BMJ Open Sport Exerc Med.* 2016;2(1):e000060, with permission from BMJ Publishing Group Ltd.

CLINICAL PREPARATION OF PLATELET-RICH PLASMA

PRP for the majority of clinical applications is in the autologous form although some recombinant forms are becoming more readily available. The ease and speed at which autologous PRP is prepared is one of its great advantages, and there are many different commercially available PRP systems. These can be broadly categorized into three techniques: plateletpheresis (autologous selective filtration), standard cell separators, and gravitational separation (centrifuge system). In the authors' experience, preparation is most commonly achieved through centrifuging anticoagulated whole blood resulting in gravitational separation of the blood into layers due to the variation in the specific gravity of its components (Figure 8.1). This involves four key steps as follows:

1. Obtaining patient blood.
   - Patient venepuncture with blood collection in a tube that comes preprepared with anticoagulation (Figure 8.2)
2. Centrifugation—this separates the blood into three layers (Figure 8.3):
   - Hematocrit: red blood cells
   - Buffy coat: leukocytes and platelets
   - Plasma
3. Selective discarding of unwanted content.
   - This step is used to remove the unwanted red cell content ± the platelet and leucocyte-poor plasma

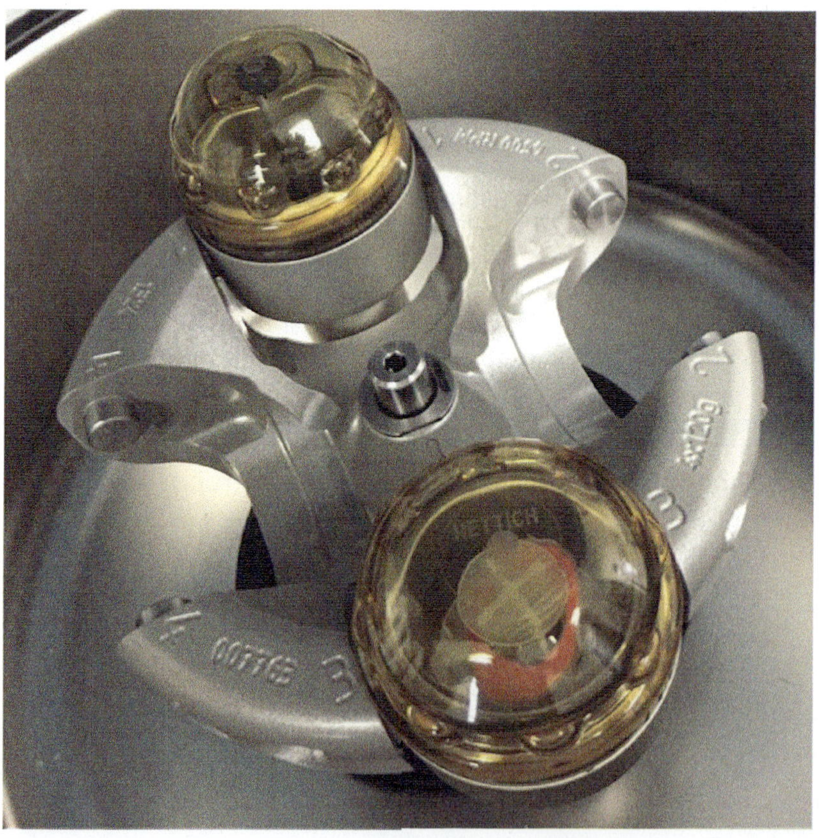

Figure 8.1. An example of a table top centrifuge machine for platelet-rich plasma preparation.

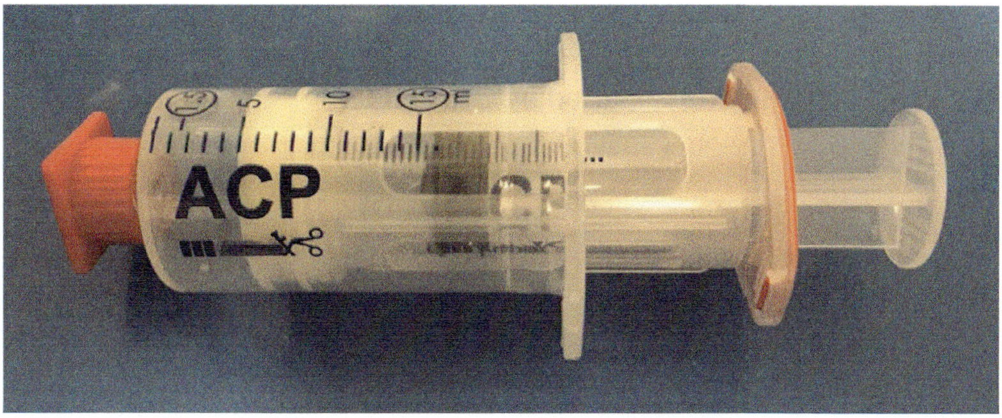

Figure 8.2. The Arthrex ACP (autologous conditioned plasma) Double syringe system used for platelet-rich plasma preparation.

4. Application of PRP.
   - Having said this, similar to the classification systems described above, there is marked variation in the preparation of PRP. Protocols vary in terms of the volume of blood taken, machines/systems used, anticoagulant, rate and duration of spins, and whether one or two spins are used. The exact technique of preparation is largely dependent on the manufacturer's specifications of each system used. A systematic review by Chahla et al[38] assessed the PRP processing protocols within the literature, and some of the processing characteristics are summarized in Table 8.2.
   - The centrifuge systems are small enough for storage in clinical areas or operating theatres, and the PRP can be ready to use within 15 minutes (spin time dependent) of obtaining the patient's blood. If a PRP gel is desired, this can be achieved with the addition of calcium (± thrombin), although further time is required for gelation to occur.[39] In most cases, the PRP obtained is used immediately, although it is possible to freeze or freeze dry samples for later use. With both methods, platelet and growth factor counts decrease over time, but the freeze-dried technique shows better preservation with growth factor levels being only slightly reduced from baseline at 8 weeks.[40]
   - To the authors knowledge, no recombinant PRP preparations exist commercially. However, some of their constituents are readily available: rhPDGF and rhBMP.

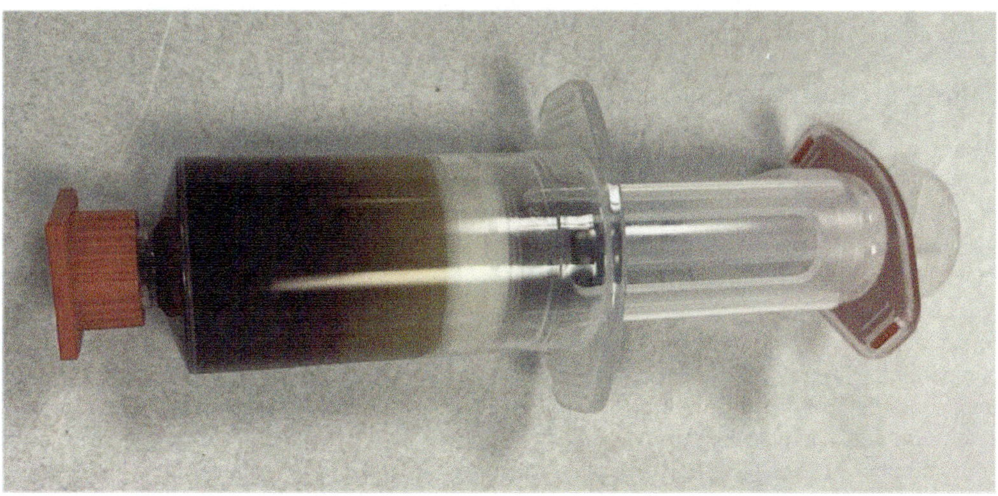

Figure 8.3. Blood sample following initial centrifuge, with blood separating into three layers.

TABLE 8.2 Summary of Platelet-Rich Plasma Processing Characteristics Within the Literature as Reported by Chahla et al

Processing Characteristic	Value
Median blood volume extracted	51 mL (8-450 mL)
Most common anticoagulant	Acid citrate dextrose solution A
Percentage of studies using centrifuge process	95%
Median rate for first spin	1,500 rpm (120-5,800 rpm)
Median first spin time	14 min (3-15 min)
Percentage of studies performing second spin	20%
Median volume of platelet-rich plasma produced	5 mL (2-30 mL)

Data from Chahla J, Cinque ME, Piuzzi NS, et al. A call for standardization in platelet-rich plasma preparation protocols and composition reporting: a systematic review of the clinical orthopaedic literature. *J Bone Joint Surg Am.* 2017;99(20):1769-1779.

PLATELET-RICH PLASMA IN NON–FRACTURE-RELATED BONE HEALING

Given the potential bone healing properties of PRP, there has been significant interest in its use as an adjunct to encourage bony union in a nonfracture setting. Some evidence exists in the use of PRP in osteotomy healing. In 2007, Dallari et al[41] reported the results of their three-arm RCT. They looked at tibial healing following high tibial osteotomy, comparing the osteogenic potential of lyophilized bone chips combined with platelet gel (group A) or with platelet gel and bone marrow stromal cells (group B), with that of lyophilized bone chips alone (group C). Groups A and B showed significantly increased osteoblasts and osteoid at 6 weeks, increased bone chip apposition, and increased osseointegration at 6 weeks and 1 year. The addition of the bone marrow stromal cells did contribute to significantly higher revascularization. Subsequent to this, Peerbooms et al[42] performed a retrospective observational study also looking at the addition of PRP to bone chips in high tibial osteotomies. Although not all statistically significant, they reported lower bone density at the osteotomy site at all three time points (1, 6, and 12 weeks) in the PRP group, indicating no benefit and a potential inhibitory effect. Further to this, there is some in vivo and vitro evidence exploring the potential use of PRP in spinal fusion surgery and ankle arthrodesis.

Spinal Fusion surgery

Several studies have examined the use of PRP as an adjunct to spinal fusion surgery. This includes exploratory work assessing the potential benefits of PRP in the setting of spinal fusion in a rat model. Kamoda et al[43] assessed the impact of PRP addition to hydroxyapatite for spinal interbody fusion in Sprague-Dawley rats. They identified significant differences in the fusion rate between those where both PRP and hydroxyapatite was used versus hydroxyapatite alone. In 2013, further work from Kamoda et al[44] then explored the potential role of PRP in posterolateral lumbar fusion in a larger group of rats. They again identified a higher proportion of fusion in the PRP group compared to controls. They also found higher levels of bone formation in the PRP group but no impact on the proportion of inflammatory neurons present in the dorsal root ganglion (an indicator of potential neuropathic pain stimulation).

A number of clinical studies have also addressed the use of PRP as an adjunct to aid bony union in spinal fusion.[45,46] Overall, these studies remain largely observational in nature meaning the ability to draw conclusions regarding a causative effect for PRP on bony healing is limited. There have, however, been two small RCTs performed in this area. In 2011, Sys et al[47] examined the potential benefit of PRP addition to iliac crest autograft in posterior lumbar interbody fusion for 40 patients (20 intervention: 20 control) at a single center recruited over an 18-month period. There was no sample size calculation performed, and no primary outcome was identified. Platelet concentrations in the PRP group were not reported. Overall, there were no significant differences found between the intervention and control groups in relation to their patient-reported outcome measures out to 2 years (Short Form-36, Oswestry Disability Index, and Visual Analogue Scale scores) or computed tomography radiographic fusion at 3, 6, and 12 months. In 2019 Kubota et al[48] also performed an RCT to examine the potential benefit of PRP addition to autologous bone grafting (ABG), this time in the setting of posterolateral lumbar fusion surgery. They randomized 62 patients (31 intervention: 31 control) at a single center over a 6-year period. Again, no sample size calculation was performed or primary outcome identified. Platelet concentrations in the PRP group were on average 7.7 times higher than that of autologous blood, alongside identified higher concentrations of the growth factors PDGF-AA, PDGF-BB, PDGF-AB, and TGF-β. Overall, they identified a significantly greater rate of bone fusion in the PRP group versus the control group (93.7% vs 74.2%, $P = .012$), a greater area of bone union (572 vs 367 mm^2, $P = .02$), as well as a shorter period until bone union (7.8 vs 9.4 months, $P = .012$) for PRP versus controls. There were no significant differences in pain score between groups.

One of the proposed reasons for difference in outcome between the two trials is the potential difference in platelet concentration between the two studies. In 2020, this is supported by a recent systematic review by Manini et al,[46] where they found that platelet concentration within PRP had a major impact on successful spinal fusion, with much higher fusion rates versus control (odds ratio 4.35, 95% CI 2.13-8.83) for studies that used high platelet concentrations (greater than or equal to five times higher than autologous blood), compared to those with lower platelet concentrations or those that did not report platelet concentration (odds ratio 0.55, 95% CI 0.36-0.83). As previously described, there remains much debate in the literature regarding optimal PRP concentrations, in particular in relation to overall volume and proportion of leukocytes contained within the medium.[49]

With regard to the overall effect of PRP on spinal fusion surgery, in 2020, a systematic review by Cai et al[45] has summarized the latest evidence. This included 10 studies and 566 participants, with three different types of PRP utilized. They identified several significant differences in the methods of PRP preparation, activation, and formulation across the studies. The risk of bias for the majority of included evidence was high. Overall, they identified no significant difference in fusion rate for addition of PRP versus controls (risk ratio 0.96, 95% CI 0.88-1.05) from six eligible studies. There was also no significant difference for pain scores or complication rates between the groups. They concluded that current evidence did not support the routine use of PRP for spinal fusion surgery but that further research in the form of high-quality RCTs was required for additional evaluation.

Foot and Ankle Arthrodesis

The rationale for use of PRP in foot and ankle (F&A) arthrodesis has been supported by the clinical correlation identified between the level of growth factors present at the fusion site (PDGF and VEGF) of healed and nonhealed diabetic hindfoot arthrodesis patients.[50] Diabetic patients are a particular group of interest when undergoing F&A surgery due to the established risk of nonunion in this setting.[51,52] As well as reduced growth factor expression, diabetes has also been associated with reduced collagen proliferation and increased expression of advanced glycation end products.[53,54] PRP therefore provides a potential vehicle for a targeted concentration of growth factors and other bioactive proteins that attenuate the negative sequelae of hyperglycemia to aid nonfracture bone healing in this setting.

In 2009, the potential benefit of PRP addition to arthrodesis in diabetic patients has been explored by Pinzur.[55] He examined 44 high-risk diabetic patients undergoing arthrodesis in the setting of Charcot neuroarthropathy, a chronic condition typically seen as end-stage disease of poorly controlled diabetes. All 44 patients (46 feet) underwent injection of PRP and bone marrow aspirate at the time of wound closure, with surgical management performed using a ring external fixator. Forty-two out of the 46 feet (91.3%) had achieved bony union at a mean of 26 months following surgery. Though there was no control group, the union rate achieved does appear to be favorable compared to the associated literature—with 86% reported in a recent systematic review.[56]

The role of PRP in F&A surgery has also been analyzed in the setting of syndesmotic fusion for total ankle replacement (TAR). In 2005, Barrow and Pomeroy[57] performed a retrospective cohort study of syndesmosis fusion with and without PRP for 20 patients undergoing TAR. They identified a significantly greater fusion rate with the addition of PRP to the fusion site versus controls (100% vs 62%, respectively, $P = .001$). In 2005, these findings were supported by Coetzee et al[58] who again examined syndesmotic fusion in TAR, with 66 patients in the PRP group and 114 patients in the control group. They also identified a statistically significant improvement in time to fusion and absence of nonunion/delayed union in the PRP group.

As well as in clinical application of PRP, there has also been clinical interest expressed in the use of PDGF, one of the main bioactive constituents of PRP, when considering F&A arthrodesis. In 2011, DiGiovanni et al[59] explored the use of recombinant PDGF (rhPDGF-BB) combined with beta-tricalcium phosphate (β-TCP) compared to ABG in the form of a randomized controlled feasibility trial for 20 patients undergoing F&A fusions. The primary outcome was radiographic union identified by a radiologist blinded to the treatment intervention. Secondary outcomes including PROMs (patient reported outcome measure) were also performed. In this small study, no formal between group analyses were performed, but there was a trend toward better radiographic bony union between the intervention and control groups at 36 weeks (77% [10/13] vs 50% [3/6], respectively). A further larger follow-up RCT was then performed by the same group of 434 patients that underwent arthrodesis with either rhPDGF-BB and β-TCP (intervention) or ABG (control).[60] The primary outcome was radiographic union according to computed tomography at 6 months, where they identified a statistically significant difference in the rate of bony union for the intervention group versus controls (66.5% vs 62.6%, respectively, $P < .05$). There was also a statistically significantly higher clinically determined union rate in the intervention group (88.3% vs 87.2% respectively, $P < .05$). It is, however, important to note that the differences in both outcomes were small, and of uncertain clinical significance, although there was also a better safety profile identified in the intervention group. Cost analyses were not performed.

The case for use of rhPDGF and β-TCP has also been strengthened by a further RCT examining its use in ankle and hindfoot arthrodesis, where again better fusion rates were seen compared to control (ABG), although this time with a significantly greater magnitude of difference (84% fusion at 24 months for intervention, vs 65% for controls, $P < .001$).[61]

Overall, there is scientific rationale for the use of PRP in F&A surgery, and in particular diabetic patients, although the evidence is largely of low quality. There is higher-level evidence available to suggest a positive effect of rhPDGF and β-TCP on bony fusion rates for F&A arthrodesis. Larger studies including health economic analyses are, however, still required before widespread clinical use can be recommended. The success of these studies has in turn helped to demonstrate the efficacy of PDGF in F&A surgery and were instrumental in the development of a combination product, recombinant rhPDGF bb + β-TCP. This has been subsequently FDA approved for F&A indications (Augment bone Graft, Wright Medical Group) for use as an alternative to autograft in arthrodesis (ie, fusion procedures) of the ankle and/or hindfoot that require the need for supplemental graft materials.

PLATELET-RICH PLASMA IN ACUTE FRACTURE MANAGEMENT

The use of PRP in the management of acute fractures has been investigated in a number of animal studies. These studies included direct addition of PRP alone or within a scaffold. Simman et al[62] investigated the effects of PRP on long bone healing in rats and demonstrated that PRP accelerates bone fracture healing in rat femurs via modulation of TGF-β1 and BMP-2 growth fracture expression. Guzel et al[63] reported significantly ($P < .05$) higher histological and biomechanical bone healing as well as increased bone strength when PRP was applied to simulated femoral fractures in rats. Also in rats, Rai et al[64] created femoral fractures with segmental critical-sized defects and found that the addition of PRP to a polycaprolactone TCP scaffold produced increased torsional stiffness at 12 weeks postsurgery and lower nonunion rates than those treated with an empty scaffold. In a rabbit model, Kasten et al[65] found improved diaphyseal bone healing with a calcium-deficient hydroxyapatite scaffold and PRP. In rabbits, Xie et al[66] constructed a critical defect in the radius of 45 New Zealand white rabbits. Four treatment groups were examined: group A, empty bone defect; group B, PRP; group C, autogenous bone particles + bone mesenchymal stem cells on the left radius; and group D, autogenous bone particles + PRP + bone mesenchymal stem cells on the right radius. X-ray, histology, and histomorphometry data revealed that the area of the newly formed bone was larger in group D. In addition, PRP could improve cell proliferation, osteogenic differentiation, and the release of growth factors (GFs), TGF-β1, and PDGF-AB. In sheep, Sarkar et al[67] created a critical-sized defect within the tibial diaphysis which was then treated with PRP in a collagen carrier or with collagen alone. Contrary to the results of other animal studies, Sarkar et al[67] reported that bone volume, mineral density, mechanical rigidity, and histology of the newly formed bone in the defect did not differ significantly between the PRP treated and the control group, and no effect of PRP upon bone formation was observed.

In hip fractures, Griffin et al[68] performed an RCT with the injection of PRP into the fracture site of intracapsular hip fractures undergoing internal fixation. The primary outcome measure was the proportion of patients undergoing revision within 1 year of injury, for which there was an absolute risk reduction of 5.6% in favor of PRP, but this was not significant ($P = .569$). In contrast, a similar single center RCT in Egypt reported an increased rate of radiological union and a lower rate of fixation failure in the PRP group.[69] For the management of diaphyseal femur fractures treated with intramedullary nailing, Singh et al[70] found PRP to have no effect on fracture healing. PRP and a matrix scaffold provided by fibrin membrane may provide an artificial hematoma effect in the initial phase of healing in open fractures or intramedullary nailing that have required open reduction.

An RCT by Liebergall et al[71] reported an improved time to union (1.5 vs 3 months) in distal tibial fractures managed with fixation supplemented with a composite graft of PRP, MSCs in suspension from bone marrow aspirate, and demineralized bone matrix (DBM) delivered to the fracture site. Regarding the treatment of calcaneal fractures, Wei et al[72] performed a three-arm RCT in patients with displaced type III calcaneal fractures who underwent open reduction and internal fixation and additionally received autograft alone, allograft + PRP, or allograft alone. At 24 and 72 months postoperatively, statistically significant ($P < .05$) differences existed clinically and radiologically in favor of the autograft and allograft + PRP groups. The addition of PRP to allograft was shown to be as effective as autograft in these fractures.

Namazi and Mehbudi[73] looked at the use of intra-articular PRP injections in the management of intra-articular distal radius fractures. This was a small cohort RCT in which the fractures were treated with closed reduction and percutaneous fixation, with the treatment group receiving the PRP injection. They focused on pain and activity scores rather than bony union/fracture healing, finding a significant difference in favor of PRP postoperatively. Additionally, there was a significant difference in flexion at 3 months, but this difference was not retained at longer follow-up.

Overall, there does not appear to be clear evidence to support the use of PRP in the routine management of acute fractures. There are still some conflicting results in both the animal and clinical human studies indicating that further research is required. While the results of a number of RCTs have been published, many of these have small sample sizes raising the possibility of statistical error.

Treatment of Patients at Increased Risk of Nonunion

Certain patient groups are at an increased risk of a delayed or nonunion as a result of comorbidities. These patients provide surgeons with significant treatment challenges, and if union is not achieved with the initial intervention, there is often a significant impact on patient morbidity and also health care costs. There has been some basic science and patient-based PRP research focused specifically on the acute fracture management in those with a higher risk of nonunion.

In a diabetic Wistar rat femur fracture model, PRP delivery at the fracture site normalized early cell proliferation and chondrogenesis and improved mechanical strength.[74] Mariano et al[75] demonstrated PRP to significantly enhance bone formation and healing in critical-sized defects in diabetic rats. Similarly, in osteoporotic rats, Chen et al[76] found that medium concentration PRP ($2.65 \pm 0.2 \times 10^9$/mL) was effective in inducing proliferation and osteogenic differentiation of MSCs and in promoting femoral fracture healing. They did, however, find that high-concentration ($8.21 \pm 0.4 \times 10^9$/mL) PRP inhibited osteogenic differentiation and callus remodeling.

Rodriguez-Collazo and Urso[77] investigated the healing rates in distal tibial fractures treated with an Ilizarov fixator together with combined DBM, PRP, and bone marrow aspirate concentrate (BMAC) in patients with significant comorbidities (diabetes, smoking, obesity, and renal disease). They observed faster bone healing but no difference in nonunion rates in those treated with DBM + BMAC + PRP versus DBM alone. Similarly, although not necessarily in "high-risk" patients, Lee et al[78] showed that the injection of BMAC and PRP at the osteotomy site in patients undergoing bilateral tibial lengthening produced faster healing at each cortex and earlier weight bearing. In both of these studies and that previously mentioned by Liebergall et al,[71] it is difficult to conclude whether BMAC or PRP was the influencing factor in these cases; furthermore, the results of all three studies are based on small cohorts (10-12 patients per cohort: treatment and control).

Despite positive results of PRP in osteoporotic and diabetic rats, the isolated effect of PRP in those patients who are at an increased risk of nonunion remains unclear. It does, however, appear to be of benefit when used in conjunction with concentrated bone marrow aspirate.

Platelet-Derived Growth Factor in Acute Fracture Management

With the interest in rhPDGF in F&A surgery, it is plausible that it may have a benefit in acute fracture management; however, less evidence currently exists in the literature. Bordei[22] investigated the effect of locally applied PDGF in fracture healing in a rat model and found that PDGF stimulates osteoblasts and increases bone formation, with radiological evidence of enhanced bony healing. Additionally Al-Zube et al[79] showed rhPDGF-BB to significantly improve fracture healing in diabetic rats. In a pilot clinical RCT, Christersson et al[80] locally administered rhPDGF-BB and an osteoconductive scaffold (β-TCP) (Augment Bone Graft, Wright Medical Group) in acute wrist fractures, but detected no reduction in healing time. To the authors' knowledge, there is no further clinical data looking specifically at recombinant PDGF in the acute fracture setting.

PLATELET-RICH PLASMA IN THE MANAGEMENT OF NONUNIONS

Throughout history, treatment of fracture nonunion has remained a focus of interest and research to the medical community. Even with appropriate management, nonunion has not been eradicated and can lead to significant physical and psychological detriment to the patient, as well as the larger socioeconomic impact it places on society. In the UK, the average cost of long bone fracture nonunion treatment is £29,204 per patient and in Canada, 67% to 97% of costs associated with tibial fractures were specifically related to nonunion.[81] In 1986, the FDA defined a nonunion as follows: *"A fracture that is a minimum of 9 months post occurrence and is not healed and has not shown radiographic progression for 3 months" (FDA 1986).*[82] There is, however, no fixed standardized system that exists in the literature to define a nonunion and other descriptive terms often exist: hypertrophic, atrophic, oligotrophic, septic, pseudoarthrosis, among others.

The "gold standard" for surgical treatment of long bone nonunion is the use of ABG.[83] However, there are a number of potential negative aspects of utilizing autograft which include cost, limited supply for large defects, donor site morbidity, and increased surgical time required. Several studies have therefore looked at the other options available, including "growth factors," such as PRP.

Platelet-Rich Plasma Used in Isolation

Say et al[84] examined the effect of percutaneous application of PRP to 20 patients with aseptic delayed union (8 patients) or nonunion (12 patients) of tibia or femoral fractures. A total of three PRP doses were administered under fluoroscopic control at intervals of 1 week at a median of 6 to 8 months post fracture. No complications were seen attributable to the use of PRP, but 11 cases did not unite and went on to require revision surgery and bone graft. Tawfik et al[85] conducted a similar study on 20 patients with clinical and radiological signs of nonunion at a median of 8 months post injury. Orthogonal serial follow-up radiographs were performed following PRP injection at 6 weeks post injection and then every 4 weeks until healing was confirmed. They found that there was evidence of callus formation seen in 85% of patients by the end of the 17th week postintervention and that the remaining three patients failed to unite within the 24-week follow-up study period.

Duramaz et al[86] retrospectively studied 14 consecutive patients with femoral or tibial nonunion that had been treated by percutaneous PRP application. They compared outcomes with a matched cohort of 15 patients who had undergone exchange nailing and found the PRP group to have a statistically significantly lower procedure time (as would be expected), with a mean time of 16 versus 66 minutes. They also found a lower time to union in the PRP group with 16.71 ± 2.4 weeks compared to 19.07 ± 3.67 weeks ($P = .053$). No significant difference, however, was seen in the overall rate of union of each group.

With a larger series, in 2015, Malhotra et al[87] studied 94 patients with established nonunion. This was a prospective case series with no control group. The authors injected 15 to 20 mL of autologous PRP ($>2 \times 10^6/\mu L$) under image intensifier control to the site of established long bone fractures. There was a wide variation in the bone that was nonunited: 35 tibias, 30 femurs, 11 humeri, 4 radii, 12 ulnas, and 2 with both radius and ulna were included. Eighty-two patients had their fractures united at the end of 4 months following application of PRP. Thirty-four patients showed bridging trabeculae at the end of the second month, while 41 patients showed similar findings at the end of the third month. Twelve patients did not show any sign of union at 4 months and were deemed as failures. No complications pertaining to the injection of PRP were reported.

Kaushik et al[88] conducted a study looking at 20 patients with delayed or nonunion of long bones between 2018 and 2019. They treated the patients with isolated PRP injections with no surgical intervention and found that at study follow-up, 65% showed good callus formation and benefitted from the injection but 35% did not and required further surgical intervention.

In summary, although laboratory research would suggest PRP in isolation may play a role in the treatment of nonunion, the clinical evidence is currently equivocal at best. Slightly more robust clinical evidence exists for its use in conjunction with bone graft, but higher-quality papers with homogeneity of subject matter and PRP concentration, etc., are still needed before more definitive conclusions can be drawn.

Platelet-Rich Plasma and Bone Graft

Ghaffarpasand et al[89] performed a randomized controlled double-blind clinical trial looking at 75 adult patients being treated for long bone nonunion. They studied two groups who were assigned to receive either 5 mL PRP or 5 mL normal saline at the time of surgery and autologous bone grafting. Interestingly, application of PRP in this study showed a significantly higher union rate of 81.1% versus 55.3% with a decreased time to union and was associated with less pain in the recovery period.

Chu et al[90] constructed a study over approximately a 2-year period enrolling 60 patients with nonunions that went onto be treated by ABG, ABG + PRP, or ABG + PRP and extracorporeal shock wave therapy. Results for 55 of the patients were available at follow-up, with the results showing promise for the use of ABG + PRP in the nonunion setting. The addition of extracorporeal shock wave therapy was also shown to be slightly beneficial but did not reach statistical significance.

Zhang et al[91] performed a study where 47 patients with long bone fracture nonunions were randomly divided into two groups: monotherapy group ($n = 22$) and combination group ($n = 25$). In the monotherapy group, autologous bone marrow MSC transplantation was performed at the bone nonunion site. In the combination group, autologous platelet-rich plasma combined with bone marrow MSC transplantation was implemented in the nonunion site. Callus score, clinical healing time, local complications, and limb function grade were recorded and compared between the two groups. The healing properties and limb function in the combination group were significantly superior to those in the monotherapy group (healing time: [4.2 ± 1.5] vs [5.6 ± 1.1] months, $P < .05$; healing rate: 92% vs 86%, $P < .05$; callus score: 2.74 ± 0.36 vs 2.32 ± 0.53, $P < .05$; limb function recovery rate: 77% vs 84%, $P < .05$).

Roffi et al[92] performed a systematic review of the literature regarding PRP and bone defects and found 64 appropriate papers. Forty-five were preclinical in vivo studies and 19 were clinical studies. Forty-five studies were based on animal models. Of the animal studies, delivery mode of PRP was percutaneous in three papers, while the remainder involved surgical application of the PRP. Sixteen percent of articles detailed the effect of PRP alone, while 84% involved the effect of PRP mixed with other materials (53% with 3D scaffolds, autograft in 23.5%, and 23.5% with powders, granules, or pastes). The rest involved allograft or xenograft. PRP concentration was reported in 71% of studies but was found to be heterogeneous throughout.

Eleven of the identified clinical papers focused on the use of PRP in nonunion. Four of these papers used a minimally invasive approach with percutaneous injection of PRP and six as a topical enhancer during revision surgery. One paper reported the comparison of both. Overall, a potential benefit of PRP use was seen in several papers in each setting, but significant heterogeneity in the literature was identified. All but one of the studies that their search synthesized considered patients affected by delayed or nonunion in different anatomical regions pooled together (mainly humerus, femur, and tibia), thus again decreasing the homogeneity and comparability of data. The lack of well-designed RCTs investigating PRP in the setting of nonunion remains problematic when considering more widespread use in clinical practice.

Despite its potential promise, the level of research regarding PRP and nonunion remains at best small case series and cohort studies. Conflicts in the literature can also potentially be explained by absence of a consensus about how to prepare the PRP, variation in cell count, and in application technique as previously described.

COMPLICATIONS

Overall, the complication profile associated with PRP use appears to be very low. In the autologous form, with injection of the patient's own blood, the chance of an allergic reaction to PRP is very unlikely. Additionally, the authors identified no evidence to suggest that the use of PRP increased infection risk. There is some evidence that PRP may indeed have an inhibitory effect on bacterial growth, particularly within the first 1 to 2 hours after initiating treatment.[93] The possibility of patients developing an infection exists with all invasive procedures, and so meticulous aseptic technique should be utilized in the preparation and insertion of PRP.

CONCLUSIONS

The potential treatment efficacy of PDGF, one of the main constituents of PRP, has been explored in a limited setting. Currently, evidence primarily pertains to in vivo studies and those investigating nonfracture bone healing, where a general support for potential benefit has been identified. There is, however, little available research to address the potential benefits of PDGF use in the fracture setting (either acutely or in cases of nonunion/delayed union), and this remains an interesting area for future clinical studies (Figure 8.4A-F).

Regarding PRP, there is sufficient evidence from use in in vitro and in vivo nonclinical studies to support its role in all types of bone healing. This is perhaps strongest in those with potential for poor healing capacity, such as diabetics or smokers. The lack of prospective randomized

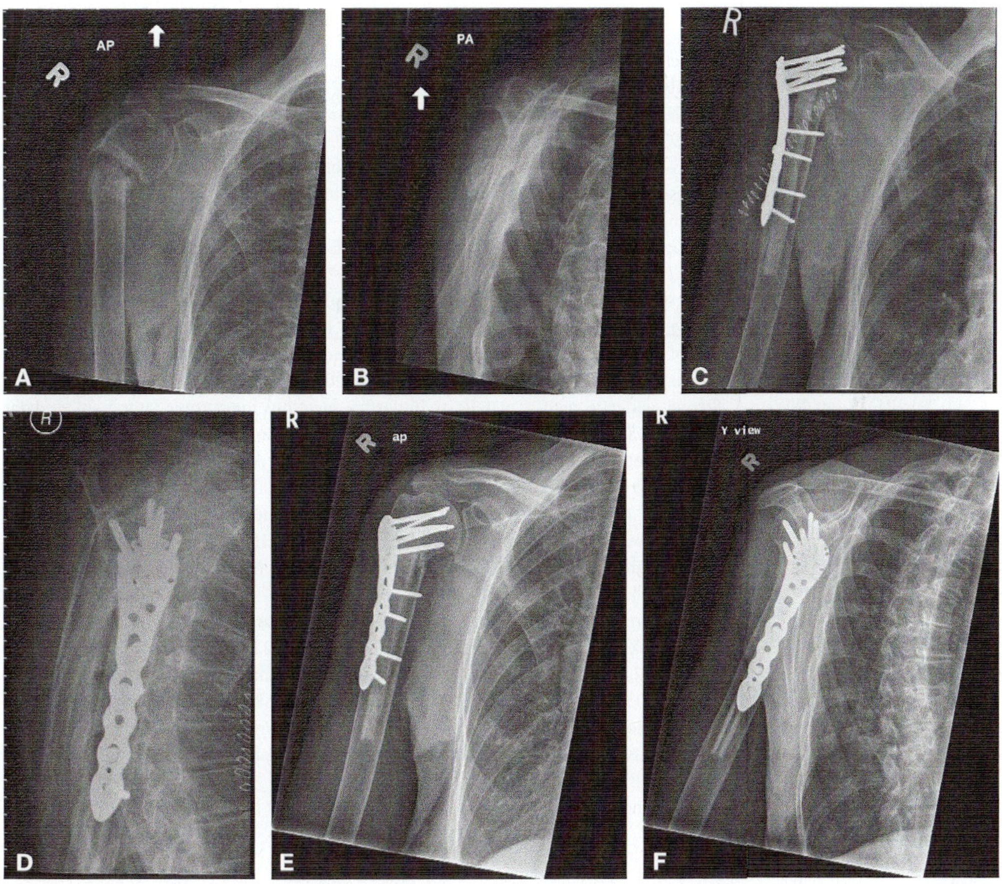

Figure 8.4. AP **(A)** and lateral **(B)** radiographs of two part proximal humerus fracture referred for pseudarthrosis at 9 months after nonoperative treatment. AP **(C)** and lateral **(D)** radiographs of proximal humerus immediately following nonunion repair with open reduction and plate fixation, use of an intramedullary fibula strut graft, and platelet-derived growth factor. AP **(E)** and lateral **(F)** radiographs of proximal humerus 9 months following nonunion repair showing fracture union.

clinical trials with robust causal evidence are, however, a clear barrier to recommending current routine use of PRP in the clinical setting, even for those with established nonunion, where the cost-effectiveness potential is significantly greater.

Widespread heterogeneity in the nomenclature, classification, and preparation of PRP in studies acts to significantly decrease the translational worth of existing research. It is imperative that future work is of sufficient methodological quality and robust design that it allows for potential integration into clinical practice. Use of minimum reporting guidelines for PRP studies, such as those developed by Murray et al,[94] are essential to ensuring that future work is published with sufficient scientific rigor. Ongoing basic science research should focus on determining the optimum consistency of PRP and delivery for clinical application, followed by evaluation in the translational setting. Given the significant potential cost associated with increasing PRP utilization, use of future health economic analyses will be an integral part of understanding clinical applicability, particularly within financially constrained health care systems.

References

1. Xu XR, Zhang D, Oswald BE, et al. Platelets are versatile cells: new discoveries in hemostasis, thrombosis, immune responses, tumor metastasis and beyond. *Crit Rev Clin Lab Sci.* 2016;53(6):409-430. doi:10.1080/10408363.2016.1200008
2. Foster TE, Puskas BL, Rodeo SA, et al. Platelet-rich plasma from basic science to clinical applications. *Am J Sports Med.* 2009;37(11):2259-2272. doi:10.1177/0363546509349921
3. Rendu F, Brohard-Bohn B. The platelet release reaction: granules' constituents, secretion and functions. *Platelets.* 2001;12(5):261-273. doi:10.1080/09537100120068170
4. Alsousou J, Thompson M, Hulley P, Noble A, Willett K. The biology of platelet-rich plasma and its application in trauma and orthopaedic surgery: a review of the literature. *J Bone Jt Surg: Ser B.* 2009;91(8):987-996. doi:10.1302/0301-620X.91B8.22546
5. Weibrich G, Kleis WKG, Hafner G, Hitzler WE. Growth factor levels in platelet-rich plasma and correlations with donor age, sex, and platelet count. *J Cranio-Maxillofacial Surg.* 2002;30(2):97-102. doi:10.1054/jcms.2002.0285
6. Marx RE. Clinical controversies in oral and maxillofacial surgery: part two platelet-rich plasma: evidence to support its use. *J Oral Maxillofac Surg.* 2004;62(4):489-496. doi:10.1016/j.joms.2003.12.003
7. Phadke A, Singh B, Bakti N. Role of platelet rich plasma in rotator cuff tendinopathy: clinical application and review of literature. *J Clin Orthop Trauma.* 2019;10(2):244-247. doi:10.1016/j.jcot.2018.10.014
8. De Vos RJ, Windt J, Weir A. Strong evidence against platelet-rich plasma injections for chronic lateral epicondylar tendinopathy: a systematic review. *Br J Sports Med.* 2014;48(12):952-956. doi:10.1136/bjsports-2013-093281
9. Zhang YJ, Xu SZ, Gu PC, et al. Is platelet-rich plasma injection effective for chronic Achilles tendinopathy? A meta-analysis. *Clin Orthop Relat Res.* 2018;476(8):1633-1641. doi:10.1007/s11999.0000000000000258
10. Ali M, Oderuth E, Atchia I, Malviya A. The use of platelet-rich plasma in the treatment of greater trochanteric pain syndrome: a systematic literature review. *J Hip Preserv Surg.* 2018;5(3):209-219. doi:10.1093/jhps/hny027
11. Liddle AD, Rodríguez-Merchán EC. Platelet-rich plasma in the treatment of patellar tendinopathy. *Am J Sports Med.* 2015;43(10):2583-2590. doi:10.1177/0363546514560726
12. Gato-Calvo L, Magalhaes J, Ruiz-Romero C, Blanco FJ, Burguera EF. Platelet-rich plasma in osteoarthritis treatment: review of current evidence. *Ther Adv Chronic Dis.* 2019;10:1-18. doi:10.1177/2040622319825567
13. Martinez-Zapata MJ, Martí-Carvajal AJ, Solà I, et al. Autologous platelet-rich plasma for treating chronic wounds. *Cochrane Database Syst Rev.* 2016;2016(5):CD006899. doi:10.1002/14651858.CD006899.pub3
14. Zaffagnini S, Poggi A, Reale D, Andriolo L, Flanigan DC, Filardo G. Biologic augmentation reduces the failure rate of meniscal repair: a systematic review and meta-analysis. *Orthop J Sport Med.* 2021;9(2):232596712098162. doi:10.1177/2325967120981627
15. Järvinen TAH. Neovascularisation in tendinopathy: from eradication to stabilisation? *Br J Sports Med.* 2020;54(1):1-2. doi:10.1136/bjsports-2019-100608
16. Cook JL, Rio E, Purdam CR, Docking SI. Revisiting the continuum model of tendon pathology: what is its merit in clinical practice and research? *Br J Sports Med.* 2016;50(19):1187-1191. doi:10.1136/bjsports-2015-095422
17. Farahat MN, Yanni G, Poston R, Panayi GS. Cytokine expression in synovial membranes of patients with rheumatoid arthritis and osteoarthritis. *Ann Rheum Dis.* 1993;52(12):870-875. doi:10.1136/ard.52.12.870
18. Marques LF, Stessuk T, Camargo ICC, Sabeh Junior N, Dos SL, Ribeiro-Paes JT. Platelet-rich plasma (PRP): methodological aspects and clinical applications. *Platelets.* 2015;26(2):101-113. doi:10.3109/09537104.2014.881991
19. Slater M, Patava J, Kingham K, Mason RS. Involvement of platelets in stimulating osteogenic activity. *J Orthop Res.* 1995;13(5):655-663. doi:10.1002/jor.1100130504

20. Georgakopoulos I, Tsantis S, Georgakopoulos P, et al. The impact of Platelet Rich Plasma (PRP) in osseointegration of oral implants in dental panoramic radiography: texture based evaluation. *Clin Cases Miner Bone Metab.* 2014;11(1):59-66. doi:10.11138/ccmbm/2014.11.1.059
21. Hart CE, Bailey M, Curtis DA, et al. Purification of PDGF-AB and PDGF-BB from human platelet extracts and identification of all three PDGF dimers in human platelets. *Biochemistry.* 1990;29(1):166-172. doi:10.1021/bi00453a022
22. Bordei P. Locally applied platelet-derived growth factor accelerates fracture healing. *J Bone Joint Surg Br.* 2011;93-B(12):1653-1659. doi:10.1302/0301-620X.93B12.27244
23. Lebaron RG, Athanasiou KA. Extracellular matrix cell adhesion peptides: functional applications in orthopedic materials. *Tissue Eng.* 2000;6(2):85-103. doi:10.1089/107632700320720
24. Linkhart TA, Mohan S, Baylink DJ. Growth factors for bone growth and repair: IGF, TGFβ and BMP. *Bone.* Vol. 19 Elsevier Inc.; 1996:S1-S12. doi:10.1016/S8756-3282(96)00138-X
25. Kalén A, Wahlström O, Linder CH, Magnusson P. The content of bone morphogenetic proteins in platelets varies greatly between different platelet donors. *Biochem Biophys Res Commun.* 2008;375(2):261-264. doi:10.1016/j.bbrc.2008.08.014
26. Giustina A, Mazziotti G, Canalis E. Growth hormone, insulin-like growth factors, and the skeleton. *Endocr Rev.* 2008;29(5):535-559. doi:10.1210/er.2007-0036
27. Wildemann B, Schmidmaier G, Ordel S, Stange R, Haas NP, Raschke M. Cell proliferation and differentiation during fracture healing are influenced by locally applied IGF-I and TGF-β1: comparison of two proliferation markers, PCNA and BrdU. *J Biomed Mater Res: Part B Appl Biomater.* 2003;65(1):150-156. doi:10.1002/jbm.b.10512
28. Niu T, Rosen CJ. The insulin-like growth factor-I gene and osteoporosis: a critical appraisal. *Gene.* 2005;361(1-2): 38-56. doi:10.1016/j.gene.2005.07.016
29. Tsiridis E, Upadhyay N, Giannoudis P. Molecular aspects of fracture healing: which are the important molecules? *Injury.* 2007;38(Suppl 1):S11-S25. doi:10.1016/j.injury.2007.02.006
30. Gerber HP, Vu TH, Ryan AM, Kowalski J, Werb Z, Ferrara N. VEGF couples hypertrophic cartilage remodeling, ossification and angiogenesis during endochondral bone formation. *Nat Med.* 1999;5(6):623-628. doi:10.1038/9467
31. Bai Y, Li P, Yin G, et al. BMP-2, VEGF and bFGF synergistically promote the osteogenic differentiation of rat bone marrow-derived mesenchymal stem cells. *Biotechnol Lett.* 2013;35(3):301-308. doi:10.1007/s10529-012-1084-3
32. Dohan Ehrenfest DM, Rasmusson L, Albrektsson T. Classification of platelet concentrates: from pure platelet-rich plasma (P-PRP) to leucocyte- and platelet-rich fibrin (L-PRF). *Trends Biotechnol.* 2009;27(3):158-167. doi:10.1016/j.tibtech.2008.11.009
33. Magalon J, Chateau AL, Bertrand B, et al. DEPA classification: a proposal for standardising PRP use and a retrospective application of available devices. *Exerc Med.* 2016;2:60. doi:10.1136/bmjsem-2015-000060
34. Mishra A, Harmon K, Woodall J, Vieira A. Sports medicine applications of platelet rich plasma. *Curr Pharm Biotechnol.* 2012;13(7):1185-1195. doi:10.2174/138920112800624283
35. Delong JM, Russell RP, Mazzocca AD. Platelet-rich plasma: the PAW classification system. *Arthrosc: J Arthrosc Relat Surg.* 2012;28(7):998-1009. doi:10.1016/j.arthro.2012.04.148
36. Mautner K, Malanga GA, Smith J, et al. A call for a standard classification system for future biologic research: the rationale for new PRP nomenclature. *PM R.* 2015;7(4):S53-S59. doi:10.1016/j.pmrj.2015.02.005
37. Lana JFSD, Purita J, Paulus C, et al. Contributions for classification of platelet rich plasma: proposal of a new classification: MARSPILL. *Regen Med.* 2017;12(5):565-574. doi:10.2217/rme-2017-0042
38. Chahla J, Piuzzi NS, Mannava S, et al. A call for standardization in platelet-rich plasma preparation protocols and composition reporting: a systematic review of the clinical orthopaedic literature mark. *Artic J Bone Jt Surg.* 2017;99(20):1769-1779. doi:10.2106/JBJS.16.01374
39. Jo CH, Roh YH, Kim JE, Shin S, Yoon KS. Optimizing platelet-rich plasma gel formation by varying time and gravitational forces during centrifugation. *J Oral Implantol.* 2013;39(5):525-532. doi:10.1563/AAID-JOI-D-10-00155
40. Shiga Y, Kubota G, Orita S, et al. Freeze-dried human platelet-rich plasma retains activation and growth factor expression after an eight-week preservation period. *Asian Spine J.* 2017;11(3):329-336. doi:10.4184/asj.2017.11.3.329
41. Dallari D, Savarino L, Stagni C, et al. Enhanced tibial osteotomy healing with use of bone grafts supplemented with platelet gel or platelet gel and bone marrow stromal cells. *J Bone Jt Surg.* 2007;89(11):2413-2420. doi:10.2106/JBJS.F.01026
42. Peerbooms JC, Colaris JW, Hakkert AA, et al. No positive bone healing after using platelet rich plasma in a skeletal defect. An observational prospective cohort study. *Int Orthop.* 2012;36(10):2113-2119. doi:10.1007/s00264-012-1603-9
43. Kamoda H, Yamashita M, Ishikawa T, et al. Platelet-rich plasma combined with hydroxyapatite for lumbar interbody fusion promoted bone formation and decreased an inflammatory pain neuropeptide in rats. *Spine (Phila Pa 1976).* 2012;37(20):1727-1733. doi:10.1097/BRS.0b013e31825567b7
44. Kamoda H, Ohtori S, Ishikawa T, et al. The effect of platelet-rich plasma on posterolateral lumbar fusion in a rat model. *J Bone Joint Surg Am.* 2013;95(12):1109-1116. doi:10.2106/JBJS.L.00320
45. Cai Y, Tian T-Z, Chen L-Y, et al. The effect of platelet-rich plasma on the fusion rate and clinical outcome of spinal fusion surgery: a systematic review and meta-analysis. Tambella AM, ed. *PLoS One.* 2020;15(12):e0243204. doi:10.1371/journal.pone.0243204

46. Manini DR, Shega FD, Guo C, Wang Y. Role of platelet-rich plasma in spinal fusion surgery: systematic review and meta-analysis. *Adv Orthop.* 2020;2020:1-8. doi:10.1155/2020/8361798
47. Sys J, Weyler J, Van Der Zijden T, Parizel P, Michielsen J. Platelet-rich plasma in mono-segmental posterior lumbar interbody fusion. *Eur Spine J.* 2011;20(10):1650-1657. doi:10.1007/s00586-011-1897-0
48. Kubota G, Kamoda H, Orita S, et al. Platelet-rich plasma enhances bone union in posterolateral lumbar fusion: a prospective randomized controlled trial. *Spine J.* 2019;19(2):e34-e40. doi:10.1016/j.spinee.2017.07.167
49. Straum OK. The optimal platelet concentration in platelet-rich plasma for proliferation of human cells in vitro-diversity, biases, and possible basic experimental principles for further research in the field: a review. *PeerJ.* 2020;8:e10303. doi:10.7717/peerj.10303
50. Verma R, Koerner J, Breitbart E, et al. Correlation of growth factor levels at the fusion site of diabetic patients undergoing hindfoot arthrodesis and clinical outcome. *Curr Orthop Pract.* 2011;22(3):251-256. doi:10.1097/BCO.0b013e318212584c
51. Lavery LA, Lavery DC, Green T, et al. Increased risk of nonunion and Charcot arthropathy after ankle fracture in people with diabetes. *J Foot Ankle Surg.* 2020;59(4):653-656. doi:10.1053/j.jfas.2019.05.006
52. Shibuya N, Humphers JM, Fluhman BL, Jupiter DC. Factors associated with nonunion, delayed union, and malunion in foot and ankle surgery in diabetic patients. *J Foot Ankle Surg.* 2013;52(2):207-211. doi:10.1053/j.jfas.2012.11.012
53. Macey LR, Kana SM, Jingushi S, Terek RM, Borretos J, Bolander ME. Defects of early fracture-healing in experimental diabetes. *JBJS.* 1989;71(5).
54. Cortizo AM, Lettieri MG, Barrio DA, Mercer N, Etcheverry SB, McCarthy AD. Advanced glycation end-products (AGEs) induce concerted changes in the osteoblastic expression of their receptor RAGE and in the activation of extracellular signal-regulated kinases (ERK). *Mol Cell Biochem.* 2003;250(1-2):1-10. doi:10.1023/A:1024934008982
55. Pinzur MS. Use of platelet-rich concentrate and bone marrow aspirate in high-risk patients with Charcot arthropathy of the foot. *Foot Ankle Int.* 2009;30(2):124-127. doi:10.3113/FAI.2009.0124
56. Ha J, Hester T, Foley R, et al. Charcot foot reconstruction outcomes: a systematic review. *J Clin Orthop Trauma.* 2020;11(3):357-368. doi:10.1016/j.jcot.2020.03.025
57. Barrow CR, Pomeroy GC. Enhancement of syndesmotic fusion rates in total ankle arthroplasty with the use of autologous platelet concentrate. *Foot Ankle Int.* 2005;26(6):458-461. doi:10.1177/107110070502600606
58. Coetzee JC, Pomeroy GC, Watts JD, Barrow C. The use of autologous concentrated growth factors to promote syndesmosis fusion in the agility total ankle replacement. A preliminary study. *Foot Ankle Int.* 2005;26(10):840-846. doi:10.1177/107110070502601009
59. DiGiovanni CW, Baumhauer J, Lin SS, et al. Prospective, randomized, multi-center feasibility trial of rhPDGF-BB versus autologous bone graft in a foot and ankle fusion model. *Foot Ankle Int.* 2011;32(4):344-354. doi:10.3113/FAI.2011.0344
60. DiGiovanni CW, Lin SS, Baumhauer JF, et al. Recombinant human platelet-derived growth factor-BB and beta-tricalcium phosphate (rhPDGF-BB/β-TCP): an alternative to autogenous bone graft. *J Bone Jt Surg.* 2013;95(13):1184-1192. doi:10.2106/JBJS.K.01422
61. Daniels TR, Younger ASE, Penner MJ, et al. Prospective randomized controlled trial of hindfoot and ankle fusions treated with rhPDGF-BB in combination with a β-TCP-collagen matrix. *Foot Ankle Int.* 2015;36(7):739-748. doi:10.1177/1071100715576370
62. Simman R, Hoffmann A, Bohinc RJ, Peterson WC, Russ AJ. Role of platelet-rich plasma in acceleration of bone fracture healing. *Ann Plast Surg.* 2008;61(3):337-344. doi:10.1097/SAP.0b013e318157a185
63. Guzel Y, Karalezli N, Bilge O, et al. The biomechanical and histological effects of platelet-rich plasma on fracture healing. *Knee Surgery, Sport Traumatol Arthrosc.* 2015;23(5):1378-1383. doi:10.1007/s00167-013-2734-2
64. Rai B, Oest ME, Dupont KM, Ho KH, Teoh SH, Guldberg RE. Combination of platelet-rich plasma with polycaprolactone-tricalcium phosphate scaffolds for segmental bone defect repair. *J Biomed Mater Res Part A.* 2007;81A(4):888-899. doi:10.1002/jbm.a.31142
65. Kasten P, Vogel J, Geiger F, Niemeyer P, Luginbühl R, Szalay K. The effect of platelet-rich plasma on healing in critical-size long-bone defects. *Biomaterials.* 2008;29(29):3983-3992. doi:10.1016/j.biomaterials.2008.06.014
66. Xie H, Cao L, Ye L, et al. Autogenous bone particles combined with platelet-rich plasma can stimulate bone regeneration in rabbits. *Exp Ther Med.* 2020;20(6):279. doi:10.3892/etm.2020.9409. PMID: 33200004; PMCID: PMC7664605.
67. Sarkar MR, Augat P, Shefelbine SJ, et al. Bone formation in a long bone defect model using a platelet-rich plasma-loaded collagen scaffold. *Biomaterials.* 2006;27(9):1817-1823. doi:10.1016/j.biomaterials.2005.10.039
68. Griffin XL, Achten J, Parsons N, Costa ML. Platelet-rich therapy in the treatment of patients with hip fractures: a single centre, parallel group, participant-blinded, randomised controlled trial. *BMJ Open.* 2013;3(6):e002583. doi:10.1136/bmjopen-2013-002583
69. Samy AM. The role of platelet rich plasma in management of fracture neck femur: new insights. *Int Orthop.* 2016;40:1019-1024. doi:10.1007/s00264-015-2844-1
70. Singh R, Rohilla R, Gawande J, Kumar SP. To evaluate the role of platelet-rich plasma in healing of acute diaphyseal fractures of the femur. *Chinese J Traumatol - English Ed.* 2017;20(1):39-44. doi:10.1016/j.cjtee.2016.03.007
71. Liebergall M, Schroeder J, Mosheiff R, et al. Stem cell-based therapy for prevention of delayed fracture union: a randomized and prospective preliminary study. *Mol Ther.* 2013;21(8):1631-1638. doi:10.1038/mt.2013.109

72. Wei L-C, Lei G-H, Sheng P, et al. Efficacy of platelet-rich plasma combined with allograft bone in the management of displaced intra-articular calcaneal fractures: a prospective cohort study. *J Orthop Res.* 2012;30(10):1570-1576. doi:10.1002/jor.22118
73. Namazi H, Mehbudi A. Investigating the effect of intra-articular PRP injection on pain and function improvement in patients with distal radius fracture. *Orthop Traumatol Surg Res.* 2016;102(1):47-52. doi:10.1016/j.otsr.2015.11.002
74. Gandhi A, Dumas C, O'Connor JP, Parsons JR, Lin SS. The effects of local platelet rich plasma delivery on diabetic fracture healing. *Bone.* 2006;38(4):540-546. doi:10.1016/j.bone.2005.10.019
75. Mariano R, Messora M, de Morais A, et al. Bone healing in critical-size defects treated with platelet-rich plasma: a histologic and histometric study in the calvaria of diabetic rat. *Oral Surgery, Oral Med Oral Pathol Oral Radiol Endodontology.* 2010;109(1):72-78. doi:10.1016/j.tripleo.2009.08.003
76. Chen L, Yang X, Huang G, et al. Platelet-rich plasma promotes healing of osteoporotic fractures. *Orthopedics.* 2013;36(6):e687-e694. doi:10.3928/01477447-20130523-10
77. Rodriguez-Collazo ER, Urso ML. Combined use of the Ilizarov method, concentrated bone marrow aspirate (cBMA), and platelet-rich plasma (PRP) to expedite healing of bimalleolar fractures. *Strategies Trauma Limb Reconstr.* 2015;10(3):161-166. doi:10.1007/s11751-015-0239-x
78. Lee H-W, Choi K-H, Kim J-Y, Yang I, Noh K-C. Prospective clinical research of the efficacy of platelet-rich plasma in the outpatient-based treatment of rotator cuff tendinopathy. *Clin Shoulder Elb.* 2019;22(2):61-69. doi:10.5397/cise.2019.22.2.61
79. Al-Zube L, Breitbart EA, O'Connor JP, et al. Recombinant human platelet-derived growth factor BB (rhPDGF-BB) and beta-tricalcium phosphate/collagen matrix enhance fracture healing in a diabetic rat model. *J Orthop Res.* 2009;27(8):1074-1081. doi:10.1002/jor.20842
80. Christersson A, Sandén B, Larsson S. Prospective randomized feasibility trial to assess the use of rhPDGF-BB in treatment of distal radius fractures. *J Orthop Surg Res.* 2015;10(1):37. doi:10.1186/s13018-015-0174-z
81. Hak DJ, Fitzpatrick D, Bishop JA, et al. Delayed union and nonunions: epidemiology, clinical issues, and financial aspects. *Injury.* 2014;45(Suppl 2):S3-S7. doi:10.1016/j.injury.2014.04.002
82. Frölke J, Patka P. Definition and classification of fracture non-unions. *Injury.* 2007;38(Suppl 2):S19-S22.
83. Bauer TW, Muschler GF. Bone graft materials: an overview of the basic science. In: *Clinical Orthopaedics and Related Research.* Lippincott Williams and Wilkins; 2000:10-27. doi:10.1097/00003086-200002000-00003
84. Say F, Türkeli E, Bülbül M. Is platelet-rich plasma injection an effective choice in cases of non-union? *Acta Chir Orthop Traumatol Cech.* 2014;81(5):340-345.
85. Tawfik A, Kamel N. Assessment of autologous platelet gel injection in nonunited long bones. *Egypt J Haematol.* 2017;42(1):31. doi:10.4103/1110-1067.206430
86. Duramaz A, Ursavaş HT, Bilgili MG, Bayrak A, Bayram B, Avkan MC. Platelet-rich plasma versus exchange intramedullary nailing in treatment of long bone oligotrophic nonunions. *Eur J Orthop Surg Traumatol.* 2018;28(1):131-137. doi:10.1007/s00590-017-2024-7
87. Malhotra R, Kumar V, Garg B, et al. Role of autologous platelet-rich plasma in treatment of long-bone nonunions: a prospective study. *Musculoskelet Surg.* 2015;99(3):243-248. doi:10.1007/s12306-015-0378-8
88. Kumar Kaushik S, Khan A, Mathur M, Jaiswal M, Jadon D. Role of PRP injection in delayed union and non union of long bone fractures. *Indian J Orthop Surg.* 2020;6(1):35-40. doi:10.18231/j.ijos.2020.007
89. Ghaffarpasand F, Shahrezaei M, Dehghankhalili M. Effects of platelet rich plasma on healing rate of long bone non-union fractures: a randomized double-blind placebo controlled clinical trial. *Bull Emerg Trauma.* 2016;4(3):134-140.
90. Chu W. Treatment of nonunion with autologous bone transplantation combined with platelet-rich plasma and extracorporeal shock wave. *Zhongguo Gu Shang.* 2019;32(5):434-439. doi:10.3969/j.issn.1003-0034.2019.05.009
91. Zhang S, Zhang T, Fu G-H, et al. Therapeutic effect of autologous platelet rich plasma combined with bone marrow mesenchymal stem cell transplantation on long shaft fracture bone nonunion. *Chinese J Tissue Eng Res.* 2017;21(29):4716-4721. doi:10.3969/j.issn.2095-4344.2017.29.021
92. Roffi A, Di Matteo B, Krishnakumar GS, Kon E, Filardo G. Platelet-rich plasma for the treatment of bone defects: from pre-clinical rational to evidence in the clinical practice. A systematic review. *Int Orthop.* 2017;41(2):221-237. doi:10.1007/s00264-016-3342-9. PMID: 27888295.
93. Mariani E, Filardo G, Canella V, et al. Platelet-rich plasma affects bacterial growth in vitro. *Cytotherapy.* 2014;16(19):1294-1304. doi:10.1016/j.jcyt.2014.06.003
94. Murray IR, Geeslin AG, Goudie EB, Petrigliano FA, LaPrade RF. Minimum information for studies evaluating biologics in orthopaedics (MIBO): platelet-rich plasma and mesenchymal stem cells. *J Bone Jt Surg Am.* 2017;99(10):809-819. doi:10.2106/JBJS.16.00793

9 Osteoinductive Substrates and Other Growth Factors

Anna J. L. Lodewijks, Taco J. Blokhuis, and Martijn Poeze

REVIEW BASIC BIOLOGY OF INDUCTIVE FACTORS

History of Osteoinduction and Inductive Factors

In fracture healing osteogenesis, the formation of bony tissue from progenitor cells is key. The proliferation and differentiation of mesenchymal stem cells (MSCs) to become osteogenic cells and form bone is promoted by growth factors.[1] Osteoinduction was first described by Charles Brenton Huggins in 1931, when epithelium of the bladder was transplanted to the abdominal wall in dogs and lead to heterotopic ossification, and osteoinduction was objectified by an increase of phosphatase activity.[2,3] Huggins[4,5] then further studied the effect of chemicals on cell behavior, which interestingly also lead to the discovery that cancerous cells can be affected by hormones for which he received the Nobel Prize in Physiology or Medicine in 1966. Heterotopic ossification was studied in the following years by Marshall R. Urist, an American orthopedic surgeon, who studied bone homeostasis and osteoinduction extensively.[6-9] He found in 1965 that decalcified bone matrix (DBM) implanted in nonskeletal tissue of animals lead to the formation of cartilage and bone on these tissues, which he called autoinduction. It was suggested that surrounding stem cells at the site of DBM implantation differentiated into osteogenic progenitor cells because of contact with the implanted DBM by a signaling pathway.[10]

Friedenstein[11] defined osteoinduction in 1968 as: "Induction of undifferentiated inducible osteoprogenitor cells that are not yet committed to the osteogenic lineage to form osteoprogenitor cells." Later Wilson-Hench[12] defined it in 1987 as a process that induced osteogenesis. This is the currently used definition.

What all these definitions have in common is that osteoinduction is defined as a process where undifferentiated stem cells are activated in a way that these cells will differentiate into osteogenic (progenitor) cells and form ectopic bone tissue. For this process, multiple osteoinductive (growth) factors are necessary for bone homeostasis and fracture healing. An osteoinductive factor is defined by a factor by which osteogenesis is induced, that is, the formation of ectopic bone tissue when expressed. This definition is in line with research of Lacroix conducted as early as in 1945, where it was hypothesized that a substance or group of substances was responsible for the process of osteogenesis. Lacroix suggested that this substance would be called "*Osteogenin*."[13]

Bone morphogenetic proteins (BMPs) are one of the most well-known osteoinductive factors. BMPs are growth factors of the transforming growth factor-beta (TGF-β) group. These glycoproteins were discovered by Urist in 1971 when studying the osteoinductive properties in DBM.[14] In the following years, BMPs were sequenced and cloned further. In 1988, Wozney et al[15] published the first results of the use of BMPs in a clinical setting for tibial nonunion. Today, 20 types of BMPs have been discovered. Two of these are Food and Drug Administration (FDA) approved for use in the clinical setting in fracture and long bone nonunion treatment, BMP-2 and BMP-7, or osteogenic protein-1.[16]

Pathways in Osteogenesis and the Effect of Osteoinductive Factors

The formation of new bone is a process that consists of multiple phases, and several pathways are involved. First, MSCs need to be recruited. These stem cells then need to differentiate into osteoblasts, and last, bone needs to be formed. Osteoinductive factors affect all three of these phases and play a part in multiple different pathways.[3]

The complete pathway of MSC recruitment and homing is not completely known, though several studies have shown activation of certain pathways and enhanced expression of growth factors and cytokines as key players in this process of recruitment and homing (Figure 9.1). Growth factors from the TGF-β superfamily, including BMPs, platelet-derived growth factor (PDGF), insulin-like growth factor (IGF), and vascular endothelial growth factor (VEGF), as well as cytokines, like tumor necrosis factor-alpha, receptor activator of nuclear factor kappa-B ligand (RANKL), osteoprotegerin, stromal cell–derived factor-1 (SDF-1), and multiple interleukins (ILs), are associated with chemotaxis of MSCs.[3,17-20]

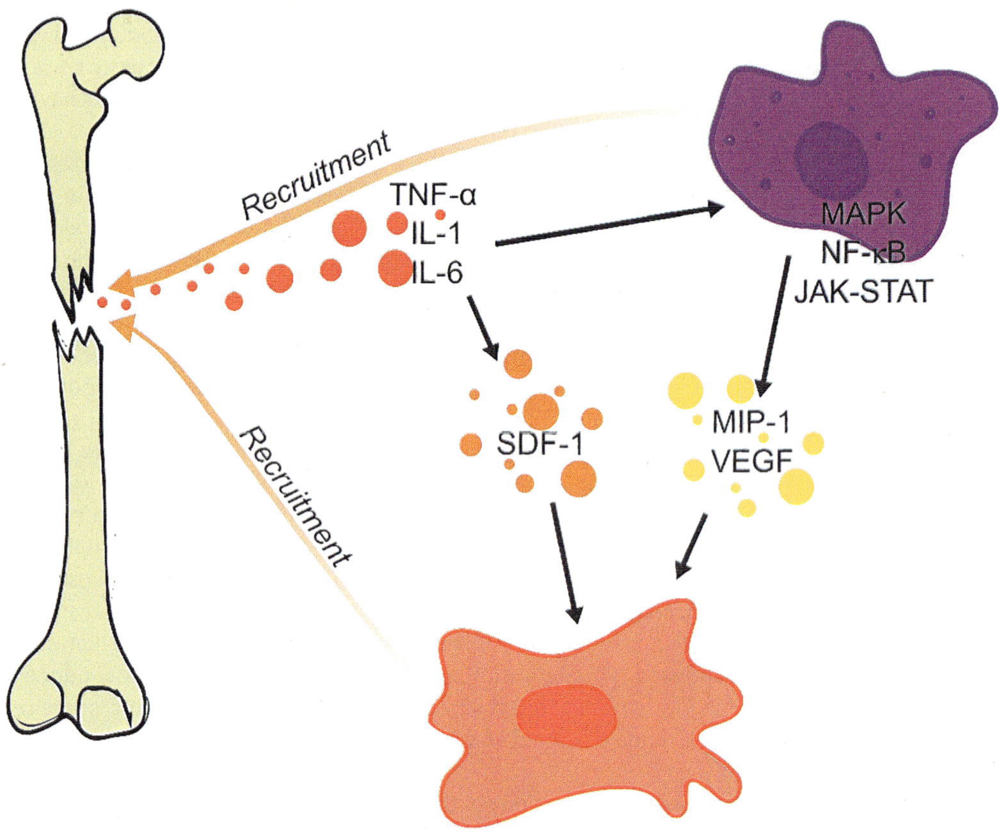

Figure 9.1. Schematic illustration shows a brief overview of mesenchymal stem cell (MSC) recruitment and involved growth factors and cytokines. Purple cell represents a macrophage with its pathways involved in cell recruitment and homing. The red cell represents a MSC. The fracture hematoma leads to the secretion of cytokines, which activates white blood cells directly and MSCs through the upregulation of SDF-1. IL, interleukin; JAK-STAT, Janus kinase-signal transducer and activator of transcription; MAPK, mitogen-activated protein kinase; MIP-1, macrophage inflammatory protein-1; NF-κB, nuclear factor kappa-B; SDF-1, stromal cell–derived factor-1; TNF-α, tumor necrosis factor-alpha; VEGF, vascular endothelial growth factor.

The first step in fracture healing is an inflammatory response. With this response, cytokines like tumor necrosis factor-alpha and IL-1 and -6 are expressed in the fracture hematoma. These cytokines bind with their receptors on macrophages and other white blood cells, instigating chemotaxis of stem cells and osteoprogenitor cells to the fracture site. Three pathways that are most prominent in chemotaxis and homing of MSCs: the mitogen-activated protein kinase (MAPK), nuclear factor kappa-B, and Janus kinase-signal transducer and activator of transcription (STAT) pathway. When these pathways are activated, they lead to attraction and activation of more inflammatory cells.[21] These inflammatory cells then secrete other factors, such as macrophage inflammatory proteins and VEGF, that can bind to MSC receptors. Macrophage inflammatory protein-1 is associated mostly with MSC recruitment.[17,22]

On the surface of MSCs, CXC and CC motif receptors (CXCRs, CCRs) are expressed. These will bind CXC motif ligands (CXCLs), which are essential proteins in MSC recruitment. In the homing process of MSCs, the CXCR-4 receptor is the most prominent receptor for chemoattraction on MSCs. This receptor binds the cytokine SDF-1, also known as CXCL12.[23] Though this chemokine is not specific for the process of osteogenesis, SDF-1 is expressed in tissue damage, causing a local increase when, for instance, a fracture is sustained.[24]

For an MSC to differentiate into osteogenic cells, transcription factors need to be expressed. Some of the key transcription factors are Runt-related transcription factor 2 (Runx2), Osterix (Osx), and activating transcription factor 4.[25-27] The expression of transcription factors for osteogenic differentiation of MSCs is mainly instigated by two pathways, the TGF-β/Sma and Mad-related protein (SMAD) signaling pathway and the Wingless and integration-1 (Wnt) pathway. Osteoinductive factors play a vital role in the activation of these pathways.[28,29]

In 1972, Todaro and Huebner[30] studied RNA tumor viruses, which lead to the hypothesis of oncogenes being a component of these viruses that induced carcinogenesis when expressed. In 1989, Bishop and Varmus received the Nobel Prize in Physiology or Medicine for the discovery in 1976 that a single viral gene, the cytoplasmic tyrosine kinase Src, produced an altered cellular protein that was responsible for malignant degeneration of cells when infected by avian sarcoma virus.[31] This was the start of the research toward the identification of TGF-β later in the beginning of the 1980s. TGFs were discovered at the end of the 70s after research suggested that viruses were able to transform cells by the excretion of growth factors that were similar to epidermal growth factor (EGF). In 1978, de Larco et al[32] found that TGFs were able to promote increased growth of fibroblasts in vitro and decreased growth when TGFs were removed. The fact that the effect of TGFs was reversible suggested that they had an effect early in the signaling pathways. These pathways were later studied to be SMAD signaling pathways in the late 1990s.[31]

BMPs function by activation of the TGF-β/SMAD pathway. BMP binds serine/threonine kinase receptors, type I and type II. These two receptors form a heteromeric complex by phosphorylation upon binding of the BMP, which is then able to phosphorylate downstream signaling molecules. In the BMP signaling pathway, transcription factors like receptor-regulated SMADs or R-SMADs are involved. In osteogenesis, these are SMAD1, 5, and 8. When phosphorylated, the R-SMAD will then bind with a co-SMAD; in osteogenesis, this is most often SMAD4. This newly formed complex then transports to the nucleus and regulates gene expression. The receptors also act in non-SMAD pathways; these are mainly MAPK or phosphoinositide 3-kinase/protein kinase B (PI3K/AKT) pathways.[33-35] Three MAPK pathways with different effects when activated are involved in osteogenesis, JUN N-terminal kinases (JNKs) extracellular signal–related kinases, and p38 MAPKs (p38).[36]

The Wnt signaling pathway was discovered in the late 20th century. Wnt ligands are defined by being cysteine-rich proteins.[37] The first mammalian Wnt gene was discovered by Nusse et al[38] in 1982 and was initially called integration 1 (int1) as a proto-oncogene expressed in mice infected with the mouse mammary tumor virus. This study was conducted after it was found that certain strains of laboratory mice were prone to breast cancer in 1936 and a later study in 1962 that mouse mammary tumor virus, a milk-transmitted virus, was the reason for these tumors.[39-42] Normal expression of this gene was studied in 1987 and was found to be important in the development of the central nervous system and spermatogenesis.[43,44] It was then discovered that a similar gene mutation in a species of fruit flies, *Drosophila*, was already discovered and lead to these flies being wingless. This was discovered by Sharma and Chopra[45] in 1973, calling the mutation wingless or wg. The name Wnt is thus a combination of int1 and the wg mutation.

There are two main Wnt pathways, the canonical and the noncanonical pathways. The canonical pathway is β-catenin dependent, whereas the noncanonical is not. The noncanonical pathways can then be divided into two subgroups, a pathway mediated by planar cell polarity (PCP) and the Wnt/Ca^{2+} pathway.[37,46]

Wnt proteins bind to Frizzled (Fzd) receptors on the cell surface, sometimes in combination with another protein, which acts as co-receptor. In the canonical pathway low-density lipoprotein–related protein 5/6 acts as co-receptor to Fzd. Then the intracellular disheveled protein (DSH) binds the activated receptor complex, which is then able to bind a destruction complex composed of glycogen synthase kinase-3, Axin, casein kinase 1, and adenomatous polyposis coli. This complex, when not bound to DSH, phosphorylates β-catenin. Phosphorylated β-catenin will then be degraded, preventing it from entering the cell nucleus and activating gene transcription. When the destruction complex is bound, β-catenin accumulates, translocates to the nucleus, and activates gene transcription. The first noncanonical pathway, PCP, is activated by a Wnt protein binding the Fzd without lipoprotein-related protein 5/6. PCP is the process in which cells align themselves in the tissue plane and is for instance at play in the alignment of hairs on the wing of a fly.[47] This pathway continues by DSH binding to the receptor complex. This activates PCP core genes, such as Rho and JNK, which is then able to activate transcription in the nucleus. In the Wnt/Ca^{2+} pathway, calcium is released from the endoplasmic reticulum because of an increase in inositol 1,4,5-triphosphate and 1,2-diacylglycerol due to the activation of Fzd receptors. The increase of calcium leads to the activation of protein kinase C, which then activates regulatory protein, such as nuclear factor kappa B.[48]

The role of the Wnt signaling pathway in bone homeostasis was first described in the early 2000s.[25] The canonical Wnt pathway is known to promote osteogenic differentiation of MSCs by the upregulation of factors Runx2, Osx, and alkaline phosphatase (ALP).[49] BMPs have an effect on Wnt signaling.[37]

Other signaling pathways like Hedgehog and MAPK or neural epidermal growth factor-like 1 protein (NELL-1) pathway can also induce differentiation of stem cells; these, however, play a smaller role in the process. Notch is a pathway that inhibits differentiation.[25,49]

Classification of Osteoinductive Factors

Osteoinductive factors stimulate or inhibit pathways that are vital in osteogenic differentiation. BMPs are well-known osteoinductive factors that interact with important pathways, such as the TGF-β/SMAD and Wnt pathway. In addition, other factors have also been identified as osteoinductive. These factors can be classified into five categories, growth factors, cytokines, bioactive peptides, hormones, and small molecules (Figure 9.2). The division of factors into subgroups helps to differentiate the different effects and possible therapeutic properties of these factors. In this chapter, the authors will further discuss the factors that are proven or suggested to have a positive effect on bone growth at the fracture or nonunion site. Systemic osteogenic factors, such as hormones and cytokines affecting bone homeostasis, will be discussed in another chapter.

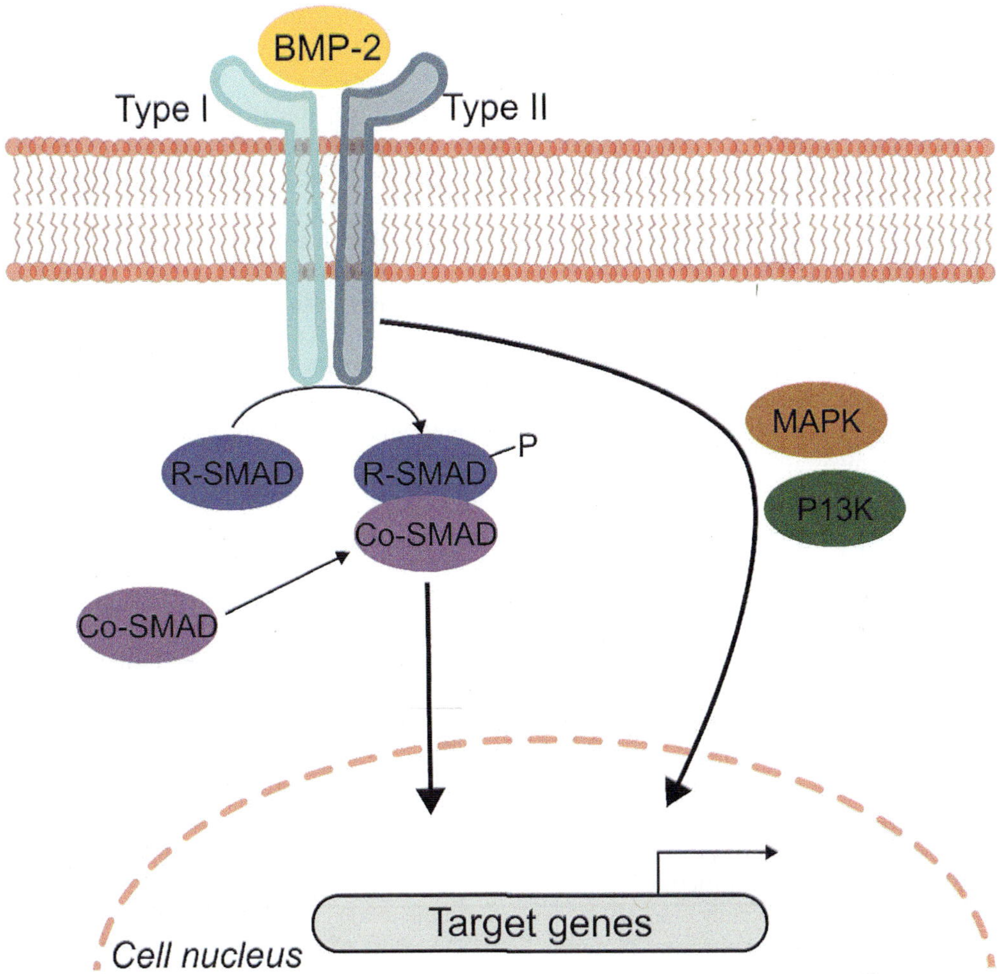

Figure 9.2. Schematic illustration shows the simplified visualization of the transforming growth factor-beta/SMAD and non-SMAD pathway. BMP-2, bone morphogenic protein-2; Co-SMAD, common-mediator Sma and Mad-related protein; MAPK, mitogen-activated protein kinase; R-SMAD, receptor activated Sma and Mad-related protein.

BONE MORPHOLOGIC PROTEINS

Available Bone Morphogenetic Proteins and Function

When Urist discovered BMPs in 1971, the pathways BMPs were involved in were still unknown. Today, 20 types of BMPs are discovered, and various functions are discovered. Additionally, BMPs are not only involved in bone formation but also play crucial roles in other pathways inducing cell growth, differentiation, and apoptosis. Knockout studies have shown that BMPs are key morphogens in embryogenesis. When lacking BMPs, severe developmental defects can occur.[50] The available BMPs in bone homeostasis can be divided in four groups, classified by function and sequence. These are the BMP-2/4 group, BMP-5/6/7/8 group, BMP-9/10 group, and BMP-12/13/14 group. BMPs are produced by the cells involved in osteogenesis. These cells can be activated by other growth factors and cytokines. For instance, studies have shown that an increase in VEGF leads to an increased secretion of BMP-2 and -4.[51]

BMPs consist of three structural parts, which in total include between 400 and 500 amino acid residues. An interesting structure in BMPs is the carboxy-terminal (C-terminal). In most BMPs, the C-terminal contains seven cysteine residues that have disulfide bonds; this is also known as the cysteine knot. This knot makes BMP capable of forming homodimers or heterodimers with other BMPs, enhancing their function.[52,53] As discussed earlier, BMPs function through the TGF-β/SMAD or non-SMAD pathways.[35] The different BMPs bind to different types of type I and type II receptors in the pathways, promoting transcription of different target genes. The BMPs that are most associated with osteogenesis are BMP-2, -4, -6, -7, and -9.[54]

Apart from the bone growth–inducing potential, BMPs have also been linked to the increase of osteoclastic differentiation and bone resorption. This process is seen in BMP-3, but it is also seen in BMP-2.[55] In vitro expression of RANKL was upregulated by BMP-2, which explains the increase of osteoclast activation.[56] The fact that BMP-2 stimulates both bone formation and resorption is interesting, indicating the limited in-depth knowledge about the precise pathways regulating homeostasis between bone formation and resorption.[57]

Clinical Applications of Bone Morphogenetic Proteins

BMPs for clinical use have first been made by the purification of BMPs in demineralized bone extracts.[15] With around 21 ng of BMP-2 in 1 g of DBM, it would take up to approximately 48 kg of DBM to get 1 mg of BMP-2 from DBM.[58] This makes the harvesting of BMPs expensive. To make BMPs more readily available, recombinant bone morphogenetic proteins (rhBMPs) were developed. The first BMPs were cloned in 1988.[15] RhBMPs were on the market and approved by the FDA 12 years later in the early 2000s. They were mostly used in spinal fusion surgery.[59] The use of rhBMPs has increased in fracture and nonunion surgical procedures later. One of the main benefits is that it can replace autografting, reducing additional surgical risks of harvesting autografts. RhBMPs are marketed as medical devices, where the rhBMPs are applied to a collagen-containing carrier matrix.[60]

At this point in time, only one rhBMP device is on the market for clinical application, which is rhBMP-2 INFUSE (Medtronic, Minneapolis, USA). Most of the indications are for spinal surgery. In fracture healing, only two devices were FDA approved. This is BMP-2 and BMP-7 (Osigraft [Olympus Biotech International]/osteogenic protein 1 [Stryker Biotech]). However, BMP-7 is not commercially available anymore. Table 9.1 shows an overview of all available BMPs and other growth factors on the market and their indications in fracture and nonunion treatment.

Side effects of local treatment with rhBMP devices reported are generally mild. Local inflammatory responses and the formation of ectopic bone are reported.[61] This ectopic bone formation has been the cause of some rare but severe complications in spinal surgery, where the localization of the product induced several incapacitating and fatal outcomes. The ectopic bone or swelling can cause nerve root compression, leading to radiating pain or loss of function. In the cervical spine, cases of spine swelling have been reported, that caused six fatalities over the years.[61]

In fracture and nonunion treatment, ectopic bone formation often does not cause problems or require addition surgery.[62] The incidence formation of ectopic bone has been related to the used dosage.[63] As mentioned earlier, BMPs also have an effect on the differentiation of osteoclasts.[57] A primate study showed bone resorption with rhBMP-2 in metaphyseal fractures before bone formation.[64] Toth et al[65] tested the effect of rhBMP on pull out force of screws; their results suggested that less force was needed to loosen a screw in bones treated with rh-BMP, though this was not significant. No cases of loss of fixation because of bone resorption have been reported.

TABLE 9.1 Osteoinductive Factors for Clinical Use, Their Function, Effect, and Indications

Classification	Factor	Brand Name (Company)	Function	Effect (In Vivo/In Vitro)	Approved Indications	Side Effects
Growth factors	Bone morphogenetic protein (BMP)-2	InductOs/INFUSE (Medtronic)	Mesenchymal stem cell (MSC) homing, osteogenic differentiation, proliferation of osteoblasts	Upregulation of osteogenic genes, such as Runx2. Bone resorption	Acute open long bone fractures with intramedullary nailing	Ectopic bone formation Local inflammatory responses Long-term effects unknown
	BMP-6	Osteogrow[a]	Osteogenesis and chondrogenesis	Upregulation of growth factors, insulin-like growth factor and epidermal growth factor Increase in bone volume in mice in combination with bisphosphonates due to activation of Wnt/β-catenin pathway	None	None yet reported in humans
	BMP-7 (osteogenic protein 1 [OP-1])	Osigraft/OP-1 (Stryker Biotech)[b]	Angiogenesis, osteogenesis, and chondrogenesis	Increase of alkaline phosphatase (ALP) and Runx2 expression	Long bone nonunion Posterolateral fusion in spinal surgery	Ectopic bone formation Local inflammatory responses Long-term effects unknown
	Platelet-derived growth factor	Augment (Wright)	MSC homing, differentiation, and angiogenesis	Activation of non-SMAD pathways	Ankle fusion	Local inflammatory responses
Peptides	P-15 (collagen type 1 peptide)	i-FACTOR (Cerapedics)	Cell attachment, osteogenic differentiation, osteointegration	Upregulation of BMP-2 and -7. Increased ALP and Runx2 activity	Long bone defects due to fracture, surgical procedures, and nonunion	Ectopic or excessive bone formation Local inflammatory responses Migration of the graft Allergic reactions

[a]Not yet available commercially; studies regarding efficacy and safety in humans not published.
[b]Not commercially available at present.

Since rhBMPs are a fairly new treatment option, long-term adverse effects are not yet known. An upregulation of BMP-2 has been found in some cancer types, raising the question whether clinical use of rhBMP-2 could induce cancer.[61] A study by Dimar et al[66] found a slight increase in the occurrence of different cancers in patients after the use of rhBMP-2 versus autografting in spinal arthrodesis at a 2-year follow-up point (3.3% vs 0.9%, P = .107). Later a meta-analysis conducted on this matter also suggested a possible increase in malignancies.[67] The rhBMP scaffold used in the study by Dimar et al[66] was rejected by the FDA because of this possible risk. Although these results were not statistically significant, it does show that more research should be conducted. A large study by Kelly et al[68] including almost 500,000 patients did actually showed a lower relative risk in the development of cancer with the use of rhBMP-2 in spinal arthrodesis in a 2- to 3-year follow-up period. Follow-up periods of studies using BMPs are relatively short. Therefore, long-term side effects, such as possible carcinogenicity, cannot be ruled out. For this lack of evidence in late complications, BMPs are discouraged to be used in the pediatric population.[69]

Bone Morphogenetic Protein-2

BMP-2 is the first BMP of the TGF-β superfamily, since BMP-1 is not part of it.[70] BMP-2 functions through the TGF-β/SMAD pathway, where the activation of the receptors upregulates activate SMAD1, 5, and 8. These SMADs then bind Co-SMAD4. This complex is then able to promote transcription of osteogenic genes.[28,29] Apart from SMAD, BMP-2 has also shown to upregulate Wnt5 and receptor tyrosine kinase–like orphan receptor 2 (Ror2), which are important factors in the noncanonical Wnt signaling pathway promoting osteoblastic differentiation.[71] The main function of BMP-2 is the differentiation from stem cells to osteoprogenitor cells and osteoblasts. The osteoblastic differentiation is mediated by Osx, a gene whose transcription is activated by Runx2. Runx2 expression is mediated by the SMAD1 pathway, which BMP-2 instigates.[53] The SMAD pathway also regulated the transcription of other factors needed in osteogenesis, like ALP and type 1 collagen. ALP is a glycoprotein that is present in many tissues, including bone. It has binding site for zinc, magnesium, and calcium and has a role in mineralization of bone tissue.[72] Expression of ALP is often used as a marker to determine osteogenic differentiation in vitro.[73]

A mice study in 2006 showed that the lack of BMP-2 is associated with delays in ossification, spontaneous fractures, and limiting the healing of fractures. What was particularly interesting in this research is that it showed that BMP-2 is important not only in bone homeostasis but also in the initiation of the healing process.[74] The addition of BMP-2 in the treatment of large bone defects or nonunion has also been studied in mice and showed to increase the capacity of bridging these defects.[75]

INFUSE (Medtronic, Minneapolis, USA), or otherwise called InductOs (Medtronic, Heerlen, The Netherlands), is the device made out of an absorbable collagen sponge with rhBMP-2 in it. It is FDA approved for tibial fractures, though the indication is very specific. The indication for use is an acute open tibial fracture (<14 days after trauma), treated with an intramedullary nail.[76,77] Thus, use in nonunion surgery is by definition off-label. If used in nonunion surgery, costs will not be covered by insurance companies, making it an expensive treatment option. The price of this device is around 3,500 dollars per box.[16]

A meta-analysis was published in 2020 including eight studies comparing rhBMPs with autologous bone grafting in long bone nonunion. In this study, they found a difference in healing time in favor of rhBMPs. Other outcome measures, such as complications, reoperations, and functional outcomes, were similar between the groups.[78] All studies were relatively small and heterogenetic, so no definite conclusions on effect size can be drawn. On the other hand, it shows that usage of BMPs in long bone nonunion is generally safe, since no serious adverse reactions are reported.

Bone Morphogenetic Protein-6

BMP-6 increases bone density when systemically administered according to a mouse model study in 2006.[79] This effect possibly occurs because BMP-6 upregulates the genes of insulin-like growth factor 1 (IGF-1) and EGF, as well as it has shown to activate the Wnt/β-catenin pathway as concluded from a study in mice.[80] A carrier device with rhBMP-6, called OSTEOGROW (Osteogrow, Zagreb, Croatia), has been produced and studied in mice. It already has been tested in mice, where it showed increased bone volume in combination with bisphosphonate.[81,82] Some studies on the application of rhBMP-6 in humans have been published.[83,84] This material is currently not available for clinical usage.

Bone Morphogenetic Protein-7

The function of BMP-7 overlaps with that of BMP-2. It plays a role in osteogenesis, upregulating Runx2, Osx, and ALP activity through the SMAD and MAPK pathway.[85] But BMP-7 also promotes chondrogenesis and angiogenesis.[53,86]

In 2001, Friedlaender et al[87] studied the use of rhBMP-7 in 122 tibial nonunion patients. No difference in union rates was found between patients treated with rhBMP-7 in a type I collagen carrier or patients treated with autologous bone grafts. This device of a collagen carrier with rhBMP-7 bound to it (Osigraft, Stryker, Michigan, USA) and was FDA approved in 2001 for long bone nonunion when other treatment options failed. It was also approved in spinal surgery in 2003 for revision posterolateral fusion.[59] Later, Stryker, however, sold the device to Olympus, after which it was withdrawn from the market in 2014.[16,60]

The price of a rhBMP-7 device was, like rhBMP-2, around 3,500 dollars.[16] In 2009, Dahabreh et al[88] published a cost-effectiveness analysis of the use of rhBMP-7 (Osigraft) in tibial nonunion. Here 27 patients were treated with either a bone autograft from the iliac crest or rhBMP-7. All patients reached union after the first surgery. The initial costs of rhBMP-7 were higher than bone autografting. However, the total costs of the treatment leveled out, due to shorter hospital stays and follow-up time.

Bone Morphogenetic Protein-9

BMP-9, also known as growth differentiation factor-2, is not available as recombinant for clinical use. Though evidence suggests that this BMP actually has the highest osteogenic potential compared to other BMPs, showing high expression of ALP.[54,89]

In the TGF-β/SMAD pathway, BMP-9 mainly stimulates type 1 receptors. It also activates the non-SMAD pathway, as BMP-2. What makes BMP-9 an especially potent signaling molecule is the ability of interacting with other pathways, such as the Wnt/catenin pathway, hedgehog signaling and IGF pathways.[53,89,90] It is therefore no surprise that BMP-9 has an effect on many processes. In fracture healing, BMP-9 activates osteogenic differentiation, proliferation, and angiogenesis.

The use of BMP-9 in fracture healing has been studied in rats. This study showed that rh-BMP-9 was capable of inducing fracture healing in critical-size defects.[91,92]

Conclusion on the Use of Bone Morphogenetic Proteins

Since the use of rhBMP-2 is only approved for acute open tibial fractures, most other uses would be off-label. Use of rhBMP in nonunion surgery is to be discouraged at this moment. The arguments against using rhBMPs, like the additional costs of off-label use and the lack of knowledge about long-term (adverse) effects, currently outweigh the possible benefits of not needing additional bone grafting in complicated fractures or nonunion surgery. The value of rhBMP in nonunion surgery, especially when treating a large bone defect nonunion, is not known. In these types of treatments, the need for an osteoinductive and osteoconductive scaffold is apparent. The benefit of the addition of rhBMPs in these highly complex cases might, however, be small.

OTHER GROWTH FACTORS

Platelet-Derived Growth Factor

PDGFs are disulfide-linked dimers that are stored in α-granules of blood platelets. The dimers are formed from four subunits, the A, B, C, and D, either as a homodimer or heterodimer.[93,94] The existence of PDGF was first discovered in the 1970s and in the 1980s as the dimeric structure known today.[95] PDGFs are similar in structure and function to VEGFs. In 2007, it was discovered that these growth factors are able to bind to each other's receptor, enabling them to have similar regulatory effects.[96] PDGF, as well as VEGF, is a factor involved in developmental processes, cell division, and chemoattraction.[95,97] Differences in activity of the growth factor have been linked with diseases, mostly cancer, when activity is enhanced.[94,98]

The general pathway of activation of PDGF in bone regeneration starts directly after sustaining an injury. With the fracture hematoma, platelets are recruited to the injured region. These platelets contain the granules that produce and release PDGF. When released, PDGF works as a chemoattractant for inflammatory cell and MSC.[97]

PDGF signaling also induces SDF-1 expression, and vice versa, which is directly responsible for the attraction and homing of MSCs[99,100] (Figure 9.3). In differentiation of MSCs, PDGF does not directly induces differentiation, but it optimizes the local environment to promote bone regeneration. It does so by increasing vascularity by stimulating VEGF and increasing the function of BMPs by upregulation of BMP receptors.[97,101,102] The clinical use of PDGF is reviewed in Chapter 8, Platelet-Rich Plasma.

Insulin-Like Growth Factor

Two types of IGFs exist, type I and type II. The pathways involved in bone homeostasis include mostly IGF-1. IGF-1 is mostly stored and secreted by the liver, though small amounts of the growth factors are also stored in bone matrix in a bound and inactive form.[103,104] Secretion and upregulation of IGF-1 are managed by the growth hormone/IGF-1 axis. Growth hormone is secreted by the pituitary gland and increases IGF-1 secretion.[105,106] In vitro IGF-1 upregulates Runx2, ALP, and type I collagen, which are all genes inducing osteoblastic differentiation.[107] It does so by activating the same non-SMAD pathways as BMPs, such as P13K/AKT, p38, and JNK.[108] A review about the osteogenic effects of IGF has been published in 2020 by Zhang et al[109] that showed that recombinant insulin-like growth factor (rhIGF) has a positive effect on bone regeneration and density and could be a good addition to surgery in the future.

Local treatment with rhIGF-1 is studied in distraction osteogenesis in sheep, where a scaffold loaded with IGF-1 and TGF-β compared to bone grafting did not show statistically significant differences in bone growth.[110] rhIGF-1 is clinically proven to stimulate cartilage repair.[111] This effect is due to the activation of transcription factors that promote chondrocyte differentiation, like SRY-box transcription factor 9 (Sox9).[106] rhIGF-1 might be an addition to bone regenerative medicine, though at this moment sufficient evidence about efficacy and safety is lacking.

Fibroblast Growth Factor

In bone regeneration, fibroblast growth factor (FGF) has a paracrine function by binding and activating the FGF tyrosine kinase receptor that activates non-SMAD pathways, like MAPK, STAT1, P13K/AKT, and p38.[112,113] It also crosstalks with the Wnt/β-catenin pathway.[114] FGF-2, -9, and -18 have shown to increase osteogenic, chondrogenic, and vascular generation in animal

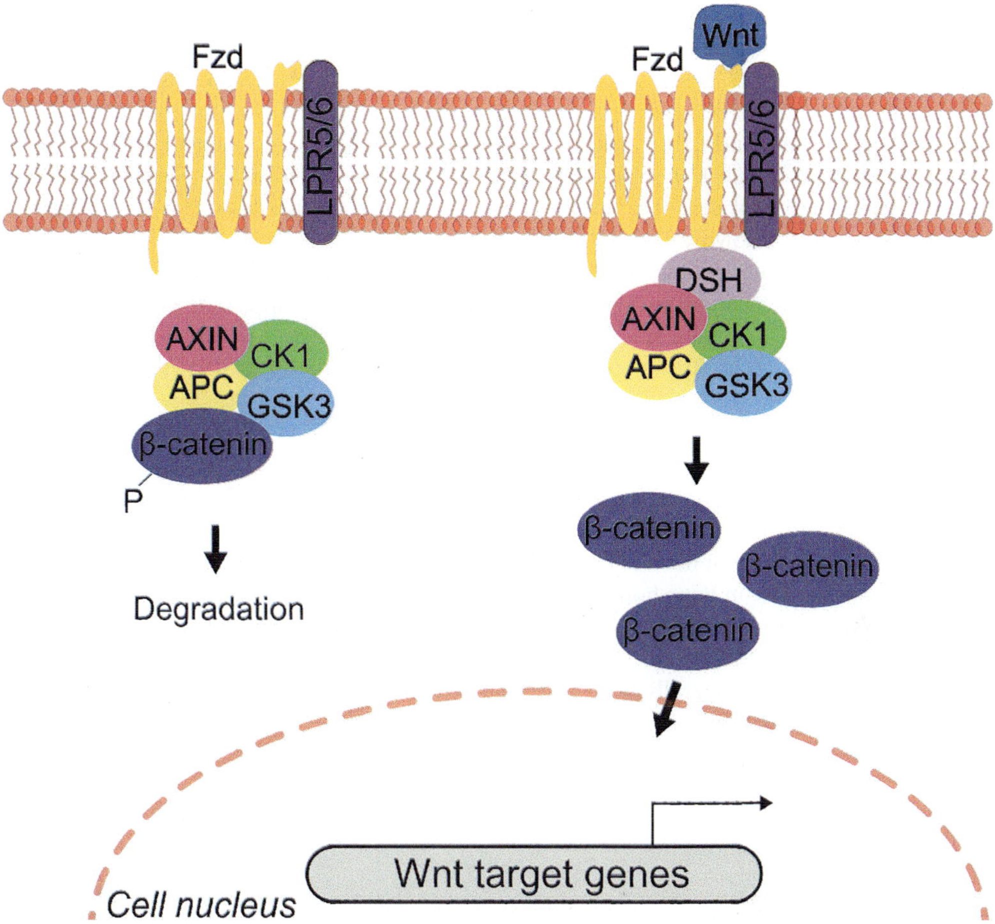

Figure 9.3. Schematic illustration shows canonical pathway Wnt signaling. Wnt binds to the receptor complex. This leads to DSH binding the destruction complex, which prevents β-catenin from being phosphorylated and degraded. The free β-catenin enters the nucleus and promotes gene transcription. APC, adenomatous polyposis coli; CK-1, casein kinase 1; DSH, disheveled protein; Fzd, frizzled receptor; GSK3, glycogen synthase kinase 3; LPR5/6, lipoprotein-related protein 5/6; Wnt, Wingless and integration-1 pathway.

models.[115-120] In rabbits treated for metaphyseal fractures with FGF-2 with gelatin hydrogel or solely gelatin hydrogel showed a significant difference in callus formation favoring FGF-2.[121] In 2010, an randomized controlled trial was performed comparing recombinant FGF (rhFGF)-2 in hydrogel in two different dosages compared to a placebo in tibial shaft fractures. Sixty patients participated in total. They found an increase in union between the FGF-2 group and placebo ($P < .05$); no difference in union was found between the two different dosages of FGF-2. Complications were similar in all groups; no serious adverse reactions were reported.[122] The positive effect of rhFGF-2 and safety have also been studied in periodontal defects and femoral head osteonecrosis.[123,124] For periodontal regeneration, rhFGF is on the market as Regroth (Kaken Pharmaceutical, Tokyo, Japan). It is not indicated for fracture of nonunion surgery as of 2025.

Epidermal Growth Factor

EGF mostly plays a role in increasing vascularity by promoting endothelial cell migration.[125] A rat model by Shen et al[126] showed that EGF-like protein-6 (EGFL6), one of the members of the

EGF superfamily, increased angiogenesis and osteogenic differentiation in distraction osteogenesis of the tibia. An upregulation of the Wnt/β-catenin pathway was observed in this study as possible explanation. More EGF-like factors have been found to have this effect, like EGFL2, 3, and 5 to 9.[127,128] Furthermore, EGF activates the same pathways of MSC differentiation as PDGF and FGF in a paracrine and endocrine manner.[129] Although EGF enhances osteogenic differentiation in the study of Shen et al,[126] a study by Matsuda et al[130] showed that it can also suppress differentiation. This suggests that EGF is an important factor in bone homeostasis. How this process is regulated, is not fully known yet.

Recombinant EGF in combination with core decompression showed increased vascularization in rats with induced femoral head necrosis compared to core decompression alone: rhEGF impregnated scaffolds also showed an increase in the healing of 4 mm rat calvarial defects compared to scaffolds alone.[131,132] The effect of recombinant EGF has not been studied in vivo in humans.

Peptides

Peptides in bone regeneration contain a wide variety of different types of peptides that can be classified into groups regarding function and origin (Figure 9.4). A peptide is a small chain of amino acids, which does not have a 3D structure like proteins. An increasing amount of peptides are known to play a role in bone homeostasis, aiding in cell attachment, and osteogenic differentiation.[133] Peptides are gaining attention, since the costs of producing peptides are generally lower than recombinant growth factors.[134,135]

Peptides are derived generally from three sources, the extracellular matrix (ECM) proteins, growth factors, and naturally occurring peptides.[134,136]

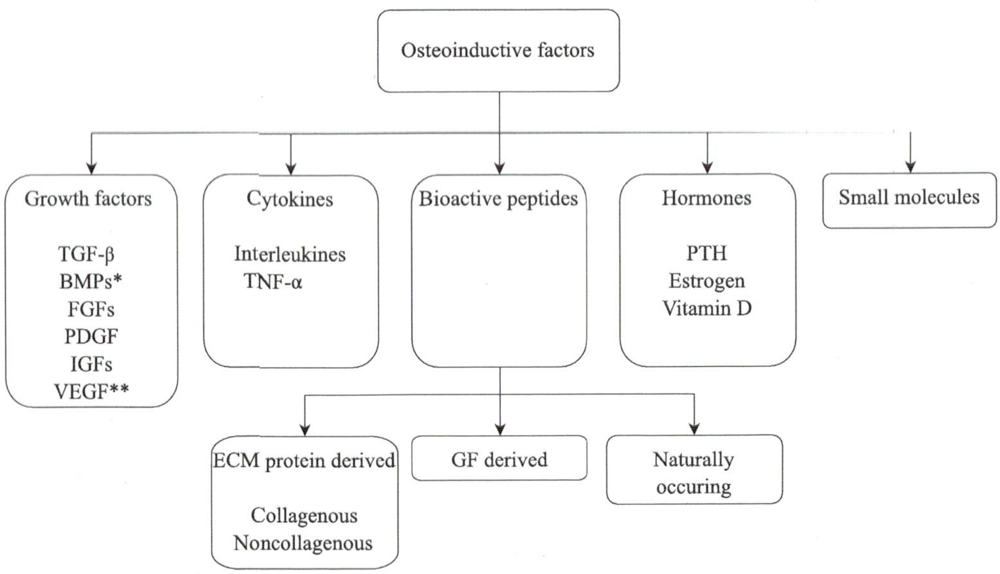

Figure 9.4. Pathway shows the classification of osteoinductive factors. *Although BMPs are part of the TGF-β superfamily, these are shown separately for illustrational purposes. **VEGF is shown because of the indispensable role in osteogenesis, though it does not directly cause mesenchymal stem cell differentiation. BMPs, bone morphogenetic proteins; FGFs, fibroblast growth factors; GF, growth factor; IGFs, insulin-like growth factors; PDGF, platelet-derived growth factor; PTH, parathyroid hormone; TGF-β, transforming growth factor-beta; TNF-α, tumor necrosis factor-alpha; VEGF, vascular endothelial growth factor.

Extracellular Matrix Peptides

Most proteins of the ECM are collagenous, of which more than 90% of ECM proteins are of the structural protein collagen type 1. Only 5% of proteins are not collagenous. Noncollagenous proteins of the ECM are among others fibronectin, vitronectin, osteocalcin, and osteonectin.[134,137,138] The ECM-derived peptides contain small domains of the ECM proteins. Their function in bone regeneration varies between cell attachment, proliferation, and osteogenic differentiation.[137] Though more ECM-derived peptides are known, focus in this section will be on some of the more well-known factors.[138]

The first ECM-derived peptide is called arginine-glycine-aspartic acid peptide (RDG). The main function of RDG is cell attachment. RDG binds the integrin receptor on the cell surface, activating focal adhesion kinase.[139] This promotes cell to cell communication and adhesion.[140] Some studies with scaffolds containing RDG showed good results regarding osteogenic and chondrogenic differentiation.[139,141] There are eight different integrin receptors that RDG is able to bind to. The activation of integrin has been linked not only to osteo- and chondrogenic differentiation but also to the degradation of cartilage. Because the precise effect of RDG is not fully known yet, it is not available for clinical use.[140,142]

One of the collagen type 1–derived peptides contains 15 amino acids and is called P-15 for that matter. It has been shown to be a potent factor in cell attachment and osteogenic differentiation of MSCs.[143,144] An in vitro study found an increase in ALP activity and BMP-2 and -7 gene expression, suggesting osteoblastic differentiation, of human osteosarcoma cells after the addition of hydrogels enhanced with P-15.[145] The P-15 is effective and available as bone grafting material in fracture and nonunion surgery.[133,146,147] It is also added to other scaffolds to promote osteointegration.[148] The P-15 biomaterial is available on the market as i-FACTOR (Cerapedics, Westminster, CO, USA). It was first indicated for spinal fusion after cervical discectomies.[149,150] In trauma surgery and orthopedics, i-FACTOR is indicated for the repair of bone defects, due to surgery, trauma, or nonunion.[151] Possible complications of the use of P-15 can be ectopic ossification, leakage of P-15, and local inflammatory responses. An increase of neuropraxia has been reported of the use of i-FACTOR in periacetabular osteotomy.[152]

Other ECM protein–derived peptides are fibronectin-mimetic protein–derived peptides, Gly-Phe-Hyp-Gly-Glu-Arg (GFOGER), and Asp-Gly-Glu-Ala (DGEA). These all show some osteogenic potential, though substantial in vivo evidence is lacking.[138]

Growth Factor–Derived Peptides

Peptides derived from growth factors retain similar functions of the original proteins.[138] BMP-2, -7, and -9–derived proteins promote osteogenesis.[136,153] Other growth factor–derived peptides, like FGF and VEGF, and also peptides derived from parathyroid hormone are involved in bone homeostasis.[154-156] Parathyroid hormone–derived peptide is FDA approved as a systemic drug in osteoporosis.[157] Growth factor–derived peptides are not available as local treatment options for fracture or nonunion treatment.

Naturally Occurring Peptides

Some of the naturally occurring peptides worth mentioning because of their osteogenic potential are osteogenic growth peptide (OGP), substance P (SP), and endothelin-1 (ET-1). Multiple reviews are published about these peptides for further reading.[133,134,137,138]

OGP was found in 1992 to enhance bone mass when it was first isolated from bone marrow.[158] It enhances the MAPK pathway and increases ALP activity.[159] In rodents, OGP increased fracture healing in three studies.[160-162] No clinical data of OGP are available.

SP is a peptide that is secreted by nerve cells and white blood cells. It has many roles in the body, among which is chemoattraction and angiogenesis.[163] It also stimulates osteogenesis.[164]

In addition, SP helps in the regulation of bone remodeling, although the pathway in which it regulates formation and degradation of bone tissue is not entirely clear yet.[165]

ET-1 was first described in 1988 as a vasoconstrictive peptide.[166] In 1997, Kasperk et al[167] found that osteoblastic cells that were stimulated with ET-1 had an increased cell proliferation. There was also an increase in ALP and type 1 collagen. Now it is known that this effect is due to an activation of the non-SMAD pathways.[168]

Small Molecules

Another emerging alternative for recombinant growth factors is small molecule drugs. They are similar in size to peptides. The growing interest in small molecules in bone regeneration is due to the fact that these are fairly easy and cheaper to manufacture than recombinant growth factors. Some small molecules are already widely available for other medical indications, for instance statins.[135,169,170] These molecules can be either naturally occurring or synthetic.[171] At this point in time, there are no small molecules on the market for bone regeneration, though some preclinical animal tests have been performed.[169] Among other statins, vitamins A, C, and D; bisphosphonates; dexamethasone; antibiotics; and immunomodulating drugs have shown in vivo to increase ALP activity.[135] Statins were found in 1999 to increase the expression of BMP-2.[172] In vitro and in vivo enhanced osteogenic differentiation of cells was seen upon stimulation with statins.[172,173] Scaffolds with statins infused are of growing interest and show good results regarding osteointegration in vitro and in vivo in animals.[174-176] Human randomized controlled trials with scaffolds loaded with simvastatin have only been performed in dental surgery, where patients treated with scaffolds with simvastatin showed a higher bone volume compared to placebo treatment after molar extraction. No differences in postoperative complaints or complications were reported.[177-179]

Vitamin D is used as an oral drug in fracture prevention in osteoporotic patients, as well as bisphosphonates.[180,181] Local treatment with vitamin D in nanoparticles or scaffolds showed an increase in ALP activity in vitro.[182,183] Bisphosphonates increase osteoprotegerin, which reduces RANKL expression. RANKL is an important stimulator of osteoclastogenesis. Through this axis, bisphosphonates can reduce bone resorption.[170] When applied locally, bisphosphonates in vitro and in vivo in animal models showed an increased osteogenic response.[184,185]

The main drawback for the use of small molecules in bone regenerative medicine is the lack of specificity of the molecules. The molecules mentioned have shown to increase ALP activity, though they also have other effects. Doxycycline, for instance, is cytotoxic depending on the dosage,[186] which also counts for statins and bisphosphonates.[173,187] Before clinical implementation of small molecules in fracture and nonunion surgery, the effects and (dose dependent) side effects should be fully understood.

CASES OF OSTEOINDUCTIVE FACTORS

RhBMP-2 in a Distal Open Tibia Fracture

The Injury

A 40-year-old patient sustained a Gustilo type 3B open distal crus fracture of the left leg after a traffic accident. The fracture was highly commuted. A computed tomography angiography showed no signs of arterial compromise.

Surgical Procedures

Acutely, an extensive débridement of the wound was performed and an external fixator was placed over the fracture. The following day, a second-look procedure and the first stage of a Masquelet procedure (MP) was performed. The external fixator was removed, and the fracture was stabilized with locking compression plates over the fibula and medial side of the tibia. Bone fragments were removed and the defect, measuring up to 11 cm, was filled with cement. The skin was closed by the plastic surgeon with a free tissue transfer using an anterior lateral thigh flap. Exactly 2 months later, the second-stage MP was performed. The cement was removed, and the void within the induced membrane was filled with bone marrow aspirate concentrate (BMAC) from the iliac crest, cancellous bone harvested from the femur using a reamer-irrigator-aspirator (RIA) combined with β-tricalcium phosphate (CERASORB, Curasan, Wake Forest, USA), and a rhBMP-2 matrix sheet (InductOs, Medtronic, UK). There was remaining malalignment of the lower leg axis after the first-stage MP; the tibia was refixed during this procedure, and an additional locking compression plate was placed on the anterolateral side of the tibia using minimally invasive plate osteosynthesis. A Z-plasty was performed on the Achilles tendon because of an equinus deformity.

Recovery

The patient made a near full recovery 1 year after the incident. The patient returned to sport (cycling) and is fully weight bearing without aid. There is a persistent slight decrease in dorsiflexion of the foot. However, this causes no problems in daily activities or sports. Control radiographs demonstrated fully incorporated grafting material into the surrounding bone, with ossification of the defect at 1-year follow-up

Learning Points

This case is a good example of the usage of the pentagon model of fracture healing. In this model, the mechanical stability, osteogenic cells, an osteoconductive scaffold, vascularity, and importantly growth factors are key in fracture healing. The mechanical stability was reached by plate fixation, osteogenic cells came from the RIA and BMAC procedure, the scaffold from the autografts, and the collagen matrix of InductOs. InductOs provided growth factors. The vascularized anterior lateral thigh flap and induced membrane provided vascularity.

This case using plate screw fixation of an acute crural fracture describes an off-label use of rhBMP-2, since the FDA approved this device only in combination with intramedullary nail fixation of the fracture. The rhBMP in this case might have been beneficial for the ossification, with very good results of bone regeneration in the defect at 1 year as shown in the radiographs in Figure 9.5. In addition, RIA and BMAC were also used to fill up the defect, which also provides osteogenic cells and growth factors. See Chapter 7 for a more extensive report on this matter.[188]

P-15 in a Nonunion After Crush Fracture of the Femur

The Injury

A 39-year-old male sustained a Gustilo type 3 open crush fracture and patella fracture of the right leg after a bicycle accident. The fractures were originally treated with plate and screw fixation. The soft tissues adequately healed without signs of infection. The patient was otherwise healthy, had an active lifestyle, and did not smoke. One year later, the patient presented himself with persistent pain and the inability to play sports. Radiographs showed limited bone growth. A positron emission tomography-computed tomography scan did not show obvious signs of infection.

Surgical Procedures

A salvage procedure in one stage was performed (Figure 9.6). The nonunion was débrided, and the defect was filled with BMAC, bioactive glass (BonAlive, Bonalive Biomaterials Ltd.), and P-15 (i-FACTOR, Cerapedics). The screws in the patella were also removed. The patient received

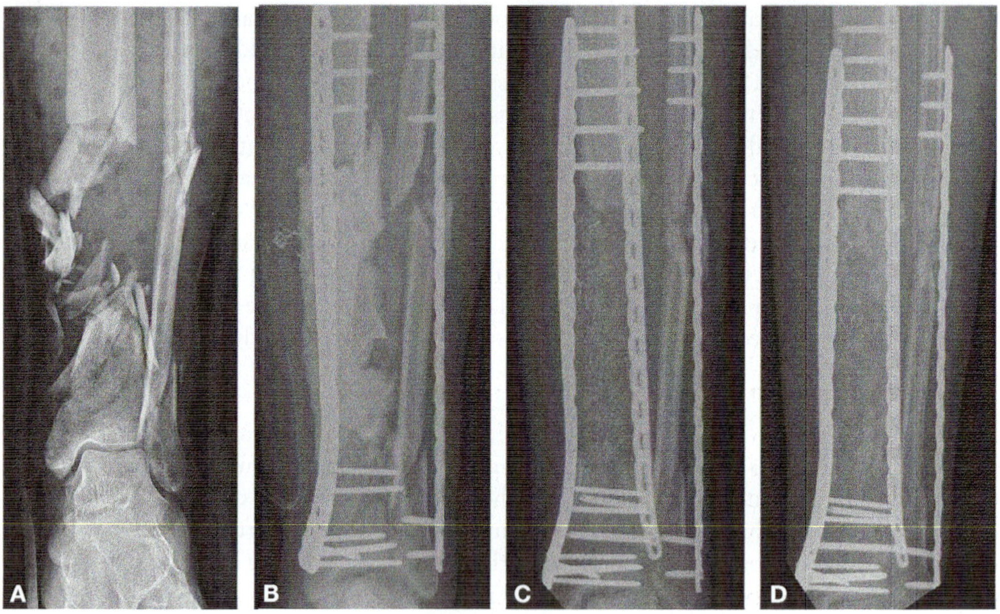

Figure 9.5. Radiographs of the left tibia at different stages in the treatment process. **A.** Radiograph in the emergency department with temporary cast splint. **B.** After the first stage Masquelet procedure (MP). **C.** Directly after the second-stage MP procedure. Grafting material is visible, in addition to revision of the plate fixation. **D.** One year after the last surgery. The grafting material is fully incorporated into the surrounding bone, and there is ossification of the defect. (Courtesy of Prof. Martijn Poeze. Department of surgery, Maastricht Universitair Medisch Centrum, The Netherlands.)

amoxicillin/clavulanic acid postoperatively until the cultures obtained during the surgery did not show any bacterial growth. A month later, the patient had a collection of fluid on the lateral side of the upper leg due to irritation and migration of the bioactive glass; this was surgically drained. Cultures of this fluid did not show infection.

Recovery

Two months after the salvage procedure, radiographs showed callus formation at the fracture site. Clinically, a hydrops of the right knee and a small dehiscence of half a centimeter of the distal part of the wound were present. Slowly the patient regained full function of his leg, and he returned to cycling 3 months after the salvage procedure. Radiographs at this point showed complete consolidation of the fracture site.

Learning Points

In this particular case, a one-stage revision procedure was performed instead of the usual two-stage MP. This approach was chosen because there were no signs of infection in the patient's history or on positron emission tomography-computed tomography. Bioactive glass was added to fill the defect in case of a potential low-grade infection. The migration of bioactive glass caused a local inflammatory reaction and fluid leakage; this complication of the product has been reported in other cases and is mentioned in the prescription.[189,190] To further fill the defect, BMAC and P-15 were added. Remarkably, full consolidation of the nonunion was reached in only 3 months. This again is a good example of a multifactorial approach of treating a nonunion, by adding an osteoinductive factor.[188,191]

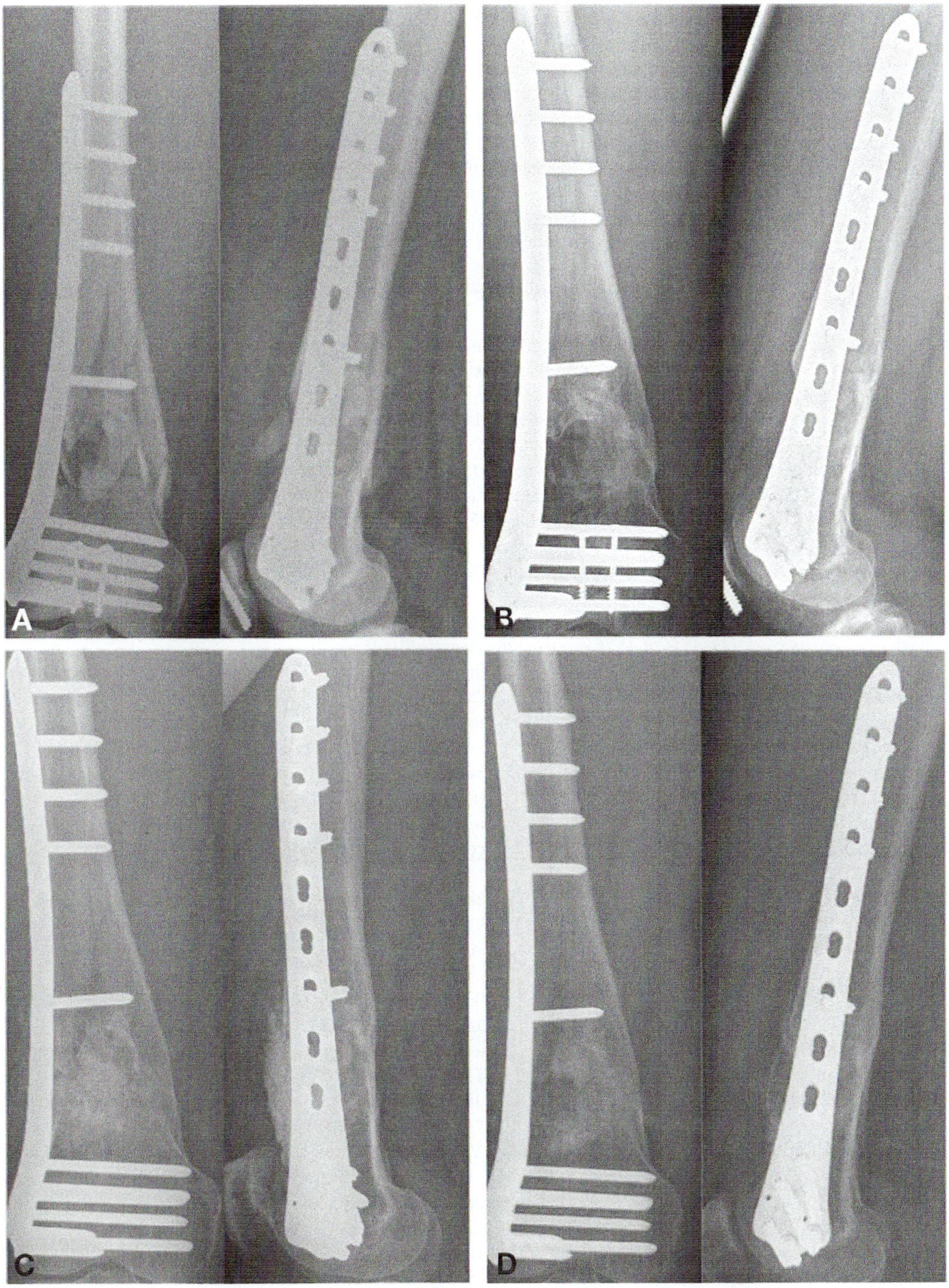

Figure 9.6. Radiographs of the right femur at different stages in the treatment process. **A.** One day after the initial plate fixation. **B.** One year postoperatively after the initial plate fixation. On the lateral side, there is some bone growth, but the majority of the fracture is still present. **C.** One day after the salvage procedure, granules of the bioactive glass are clearly visible. **D.** Three months after the salvage procedure. Consolidation of the fracture has occurred. (Courtesy of Dr. Taco Blokhuis. Department of surgery, Maastricht Universitair Medisch Centrum, The Netherlands.)

References

1. Albrektsson T, Johansson C. Osteoinduction, osteoconduction and osseointegration. *Eur Spine J*. 2001;10(Suppl 2): S96-S101. doi:10.1007/s005860100282
2. Huggins CB. The phosphatase activity of transplants of the epithelium of the urinary bladder to the abdominal wall producing heterotopic ossification. *Biochem J*. 1931;25(3):728-732. doi:10.1042/bj0250728
3. Miron RJ, Zhang YF. Osteoinduction: a review of old concepts with new standards. *J Dent Res*. 2012;91(8):736-744. doi:10.1177/0022034511435260
4. Huggins CB. *Facts*. 2022. Accessed June 13, 2022. https://www.nobelprize.org/prizes/medicine/1966/huggins/facts/
5. Huggins C. Endocrine-induced regression of cancers. *Science*. 1967;156(3778):1050-1054. doi:10.1126/science.156.3778.1050
6. Moss ML. Extraction of an osteogenic inductor factor from bone. *Science*. 1958;127(3301):755-756. doi:10.1126/science.127.3301.755
7. Levander G. On the formation of new bone in bone transplantation. *Acta Chir Scand*. 1934;74:425-426.
8. Bertelsen A. Experimental investigations into post-foetal osteogenesis. *Acta Orthop Scand*. 1944;15(2-4):139-181. doi:10.3109/17453674408991069
9. Grgurevic L, Pecina M, Vukicevic S, Marshall R. Urist and the discovery of bone morphogenetic proteins. *Int Orthop*. 2017;41(5):1065-1069. doi:10.1007/s00264-017-3402-9
10. Urist MR. Bone: formation by autoinduction. *Science*. 1965;150(3698):893-899. doi:10.1126/science.150.3698.893
11. Friedenstein AY. Induction of bone tissue by transitional epithelium. *Clin Orthop Relat Res*. 1968;59:21-37.
12. Wilson-Hench J. Osteoinduction. *Prog Biomed Eng*. 1987;4:29.
13. Lacroix P. Recent investigations on the growth of bone. *Nature*. 1945;156(3967):576-576. doi:10.1038/156576a0
14. Urist MR, Strates BS. Bone morphogenetic protein. *J Dent Res*. 1971;50(6):1392-1406. doi:10.1177/00220345710500060601
15. Wozney John M, Rosen V, Celeste Anthony J, et al. Novel regulators of bone formation: molecular clones and activities. *Science*. 1988;242(4885):1528-1534. doi:10.1126/science.3201241
16. Gillman CE, Jayasuriya AC. FDA-approved bone grafts and bone graft substitute devices in bone regeneration. *Mater Sci Eng C*. 2021;130:112466. doi:10.1016/j.msec.2021.112466
17. Maeda A. Recruitment of mesenchymal stem cells to damaged sites by plant-derived components. *Front Cell Develop Biol*. 2020;8. doi:10.3389/fcell.2020.00437
18. Meirelles Lda S, Fontes AM, Covas DT, et al. Mechanisms involved in the therapeutic properties of mesenchymal stem cells. *Cytokine Growth Factor Rev*. 2009;20(5-6):419-427. doi:10.1016/j.cytogfr.2009.10.002
19. Ponte AL, Marais E, Gallay N, et al. The in vitro migration capacity of human bone marrow mesenchymal stem cells: comparison of chemokine and growth factor chemotactic activities. *Stem Cells*. 2007;25(7):1737-1745. doi:10.1634/stemcells.2007-0054
20. Marquez-Curtis LA, Janowska-Wieczorek A. Enhancing the migration ability of mesenchymal stromal cells by targeting the SDF-1/CXCR4 axis. *Biomed Res Int*. 2013;2013:561098. doi:10.1155/2013/561098
21. Chen L, Deng H, Cui H, et al. Inflammatory responses and inflammation-associated diseases in organs. *Oncotarget*. 2017;9(6):7204-7218. doi:10.18632/oncotarget.23208
22. Bhavsar I, Miller CS, Al-Sabbagh M. Macrophage inflammatory protein-1 alpha (MIP-1 alpha)/CCL3: as a biomarker. *Gen Methods Biomarker Res Applications*. 2015;223-249. doi:10.1007/978-94-007-7696-8_27
23. Han Y, Yang J, Fang J, et al. The secretion profile of mesenchymal stem cells and potential applications in treating human diseases. *Signal Transduct Target Ther*. 2022;7(1):92. doi:10.1038/s41392-022-00932-0
24. Lau TT, Wang D-A. Stromal cell-derived factor-1 (SDF-1): homing factor for engineered regenerative medicine. *Expert Opin Biol Ther*. 2011;11(2):189-197. doi:10.1517/14712598.2011.546338
25. James AW. Review of signaling pathways governing MSC osteogenic and adipogenic differentiation. *Scientifica*. 2013;2013:684736. doi:10.1155/2013/684736
26. Cao H, Yu S, Yao Z, et al. Activating transcription factor 4 regulates osteoclast differentiation in mice. *J Clin Invest*. 2010;120(8):2755-2766. doi:10.1172/jci42106
27. Zhu K, Jiao H, Li S, et al. ATF4 promotes bone angiogenesis by increasing VEGF expression and release in the bone environment. *J Bone Miner Res*. 2013;28(9):1870-1884. doi:10.1002/jbmr.1958
28. Yuan Z, Li Q, Luo S, et al. PPARγ and Wnt signaling in adipogenic and osteogenic differentiation of mesenchymal stem cells. *Curr Stem Cell Res Ther*. 2016;11(3):216-225. doi:10.2174/1574888x10666150519093429
29. Li S-N, Wu J-F. TGF-β/SMAD signaling regulation of mesenchymal stem cells in adipocyte commitment. *Stem Cell Res Ther*. 2020;11(1):41. doi:10.1186/s13287-020-1552-y
30. Todaro GJ, Huebner RJ. N.A.S. symposium: new evidence as the basis for increased efforts in cancer research. *Proc Natl Acad Sci USA*. 1972;69(4):1009-1015. doi:10.1073/pnas.69.4.1009
31. Moses HL, Roberts AB, Derynck R. The discovery and early days of TGF-β: a historical perspective. *Cold Spring Harb Perspect Biol*. 2016;8(7):a021865. doi:10.1101/cshperspect.a021865
32. de Larco JE, Todaro GJ. Growth factors from murine sarcoma virus-transformed cells. *Proc Natl Acad Sci USA*. 1978;75(8):4001-4005. doi:10.1073/pnas.75.8.4001

33. Wrana JL, Attisano L. The Smad pathway. *Cytokine Growth Factor Rev.* 2000;11(1):5-13. doi:10.1016/S1359-6101(99)00024-6
34. Chen D, Zhao M, Mundy GR. Bone morphogenetic proteins. *Growth Factors.* 2004;22(4):233-241. doi:10.1080/08977190412331279890
35. Miyazono K, Kamiya Y, Morikawa M. Bone morphogenetic protein receptors and signal transduction. *J Biochem.* 2010;147(1):35-51. doi:10.1093/jb/mvp148
36. Derynck R, Zhang YE. Smad-dependent and Smad-independent pathways in TGF-β family signalling. *Nature.* 2003;425(6958):577-584. doi:10.1038/nature02006
37. Houschyar KS, Tapking C, Borrelli MR, et al. Wnt pathway in bone repair and regeneration—what do we know so far. *Front Cell Develop Biol.* 2019;6:00170. doi:10.3389/fcell.2018.00170
38. Nusse R, Varmus HE. Many tumors induced by the mouse mammary tumor virus contain a provirus integrated in the same region of the host genome. *Cell.* 1982;31(1):99-109. doi:10.1016/0092-8674(82)90409-3
39. Nusse R, Varmus H. Three decades of Wnts: a personal perspective on how a scientific field developed. *EMBO J.* 2012;31(12):2670-2684. doi:10.1038/emboj.2012.146
40. Korteweg R. On the manner in which the disposition to carcinoma of the mammary gland is inherited in mice. *Genetica.* 1936;18(3):350-371.
41. Lyons MJ, Moore DH. Purification of the mouse mammary tumour virus. *Nature.* 1962;194:1141-1142. doi:10.1038/1941141a0
42. Bittner JJ. Some possible effects of nursing on the mammary gland tumor incidence in mice. *Science.* 1936;84(2172):162. doi:10.1126/science.84.2172.162
43. Thomas KR, Capecchi MR. Targeted disruption of the murine int-1 proto-oncogene resulting in severe abnormalities in midbrain and cerebellar development. *Nature.* 1990;346(6287):847-850. doi:10.1038/346847a0
44. Jakobovits A, Shackleford GM, Varmus HE, et al. Two proto-oncogenes implicated in mammary carcinogenesis, int-1 and int-2, are independently regulated during mouse development. *Proc Natl Acad Sci.* 1986;83(20):7806-7810. doi:10.1073/pnas.83.20.7806
45. Sharma RP, Chopra VL. Effect of the wingless (wg1) mutation on wing and haltere development in Drosophila melanogaster. *Dev Biol.* 1976;48(2):461-465. doi:10.1016/0012-1606(76)90108-1
46. Komiya Y, Habas R. Wnt signal transduction pathways. *Organogenesis.* 2008;4(2):68-75. doi:10.4161/org.4.2.5851
47. van Amerongen R. Alternative Wnt pathways and receptors. *Cold Spring Harb Perspect Biol.* 2012;4(10):a007914. doi:10.1101/cshperspect.a007914
48. De A. Wnt/Ca2+ signaling pathway: a brief overview. *Acta Biochim Biophys Sin Shanghai.* 2011;43(10):745-756. doi:10.1093/abbs/gmr079
49. Yang K, Wang X, Zhang H, et al. The evolving roles of canonical WNT signaling in stem cells and tumorigenesis: implications in targeted cancer therapies. *Lab Investig.* 2016;96(2):116-136. doi:10.1038/labinvest.2015.144
50. Wang RN, Green J, Wang Z, et al. Bone morphogenetic protein (BMP) signaling in development and human diseases. *Genes Dis.* 2014;1(1):87-105. doi:10.1016/j.gendis.2014.07.005
51. Li B, Wang H, Qiu G, et al. Synergistic effects of vascular endothelial growth factor on bone morphogenetic proteins induced bone formation in vivo: influencing factors and future research directions. *Biomed Res Int.* 2016;2016:2869572. doi:10.1155/2016/2869572
52. Carreira AC, Alves GG, Zambuzzi WF, et al. Bone morphogenetic proteins: structure, biological function and therapeutic applications. *Arch Biochem Biophys.* 2014;561:64-73. doi:10.1016/j.abb.2014.07.011
53. Yang J, Shi P, Tu M, et al. Bone morphogenetic proteins: relationship between molecular structure and their osteogenic activity. *Food Sci Human Wellness.* 2014;3(3):127-135. doi:10.1016/j.fshw.2014.12.002
54. Cheng H, Jiang W, Phillips FM, et al. Osteogenic activity of the fourteen types of human bone morphogenetic proteins (BMPs). *J Bone Joint Surg Am.* 2003;85(8):1544-1552. doi:10.2106/00004623-200308000-00017
55. Jing Z, Liang Z, Yang L, et al. Bone formation and bone repair: the roles and crosstalk of osteoinductive signaling pathways. *Process Biochem.* 2022;118:252-262. doi:10.1016/j.procbio.2022.04.033
56. Kim RY, Oh JH, Lee BS, Seo YK, Hwang SJ, Kim IS. The effect of dose on rhBMP-2 signaling, delivered via collagen sponge, on osteoclast activation and in vivo bone resorption. *Biomaterials.* 2014;35(6):1869-1881. doi:10.1016/j.biomaterials.2013.11.029
57. Lademann F, Hofbauer LC, Rauner M. The bone morphogenetic protein pathway: the osteoclastic perspective. *Front Cell Dev Biol.* 2020;8: doi:10.3389/fcell.2020.586031
58. Pietrzak WS, Woodell-May J, McDonald N. Assay of bone morphogenetic protein-2, -4, and -7 in human demineralized bone matrix. *J Craniofac Surg.* 2006;17(1):84-90.
59. Cahill KS, Chi JH, Groff MW, McGuire K, Afendulis CC, Claus EB. Outcomes for single-level lumbar fusion: the role of bone morphogenetic protein. *Spine (Phila Pa 1976).* 2011;36(26):2354-2362. doi:10.1097/BRS.0b013e31820bc9e5
60. Marx JG, Lorio MP. Class III spine grafts. *Clinical Implementation of Bone Regeneration and Maintenance.* IntechOpen; 2019.
61. James AW, LaChaud G, Shen J, et al. A review of the clinical side effects of bone morphogenetic protein-2. *Tissue Eng Part B Rev.* 2016;22(4):284-297. doi:10.1089/ten.TEB.2015.0357

62. Garrison KR, Shemilt I, Donell S, et al. Bone morphogenetic protein (BMP) for fracture healing in adults. *Cochrane Database Syst Rev*. 2010;2010(6):CD006950. doi:10.1002/14651858.CD006950.pub2
63. Krishnan L, Priddy LB, Esancy C, et al. Delivery vehicle effects on bone regeneration and heterotopic ossification induced by high dose BMP-2. *Acta Biomater*. 2017;49:101-112. doi:10.1016/j.actbio.2016.12.012
64. Seeherman HJ, Li XJ, Bouxsein ML, Wozney JM. rhBMP-2 induces transient bone resorption followed by bone formation in a nonhuman primate core-defect model. *JBJS*. 2010;92(2).
65. Toth JM, Wang M, Patel CK, Arora A. Early term effects of rhBMP-2 on pedicle screw fixation in a sheep model: histomorphometric and biomechanical analyses. *J Spine Surg*. 2018;4(3):534-545. doi:10.21037/jss.2018.06.19
66. Dimar JRI, Glassman SD, Burkus JK, Pryor PW, Hardacker JW, Carreon LY. Clinical and radiographic analysis of an optimized rhBMP-2 formulation as an autograft replacement in posterolateral lumbar spine arthrodesis. *JBJS*. 2009;91(6):1377-1386. doi:10.2106/jbjs.H.00200
67. Carragee EJ, Chu G, Rohatgi R, et al. Cancer risk after use of recombinant bone morphogenetic protein-2 for spinal arthrodesis. *J Bone Joint Surg Am*. 2013;95(17):1537-1545. doi:10.2106/jbjs.L.01483
68. Kelly MP, Savage JW, Bentzen SM, Hsu WK, Ellison SA, Anderson PA. Cancer risk from bone morphogenetic protein exposure in spinal arthrodesis. *J Bone Joint Surg Am*. 2014;96(17):1417-1422. doi:10.2106/jbjs.M.01190
69. Rocque BG, Kelly MP, Miller JH, Li Y, Anderson PA. Bone morphogenetic protein-associated complications in pediatric spinal fusion in the early postoperative period: an analysis of 4658 patients and review of the literature. *J Neurosurg Pediatr*. 2014;14(6):635-643. doi:10.3171/2014.8.Peds13665
70. Kessler E, Takahara K, Biniaminov L, Brusel M, Greenspan DS. Bone morphogenetic protein-1: the type I procollagen C-proteinase. *Science*. 1996;271(5247):360-362. doi:10.1126/science.271.5247.360
71. Nemoto E, Ebe Y, Kanaya S, et al. Wnt5a signaling is a substantial constituent in bone morphogenetic protein-2-mediated osteoblastogenesis. *Biochem Biophys Res Commun*. 2012;422(4):627-632. doi:10.1016/j.bbrc.2012.05.039
72. Sharma U, Pal D, Prasad R. Alkaline phosphatase: an overview. *Indian J Clin Biochem*. 2014;29(3):269-278. doi:10.1007/s12291-013-0408-y
73. Trivedi S, Srivastava K, Gupta A, et al. A quantitative method to determine osteogenic differentiation aptness of scaffold. *J Oral Biol Craniofac Res*. 2020;10(2):158-160. doi:10.1016/j.jobcr.2020.04.006
74. Tsuji K, Bandyopadhyay A, Harfe BD, et al. BMP2 activity, although dispensable for bone formation, is required for the initiation of fracture healing. *Nat Genet*. 2006;38(12):1424-1429. doi:10.1038/ng1916
75. Koolen M, Longoni A, van der Stok J, der Jagt OV, Gawlitta D, Weinans H. Complete regeneration of large bone defects in rats with commercially available fibrin loaded with BMP-2. *Eur Cell Mater*. 2019;38:94-105. doi:10.22203/eCM.v038a08
76. Medtronic. *Healthcare Professionals. Infuse Bone Graft. Bone Grafting (Spine and Orthopaedic)*. Accessed June 30, 2022. https://www.medtronic.com/us-en/healthcare-professionals/products/spinal-orthopaedic/bone-grafting/infuse-bone-graft.html
77. Medtronic. Indications, *Safety, and Warnings. Infuse Bone Graft: Spine and Trauma*. Tibia trauma indications. Brief summary of indications, contraindications, and warnings for: INFUSE™ BONE GRAFT. Accessed June 30, 2022. https://www.medtronic.com/us-en/healthcare-professionals/products/spinal-orthopaedic/bone-grafting/infuse-bone-graft/indications-safety-warnings.html
78. Xie C. Meta-analysis of bone morphogenetic protein versus autologous bone grafting for limb long bone nonunion. *Chinese J Tissue Eng Res*. 2020;803-810.
79. Simic P, Culej JB, Orlic I, et al. Systemically administered bone morphogenetic protein-6 restores bone in aged ovariectomized rats by increasing bone formation and suppressing bone resorption. *J Biol Chem*. 2006;281(35):25509-25521. doi:10.1074/jbc.M513276200
80. Grasser WA, Orlic I, Borovecki F, et al. BMP-6 exerts its osteoinductive effect through activation of IGF-I and EGF pathways. *Int Orthop*. 2007;31(6):759-765. doi:10.1007/s00264-007-0407-9
81. Vukicevic S, Oppermann H, Verbanac D, et al. The clinical use of bone morphogenetic proteins revisited: a novel biocompatible carrier device OSTEOGROW for bone healing. *Int Orthop*. 2014;38(3):635-647. doi:10.1007/s00264-013-2201-1
82. Stokovic N, Ivanjko N, Erjavec I, Breski A, Peric M, Vukicevic S. Zoledronate bound to ceramics increases ectopic bone volume induced by rhBMP6 delivered in autologous blood coagulum in rats. *Biomedicines*. 2021;9(10). doi:10.3390/biomedicines9101487
83. Durdevic D, Vlahovic T, Pehar S, et al. A novel autologous bone graft substitute comprised of rhBMP6 blood coagulum as carrier tested in a randomized and controlled Phase I trial in patients with distal radial fractures. *Bone*. 2020;140:115551.
84. Chiari C, Grgurevic L, Bordukalo-Niksic T, et al. Recombinant human BMP6 applied within autologous blood coagulum accelerates bone healing: randomized controlled trial in high tibial osteotomy patients. *J Bone Miner Res*. 2020;35(10):1893-1903.
85. Chen F, Bi D, Cheng C, Ma S, Liu Y, Cheng K. Bone morphogenetic protein 7 enhances the osteogenic differentiation of human dermal-derived CD105+ fibroblast cells through the SMAD and MAPK pathways. *Int J Mol Med*. 2019;43(1):37-46. doi:10.3892/ijmm.2018.3938

86. Shen B, Wei A, Whittaker S, et al. The role of BMP-7 in chondrogenic and osteogenic differentiation of human bone marrow multipotent mesenchymal stromal cells in vitro. *J Cell Biochem.* 2010;109(2):406-416. doi:10.1002/jcb.22412
87. Friedlaender GE, Perry CR, Cole JD, et al. Osteogenic protein-1 (bone morphogenetic protein-7) in the treatment of tibial nonunions. *J Bone Joint Surg Am.* 2001;83-A(Suppl 1[Pt 2]):S151-S158.
88. Dahabreh Z, Calori GM, Kanakaris NK, Nikolaou VS, Giannoudis PV. A cost analysis of treatment of tibial fracture nonunion by bone grafting or bone morphogenetic protein-7. *Int Orthop.* 2009;33(5):1407-1414. doi:10.1007/s00264-008-0709-6
89. Mostafa S, Pakvasa M, Coalson E, et al. The wonders of BMP9: from mesenchymal stem cell differentiation, angiogenesis, neurogenesis, tumorigenesis, and metabolism to regenerative medicine. *Genes Dis.* 2019;6(3):201-223. doi:10.1016/j.gendis.2019.07.003
90. Zhang H, Wang J, Deng F, et al. Canonical Wnt signaling acts synergistically on BMP9-induced osteo/odontoblastic differentiation of stem cells of dental apical papilla (SCAPs). *Biomaterials.* 2015;39:145-154. doi:10.1016/j.biomaterials.2014.11.007
91. Nakamura T, Shirakata Y, Shinohara Y, Miron RJ, Furue K, Noguchi K. Osteogenic potential of recombinant human bone morphogenetic protein-9/absorbable collagen sponge (rhBMP-9/ACS) in rat critical size calvarial defects. *Clin Oral Investig.* 2017;21(5):1659-1665. doi:10.1007/s00784-016-1963-4
92. Nakamura T, Shirakata Y, Shinohara Y, et al. Comparison of the effects of recombinant human bone morphogenetic protein-2 and -9 on bone formation in rat calvarial critical-size defects. *Clin Oral Investig.* 2017;21(9):2671-2679. doi:10.1007/s00784-017-2069-3
93. Hock JM, Raisz LG, Canalis E. CHAPTER 11: Parathyroid hormone: anabolic and catabolic effects on bone and interactions with growth factors. In: Bilezikian JP, ed. *The Parathyroids.* 2nd ed. Academic Press; 2001:183-198.
94. Ishii Y, Hamashima T, Yamamoto S, et al. Pathogenetic significance and possibility as a therapeutic target of platelet derived growth factor. *Pathol Int.* 2017;67(5):235-246. doi:10.1111/pin.12530
95. Andrae J, Gallini R, Betsholtz C. Role of platelet-derived growth factors in physiology and medicine. *Genes Dev.* 2008;22(10):1276-1312. doi:10.1101/gad.1653708
96. Ball SG, Shuttleworth CA, Kielty CM. Vascular endothelial growth factor can signal through platelet-derived growth factor receptors. *J Cell Biol.* 2007;177(3):489-500. doi:10.1083/jcb.200608093
97. Hollinger JO, Hart CE, Hirsch SN, Lynch S, Friedlaender GE. Recombinant human platelet-derived growth factor: biology and clinical applications. *J Bone Joint Surg Am.* 2008;90(Suppl 1):48-54. doi:10.2106/jbjs.G.01231
98. Li T, Guo T, Liu H, Jiang H, Wang Y. Platelet-derived growth factor-BB mediates pancreatic cancer malignancy via regulation of the Hippo/Yes-associated protein signaling pathway. *Oncol Rep.* 2021;45(1):83-94. doi:10.3892/or.2020.7859
99. Popielarczyk TL, Huckle WR, Barrett JG. Human bone marrow-derived mesenchymal stem cells home via the PI3K-Akt, MAPK, and Jak/Stat signaling pathways in response to platelet-derived growth factor. *Stem Cells Dev.* 2019;28(17):1191-1202. doi:10.1089/scd.2019.0003
100. Bernat-Peguera A, Simón-Extremera P, da Silva-Diz V, et al. PDGFR-induced autocrine SDF-1 signaling in cancer cells promotes metastasis in advanced skin carcinoma. *Oncogene.* 2019;38(25):5021-5037. doi:10.1038/s41388-019-0773-y
101. Singhatanadgit W, Salih V, Olsen I. Up-regulation of bone morphogenetic protein receptor IB by growth factors enhances BMP-2-induced human bone cell functions. *J Cell Physiol.* 2006;209(3):912-922. doi:10.1002/jcp.20799
102. Yokota J, Chosa N, Sawada S, et al. PDGF-induced PI3K-mediated signaling enhances the TGF-β-induced osteogenic differentiation of human mesenchymal stem cells in a TGF-β-activated MEK-dependent manner. *Int J Mol Med.* 2014;33(3):534-542. doi:10.3892/ijmm.2013.1606
103. Kawai M, Rosen CJ. The insulin-like growth factor system in bone: basic and clinical implications. *Endocrinol Metab Clin N Am.* 2012;41(2):323-333, vi. doi:10.1016/j.ecl.2012.04.013
104. Laron Z. Insulin-like growth factor 1 (IGF-1): a growth hormone. *Mol Pathol.* 2001;54(5):311-316. doi:10.1136/mp.54.5.311
105. Yakar S, Isaksson O. Regulation of skeletal growth and mineral acquisition by the GH/IGF-1 axis: lessons from mouse models. *Growth Hormon IGF Res.* 2016;28:26-42. doi:10.1016/j.ghir.2015.09.004
106. Dixit M, Poudel SB, Yakar S. Effects of GH/IGF axis on bone and cartilage. *Mol Cell Endocrinol.* 2021;519:111052. doi:10.1016/j.mce.2020.111052
107. Koch H, Jadlowiec JA, Campbell PG. Insulin-like growth factor-I induces early osteoblast gene expression in human mesenchymal stem cells. *Stem Cells Dev.* 2005;14(6):621-631. doi:10.1089/scd.2005.14.621
108. Ran G, Fang W, Zhang L, et al. Polypeptides IGF-1C and P24 synergistically promote osteogenic differentiation of bone marrow mesenchymal stem cells in vitro through the p38 and JNK signaling pathways. *Int J Biochem Cell Biol.* 2021;141:106091. doi:10.1016/j.biocel.2021.106091
109. Zhang X, Xing H, Qi F, Liu H, Gao L, Wang X. Local delivery of insulin/IGF-1 for bone regeneration: carriers, strategies, and effects. *Nanotheranostics.* 2020;4(4):242-255. doi:10.7150/ntno.46408
110. Bernstein A, Mayr HO, Hube R. Can bone healing in distraction osteogenesis be accelerated by local application of IGF-1 and TGF-β1? *J Biomed Mater Res B Appl Biomater.* 2010;92B(1):215-225. doi:10.1002/jbm.b.31508

111. Wei P, Xu Y, Gu Y, Yao Q, Li J, Wang L. IGF-1-releasing PLGA nanoparticles modified 3D printed PCL scaffolds for cartilage tissue engineering. *Drug Deliv.* 2020;27(1):1106-1114. doi:10.1080/10717544.2020.1797239
112. Charoenlarp P, Rajendran AK, Iseki S. Role of fibroblast growth factors in bone regeneration. *Inflamm Regen.* 2017;37:10. doi:10.1186/s41232-017-0043-8
113. Ornitz DM, Marie PJ. Fibroblast growth factor signaling in skeletal development and disease. *Genes Dev.* 2015;29(14):1463-1486. doi:10.1101/gad.266551.115
114. Miraoui H, Marie PJ. Fibroblast growth factor receptor signaling crosstalk in skeletogenesis. *Sci Signal.* 2010;3(146). doi:10.1126/scisignal.3146re9
115. Montero A, Okada Y, Tomita M, et al. Disruption of the fibroblast growth factor-2 gene results in decreased bone mass and bone formation. *J Clin Invest.* 2000;105(8):1085-1093. doi:10.1172/jci8641
116. Behr B, Panetta NJ, Longaker MT, Quarto N. Different endogenous threshold levels of fibroblast growth factor-ligands determine the healing potential of frontal and parietal bones. *Bone.* 2010;47(2):281-294. doi:10.1016/j.bone.2010.05.008
117. Behr B, Leucht P, Longaker MT, Quarto N. Fgf-9 is required for angiogenesis and osteogenesis in long bone repair. *Proc Natl Acad Sci USA.* 2010;107(26):11853-11858. doi:10.1073/pnas.1003317107
118. Coffin JD, Florkiewicz RZ, Neumann J, et al. Abnormal bone growth and selective translational regulation in basic fibroblast growth factor (FGF-2) transgenic mice. *Mol Biol Cell.* 1995;6(12):1861-1873. doi:10.1091/mbc.6.12.1861
119. Ohbayashi N, Shibayama M, Kurotaki Y, et al. FGF18 is required for normal cell proliferation and differentiation during osteogenesis and chondrogenesis. *Genes Dev.* 2002;16(7):870-879. doi:10.1101/gad.965702
120. Su N, Jin M, Chen L. Role of FGF/FGFR signaling in skeletal development and homeostasis: learning from mouse models. *Bone Res.* 2014;2(1):14003. doi:10.1038/boneres.2014.3
121. Chen WJ, Jingushi S, Aoyama I, et al. Effects of FGF-2 on metaphyseal fracture repair in rabbit tibiae. *J Bone Miner Metab.* 2004;22(4):303-309. doi:10.1007/s00774-003-0487-6
122. Kawaguchi H, Oka H, Jingushi S, et al. A local application of recombinant human fibroblast growth factor 2 for tibial shaft fractures: a randomized, placebo-controlled trial. *J Bone Miner Res.* 2010;25(12):2735-2743. doi:10.1002/jbmr.146
123. Kitamura M, Akamatsu M, Kawanami M, et al. Randomized placebo-controlled and controlled non-inferiority phase III trials comparing trafermin, a recombinant human fibroblast growth factor 2, and enamel matrix derivative in periodontal regeneration in intrabony defects. *J Bone Miner Res.* 2016;31(4):806-814. doi:10.1002/jbmr.2738
124. Kuroda Y, Tanaka T, Miyagawa T, et al. Recombinant human FGF-2 for the treatment of early-stage osteonecrosis of the femoral head: TRION, a single-arm, multicenter phase II trial. *Regen Med.* 2021;16(6):535-548. doi:10.2217/rme-2021-0049
125. Chim SM, Qin A, Tickner J, et al. EGFL6 promotes endothelial cell migration and angiogenesis through the activation of extracellular signal-regulated kinase. *J Biol Chem.* 2011;286(25):22035-22046. doi:10.1074/jbc.M110.187633
126. Shen J, Sun Y, Liu X, et al. EGFL6 regulates angiogenesis and osteogenesis in distraction osteogenesis via Wnt/β-catenin signaling. *Stem Cell Res Ther.* 2021;12(1):415. doi:10.1186/s13287-021-02487-3
127. Hong G, Kuek V, Shi J, et al. EGFL7: master regulator of cancer pathogenesis, angiogenesis and an emerging mediator of bone homeostasis. *J Cell Physiol.* 2018;233(11):8526-8537. doi:10.1002/jcp.26792
128. Chim SM, Tickner J, Chow ST, et al. Angiogenic factors in bone local environment. *Cytokine Growth Factor Rev.* 2013;24(3):297-310. doi:10.1016/j.cytogfr.2013.03.008
129. Singh AB, Harris RC. Autocrine, paracrine and juxtacrine signaling by EGFR ligands. *Cell Signal.* 2005;17(10):1183-1193. doi:10.1016/j.cellsig.2005.03.026
130. Matsuda N, Kimar NM, Ramakrishnan PR, Cho M Il. Role of epidermal growth factor receptor in osteoblastic differentiation of rat bone marrow stromal cells. *J Bone Miner Metab.* 1996;14(3):137-145.
131. Basal O, Atay T, Ciris İ M, Baykal YB. Epidermal growth factor (EGF) promotes bone healing in surgically induced osteonecrosis of the femoral head (ONFH). *Bosn J Basic Med Sci.* 2018;18(4):352-360. doi:10.17305/bjbms.2018.3259
132. Poudel SB, Bhattarai G, Kwon TH, Lee JC. Biopotentials of collagen scaffold impregnated with plant-cell-derived epidermal growth factor in defective bone healing. *Materials (Basel).* 2023;16(9):3335.
133. Pountos I, Panteli M, Lampropoulos A, Jones E, Calori GM, Giannoudis PV. The role of peptides in bone healing and regeneration: a systematic review. *BMC Med.* 2016;14(1):103. doi:10.1186/s12916-016-0646-y
134. Visser R, Rico-Llanos GA, Pulkkinen H, Becerra J. Peptides for bone tissue engineering. *J Control Release.* 2016;244(Pt A):122-135. doi:10.1016/j.jconrel.2016.10.024
135. Balmayor ER. Targeted delivery as key for the success of small osteoinductive molecules. *Adv Drug Deliv Rev.* 2015;94:13-27. doi:10.1016/j.addr.2015.04.022
136. Wang C, Liu Y, Fan Y, Li X. The use of bioactive peptides to modify materials for bone tissue repair. *Regenerative Biomaterials.* 2017;4(3):191-206. doi:10.1093/rb/rbx011
137. Safari B, Davaran S, Aghanejad A. Osteogenic potential of the growth factors and bioactive molecules in bone regeneration. *Int J Biol Macromol.* 2021;175:544-557. doi:10.1016/j.ijbiomac.2021.02.052
138. Shekaran A, García AJ. Extracellular matrix-mimetic adhesive biomaterials for bone repair. *J Biomed Mater Res A.* 2011;96A(1):261-272. doi:10.1002/jbm.a.32979

139. Manferdini C, Trucco D, Saleh Y, et al. RGD-functionalized hydrogel supports the chondrogenic commitment of adipose mesenchymal stromal cells. *Gels*. 2022;8(6):382. doi:10.3390/gels8060382
140. Yang M, Zhang ZC, Liu Y, et al. Function and mechanism of RGD in bone and cartilage tissue engineering. *Front Bioeng Biotechnol*. 2021;9:773636. doi:10.3389/fbioe.2021.773636
141. Kim HJ, You SJ, Yang DH, Eun J. Injectable hydrogels based on MPEG–PCL–RGD and BMSCs for bone tissue engineering. *Biomater Sci*. 2020;8(15):4334-4345. doi:10.1039/D0BM00588F
142. Schaffner P, Dard MM. Structure and function of RGD peptides involved in bone biology. *Cell Mol Life Sci*. 2003;60(1):119-132. doi:10.1007/s000180300008
143. Yukna RA, Krauser JT, Callan DP, Evans GH, Cruz R, Martin M. Multi-center clinical comparison of combination anorganic bovine-derived hydroxyapatite matrix (ABM)/cell binding peptide (P-15) and ABM in human periodontal osseous defects. 6-month results. *J Periodontol*. 2000;71(11):1671-1679.
144. Green J, Schotland S, Stauber DJ, Kleeman CR, Clemens TL. Cell-matrix interaction in bone: type I collagen modulates signal transduction in osteoblast-like cells. *Am J Phys Cell Phys*. 1995;268(5):C1090-C1103.
145. Nguyen H, Qian JJ, Bhatnagar RS, Li S. Enhanced cell attachment and osteoblastic activity by P-15 peptide-coated matrix in hydrogels. *Biochem Biophys Res Commun*. 2003;311(1):179-186. doi:10.1016/j.bbrc.2003.09.192
146. Hestehave Pedersen R, Rasmussen M, Overgaard S, Ding M. Effects of P-15 peptide coated hydroxyapatite on tibial defect repair in vivo in normal and osteoporotic rats. *Biomed Res Int*. 2015;2015:253858. doi:10.1155/2015/253858
147. Spanninga BJ, Hoelen TCA, Johnson S, et al. Clinical efficacy and safety of P-15 peptide enhanced bone graft substitute in surgical bone regenerative procedures in adult maxillofacial, spine, and trauma patients: a systematic literature review. *Bone Joint Res*. 2025;14(2):77-92.
148. Fu L, Omi M, Sun M, et al. Covalent attachment of P15 peptide to Ti alloy surface modified with polymer to enhance osseointegration of implants. *ACS Appl Mater Interfaces*. 2019;11(42):38531-38536. doi:10.1021/acsami.9b14651
149. Arnold PM, Sasso RC, Janssen ME, et al. Efficacy of i-factor bone graft versus autograft in anterior cervical discectomy and fusion: results of the prospective, randomized, single-blinded Food and Drug Administration Investigational Device Exemption Study. *Spine*. 2016;41(13).
150. Thaci B, Yee R, Kim K, Vokshoor A, Johnson JP, Ament J. Cost-effectiveness of peptide enhanced bone graft i-factor versus use of local autologous bone in anterior cervical discectomy and fusion surgery. *Clinicoecon Outcomes Res*. 2021;13:681-691. doi:10.2147/ceor.S318589
151. Gomar F, Orozco R, Villar JL, Arrizabalaga F. P-15 small peptide bone graft substitute in the treatment of non-unions and delayed union. A pilot clinical trial. *Int Orthop*. 2007;31(1):93-39. doi:10.1007/s00264-006-0087-x
152. O'Brien MJM, Jones DM, Semciw AI, et al. Does the use of i-FACTOR bone graft affect bone healing in those undergoing periacetabular osteotomy (PAO) for developmental dysplasia of the hip (DDH)? A retrospective study. *J Hip Preserv Surg*. 2022;9(3):165-171. doi:10.1093/jhps/hnac027
153. Lee SJ, Won JE, Han C, et al. Development of a three-dimensionally printed scaffold grafted with bone forming peptide-1 for enhanced bone regeneration with in vitro and in vivo evaluations. *J Colloid Interface Sci*. 2019;539:468-480. doi:10.1016/j.jcis.2018.12.097
154. Chandra A, Lin T, Tribble MB, et al. PTH1–34 alleviates radiotherapy-induced local bone loss by improving osteoblast and osteocyte survival. *Bone*. 2014;67:33-40.
155. Lee JY, Choo JE, Choi YS, et al. Characterization of the surface immobilized synthetic heparin binding domain derived from human fibroblast growth factor-2 and its effect on osteoblast differentiation. *J Biomed Mater Res A*. 2007;83(4):970-979.
156. Chen T, Wang Y, Hao Z, Hu Y, Li J. Parathyroid hormone and its related peptides in bone metabolism. *Biochem Pharmacol*. 2021;192:114669. doi:10.1016/j.bcp.2021.114669
157. Rachner TD, Hofbauer LC, Göbel A, Tsourdi E. Novel therapies in osteoporosis: PTH-related peptide analogs and inhibitors of sclerostin. *J Mol Endocrinol*. 2019;62(2):R145-R154. doi:10.1530/JME-18-0173
158. Bab I, Gazit D, Chorev M, et al. Histone H4-related osteogenic growth peptide (OGP): a novel circulating stimulator of osteoblastic activity. *EMBO J*. 1992;11(5):1867-1873. doi:10.1002/j.1460-2075.1992.tb05238.x
159. Gabarin N, Gavish H, Muhlrad A, et al. Mitogenic Gi protein-MAP kinase signaling cascade in MC3T3-E1 osteogenic cells: Activation by C-terminal pentapeptide of osteogenic growth peptide [OGP(10–14)] and attenuation of activation by cAMP. *J Cell Biochem*. 2001;81(4):594-603. doi:10.1002/jcb.1083
160. Shuqiang M, Kunzheng W, Xiaoqiang D, Wei W, Mingyu Z, Daocheng W. Osteogenic growth peptide incorporated into PLGA scaffolds accelerates healing of segmental long bone defects in rabbits. *J Plast Reconstr Aesthet Surg*. 2008;61(12):1558-1560. doi:10.1016/j.bjps.2008.03.040
161. Fei Q, Guo C, Xu X, et al. Osteogenic growth peptide enhances the proliferation of bone marrow mesenchymal stem cells from osteoprotegerin-deficient mice by CDK2/cyclin A. *Acta Biochim Biophys Sin Shanghai*. 2010;42(11):801-886. doi:10.1093/abbs/gmq086
162. Zhao ZY, Shao L, Zhao HM, Zhong ZH, Liu JY, Hao CG. Osteogenic growth peptide accelerates bone healing during distraction osteogenesis in rabbit tibia. *J Int Med Res*. 2011;39(2):456-463. doi:10.1177/147323001103900213
163. Ko KR, Lee H, Han SH, et al. Substance P. A promising therapeutic target in musculoskeletal disorders. *Int J Mol Sci*. 2022;23(5):2583. doi:10.3390/ijms23052583

164. Goto T, Nakao K, Gunjigake K, Kido MA, Kobayashi S, Tanaka T. Substance P stimulates late-stage rat osteoblastic bone formation through neurokinin-1 receptors. *Neuropeptides*. 2007;41(1):25-31.
165. Li FX, Xu F, Lin X, et al. The role of substance P in the regulation of bone and cartilage metabolic activity. *Front Endocrinol (Lausanne)*. 2020;11:77. doi:10.3389/fendo.2020.00077
166. Yanagisawa M, Inoue A, Ishikawa T, et al. Primary structure, synthesis, and biological activity of rat endothelin, an endothelium-derived vasoconstrictor peptide. *Proc Natl Acad Sci*. 1988;85(18):6964-6967.
167. Kasperk CH, Börcsök I, Schairer HU, et al. Endothelin-1 is a potent regulator of human bone cell metabolism in vitro. *Calcif Tissue Int*. 1997;60(4):368-374. doi:10.1007/s002239900245
168. Sin A, Tang W, Wen CY, Chung SK, Chi KY. The emerging role of endothelin-1 in the pathogenesis of subchondral bone disturbance and osteoarthritis. *Osteoarthr Cartil*. 2015;23(4):516-524. doi:10.1016/j.joca.2014.11.002
169. Carbone EJ, Rajpura K, Jiang T, Laurencin CT, Lo KW-H. Regulation of bone regeneration with approved small molecule compounds. *Adv Regen Biol*. 2014;1(1):25276. doi:10.3402/arb.v1.25276
170. Safari B, Aghanejad A, Roshangar L, Davaran S. Osteogenic effects of the bioactive small molecules and minerals in the scaffold-based bone tissue engineering. *Colloids and Surf B Biointerfaces*. 2021;198:111462. doi:10.1016/j.colsurfb.2020.111462
171. Aravamudhan A, Ramos DM, Nip J, et al. Osteoinductive small molecules: growth factor alternatives for bone tissue engineering. *Curr Pharm Des*. 2013;19(19):3420-3428. doi:10.2174/1381612811319190008
172. Mundy G, Garrett R, Harris S, et al. Stimulation of bone formation in vitro and in rodents by statins. *Science*. 1999;286(5446):1946-1949. doi:10.1126/science.286.5446.1946
173. Pagkalos J, Cha JM, Kang Y, Heliotis M, Tsiridis E, Mantalaris A. Simvastatin induces osteogenic differentiation of murine embryonic stem cells. *J Bone Miner Res*. 2010;25(11):2470-2478. doi:10.1002/jbmr.163
174. Rezk AI, Yeon Kim J, Su Kim B, Park CH, Kim CS. De novo dual functional 3D scaffold using computational simulation with controlled drug release. *J Colloid Interface Sci*. 2022;625:12-23. doi:10.1016/j.jcis.2022.05.020
175. Zhang X, Fan J, Chen C, Aghalooc T, Lee M. Co-delivery of simvastatin and demineralized bone matrix hierarchically from nanosheet-based supramolecular hydrogels for osteogenesis. *J Mater Chem B*. 2021;9(37):7741-7750. doi:10.1039/d1tb01256h
176. Jun JH, Oh KC, Park KH, Jung N, Li J, Moon HS. Improvement of osseointegration by ultraviolet and/or simvastatin treatment on titanium implants with or without bone graft materials. *Materials (Basel)*. 2021;14(13):3707. doi:10.3390/ma14133707
177. Diniz JA, Barbirato DDS, do Nascimento EHL, et al. Tomographic evaluation of the effect of simvastatin topical use on alveolar bone microarchitecture, pain and swelling after mandibular third molar extraction: a randomized controlled trial. *Clin Oral Investig*. 2022;26(4):3533-3545. doi:10.1007/s00784-021-04322-8
178. Degala S, Bathija NA. Evaluation of the efficacy of simvastatin in bone regeneration after surgical removal of bilaterally impacted third molars-a split-mouth randomized clinical trial. *J Oral Maxillofac Surg*. 2018;76(9):1847-1858. doi:10.1016/j.joms.2018.04.035
179. Cruz R, Moraschini V, Calasans-Maia MD, et al. Clinical efficacy of simvastatin gel combined with polypropylene membrane on the healing of extraction sockets: a triple-blind, randomized clinical trial. *Clin Oral Implants Res*. 2021;32(6):711-720. doi:10.1111/clr.13740
180. Bischoff-Ferrari HA, Willett WC, Wong JB, Giovannucci E, Dietrich T, Dawson-Hughes B. Fracture prevention with vitamin D supplementation: a meta-analysis of randomized controlled trials. *JAMA*. 2005;293(18):2257-2264. doi:10.1001/jama.293.18.2257
181. Black DM, Thompson DE, Bauer DC, et al. Fracture risk reduction with alendronate in women with osteoporosis: the Fracture Intervention Trial. FIT Research Group. *J Clin Endocrinol Metab*. 2000;85(11):4118-4124. doi:10.1210/jcem.85.11.6953
182. Nah H, Lee D, Heo M, et al. Vitamin D-conjugated gold nanoparticles as functional carriers to enhancing osteogenic differentiation. *Sci Technol Adv Mater*. 2019;20(1):826-836. doi:10.1080/14686996.2019.1644193
183. Sattary M, Rafienia M, Kazemi M, Salehi H, Mahmoudzadeh M. Promoting effect of nano hydroxyapatite and vitamin D3 on the osteogenic differentiation of human adipose-derived stem cells in polycaprolactone/gelatin scaffold for bone tissue engineering. *Mater Sci Eng C Mater Biol Appl*. 2019;97:141-155. doi:10.1016/j.msec.2018.12.030
184. Wei P, Yuan Z, Jing W, et al. Strengthening the potential of biomineralized microspheres in enhancing osteogenesis via incorporating alendronate. *Chem Eng J*. 2019;368:577-588. doi:10.1016/j.cej.2019.02.202
185. Cattalini JP, Boccaccini AR, Lucangioli S, Mouriño V. Bisphosphonate-based strategies for bone tissue engineering and orthopedic implants. *Tissue Eng Part B Rev*. 2012;18(5):323-340. doi:10.1089/ten.TEB.2011.0737
186. El-Habashy S, Eltaher H, Gaballah A, Mehanna VR, El-Kamel AH. Biomaterial-based nanocomposite for osteogenic repurposing of doxycycline. *Int J Nanomedicine*. 2021;16:1103-1126. doi:10.2147/ijn.S298297
187. Pourgonabadi S, Mousavi SH, Tayarani-Najaran Z, Ghorbani A. Effect of zoledronate, a third-generation bisphosphonate, on proliferation and apoptosis of human dental pulp stem cells. *Can J Physiol Pharmacol*. 2018;96(2):137-144. doi:10.1139/cjpp-2016-0348
188. Van Vugt TAG, Geurts JAP, Blokhuis TJ. Treatment of infected tibial non-unions using a BMAC and S53P4 BAG combination for reconstruction of segmental bone defects: a clinical case series. *Injury*. 2021;52(Suppl 2):S67-S71. doi:10.1016/j.injury.2020.09.029

189. Drago L, Romanò D, De Vecchi E, et al. Bioactive glass BAG-S53P4 for the adjunctive treatment of chronic osteomyelitis of the long bones: an in vitro and prospective clinical study. *BMC Infect Dis.* 2013;13(1):584. doi:10.1186/1471-2334-13-584
190. Romanò CL, Logoluso N, Meani E, et al. A comparative study of the use of bioactive glass S53P4 and antibiotic-loaded calcium-based bone substitutes in the treatment of chronic osteomyelitis. *Bone Joint J.* 2014;96-B(6):845-850. doi:10.1302/0301-620X.96B6.33014
191. Desai P, Hasan SM, Zambrana L, et al. Bone mesenchymal stem cells with growth factors successfully treat nonunions and delayed unions. *HSS J.* 2015;11(2):104-111. doi:10.1007/s11420-015-9432-1

10 Membrane-Directed Bone Formation

William Doss and Brent Norris

INTRODUCTION

As the field of orthopedic surgery continues to evolve, so does the management of complex problems like limb salvage and preservation. Current techniques, like distraction osteogenesis and the Masquelet technique have successfully treated devastating limb injuries that would have previously been amputated. However, managing critical bone defects continues to plague orthopedic surgeons and their patients as successful outcomes are often associated with loss of function, not to mention the time and number of surgeries associated with the treatment. A critical bone defect is described as an area of missing bone that will not undergo spontaneous union without intervention, and while their size varies depending on location, it has been shown to be around 2 to 2.5 times the diameter of the affected bone.[1-3] Such defects are often the result of trauma, nonunion (with devitalized bone), chronic osteomyelitis (after aggressive resection), and neoplasm.[4]

Multiple surgical methods have been utilized in the management of these critical defects. They include distraction osteogenesis with a ring fixator, vascularized bone grafting, and the induced membrane technique, which was first described by Masquelet.[5] The goal of each of these treatments is to achieve a functional limb with bony union. This chapter will elaborate on the induced membrane technique, but the other methods should be reviewed as they are still used today to manage this complex problem.

Masqualet's landmark study published in 2000 reviewed a technique he used to manage critical bone defects in a series of patient from 1986 to 1999.[5] His method included the insertion of a cement spacer into a bone defect and subsequent removal of the cement spacer followed by autologous grafting several weeks later as a second procedure. His technique showed success in managing defects from 5 to 24 cm. The results also showed that with radical débridement, this technique could also be successful in the setting of infection.

Embarking on the route of limb salvage with the induced membrane technique is a decision that should not be entered into lightly. Multiple factors affect the success of the masquelet technique including but not limited the presence of infection, size and location of the defect, the soft tissue envelop around the defect, and probably the most important the patients physiology and/or comorbidities. One previous study demonstrated that the average hospital cost at 2 years was upwards of 155,000 U.S. dollars with an overall amputation rate of 14.5% within their cohort.[4]

The introduction of this innovative technique has opened a vast area of research into its mechanism for success. Since the original publication, the biology of the membrane has been intensely investigated, along with multiple publications demonstrating alterations in the technique to increase the rate of success in these devastating injuries and their associated critical bone defect. Further work is ongoing including ways to manage the dead space more effectively (graft cages) as well as control graft density and bioactivity, but these topics (although very intriguing) are outside the scope of this chapter.

BIOLOGY OF THE INDUCED MEMBRANE TECHNIQUE

The induced membrane has both important physical and biological properties, providing a physical barrier to contain future graft and supplying nutrient and growth factors to the implanted graft. In Masquelet's original publication, the membrane was retained because he felt removing it increased the bleeding, which could result in wound issues and potentially impairment of graft placement.[5] Further research and understanding of the membrane has shown that it has multiple properties that are fundamental to the success of a successful bony union and graft incorporation. Extensive research has demonstrated that the membrane serves several purposes: promotes neovascularization, acts as a physical barrier to contain the implanted graft, promotes endochondral ossification, stimulates gene expression for bone growth and differentiation, and has proinflammatory proteins that aide to clear persistent infection.

The creation or the induction of the membrane is based on the immune system and the strong response that occurs from exposure to a foreign body reaction. The overall goal of the body's response is to encapsulate the foreign material and shield it from the rest of the body.[6] After a cement spacer is placed, the body begins its inflammatory response. Initially blood proteins become deposited on the cement surface and created a provisional matrix.[7] As the inflammatory cascade continues, the addition of complement, interleukins, cytokines, and macrophage infiltration turn the provisional matrix to a complex structure of fibrous material.[7] This fibrous structure undergoes remodeling and changes as a function of time. Investigation into the ideal timing for the second stage of the procedure as a function of the biology of the membrane is at the center for this area of research.

As discussed, the membrane serves as important physical barrier to contain graft. Pelissier et al[8] used a rabbit model to study the cellular makeup of the graft at 2, 4, 6, and 8 weeks post implantation. At the early stage of 2 weeks, the membrane consisted of two distinct layers, an inner synovial-like epithelium and an outer fibrous layer consisting of fibroblast, myofibroblasts, and collagen fibers. At 4 weeks, the cellular makeup was similar; however, collagen fibers appeared to be arranged parallel to the spacer surface. At both 6 and 8 weeks, the edema of the synovial-like epithelium had decreased and the membrane was less cellular.[8] Another study by Wang et al[9] was also performed in rabbits. They noted the similar macrostructure of two distance layers of the membrane. Their findings showed similar results that the cellularity of membrane decreased over time but noted that the peak overall thickness of the membrane was at 2 weeks. One major difference was that they also found blood vessels were visualized along the inner membrane and peaked in volume at 4 weeks. They noted the number/volume of vessels did not decrease until around the 8-week mark.[9] The evaluation of the membrane in a human has also been demonstrated. A study by Aho et al[10] harvested a small piece of membrane during the second stage of the procedure. They included the membranes from 14 patients in which a cement spacer had been present between 1 and 33 months. The histologic evaluation showed that the younger membranes consisted of immature granulation tissue and older membranes contained more organized fibrous tissue. The membrane harvested at 4 weeks showed vascular proliferation, including multiple capillaries and small veins. They observed that this vascularity decreases over time, and at 12 weeks, the membrane exhibited less than 60% the number of vascular structures.[10]

A series of cellular signals are present and directly secreted by the membrane and surrounding bone during the maturation process. Creation of a new microcirculation and promotion of a neovascularization are important components for providing nutrients to the inserted bone graft and eventually the consolidation of the graft to the surrounding bone. The development of newly formed blood vessels is signaled by vascular endothelial growth factor (VEGF). In vivo studies in rabbits have shown that VEGF peaks between 4 and 6 weeks.[8,9] In vitro studies also demonstrate peak in VEGF between 4 and 6 weeks.[10,11] Furthermore, the level of VEGF shows a dramatic decrease at the 8-week mark.[10] Bone morphogenetic protein (BMP)-2, an osteoinductive protein, is also found in the induced membrane. It levels have been shown to rise and decrease similarly to that of VEGF. The rabbit model created by Pelissier et al[8] showed a peak BMP level at 4 weeks and a decreased to levels similar to native periosteum by 8 weeks. This is contrast to a study by Wang et al,[9] which exhibited a peak BMP level at 6 weeks. Regardless of 4 or 6 weeks, the levels taper off quickly at the 8-week mark.

Another important function of the membrane is its osteoinductive and osteogenic abilities and capabilities. Examining membranes harvested during second stage grafting showed evidence of matured lamellar bone, mesenchymal stem cells, and growth factors for osteoprogenitor cells.[10,11] It is felt that activation of the SMAD (group of cellular proteins that transfer signals to the nucleus of a cell) and mitogen-activated protein kinase pathways occur, which increases the levels of Runt-related transcription factor 2.[11,12] This is an important stimulator of bone generation.[8] Transforming growth factor-β is also a powerful stimulator of undifferentiated mesenchymal stem cells, and this is also secreted by the membrane.[13]

Polymethylmethacrylate (PMMA) is the original spacer material used by Masquelet, and similarly, many of the original in vitro studies used PMMA. The introduction of the antibiotics into PMMA (likely stimulated by the arthroplasty literature) became advantageous when treating infected nonunion. Various antibiotics have been added to the cement, and questions have been raised about the effect this addition would have on the induced membrane. Could the cement be used a vehicle to deliver medication to the local tissue and influence the development of the best membrane possible?

To answer the first question, Nau et al[14] created a study using a rat model to compare the biology and structure of the membrane using antibiotic-laden cement versus plain cement. In their study, they added vancomycin, gentamicin, and clindamycin to their cement mixtures. They isolated the membranes at 2, 4, and 6 weeks and compared them to their control. They found that gentamicin and vancomycin produce membranes more vascular and thicker than their control at both 4 and 6 weeks. They found no difference in the cellular components between the groups. In a similar study, Shah et al[15] examined whether antibiotics added to the cement space could treat infected tissue. They created a rat model where they would place clindamycin cement spacer in a rat model and add an inoculation dose of *Staphylococcus aureus*. Their findings showed that the animal treated with antibiotic cement remained without infection in 87% of animals. They concurrently examined the rate at which antibiotic was eluded from the cement and found that 28% of the added antibiotic was released within the first 6 hours and 100% released within 28 days. Further research in ongoing and including several studies out of the University of Frankfurt (Germany) that are advancing our understanding of how various antibiotics effect/influence the formation of the induced membrane. It can be said that the use of antibiotic-impregnated cement has become the standard when performing the Masquelet induced membrane technique.

During the second stage of the procedure, the defect created by the cement space is filled with bone graft. Iliac crest bone graft has long been considered the gold standard for autograft.[16] Graft from iliac crest is rich in progenitor cells, growth factors, and is easily obtained.[16] Additionally, large volumes of graft can be obtained. A study by Dhawan et al[17] demonstrated that an average of 38 cm^3 could be harvested from the posterior iliac crest. Harvesting the posterior iliac crest is demanding, and patient positioning is a challenge. Multiple complications have been described as well, including donor site pain for greater than 6 months, infection, and pelvic fracture.[18,19] In contract to the posterior iliac spine, the anterior iliac spine is easier to access, but the amount of graft harvest is considerably less and can still be associated with multiple complications as previously mentioned.

The reamer-irrigator-aspirator (RIA) is a more recent method used to the harvesting of autologous bone graft. This method consists of a single pass, intramedullary reamer connected to both saline irrigation and a suction aspirator. As the sharp reamer is passed through an intramedullary canal (usually the femur), the reaming's from the endosteum are aspirated and collected in a trap. In healthy adult patients, large volumes of bone graft can be obtained.[20] In a study by Stafford and Norris[21] where RIA was used for harvesting graft in the treatment of nonunion with the Masquelet technique, they reported an average graft volume of 47 cm^3.[21] In addition to providing a reliable larger volume of bone graft, RIA has been shown to produce less complications than iliac crest bone graft (ICBG). Complication of RIA can include excessive blood loss, heterotopic ossification, iatrogenic fracture, and anterior cortex perforation of the femur.[22] In a review by Dimitriou et al,[22] they found that overall complications of RIA in the literature were 6% and 19.37% for the iliac crest bone harvesting. The cellular biology of the collected graft has been shown to contain viable cells primed for osteosynthesis.[23] When comparing RIA to ICBG, RIA contained a higher amount of fibroblast growth factor, platelet-derived growth factor, BMP-2, and transforming growth factor-β.[24]

TECHNIQUE

Preparation for the induce membrane technique begins with patient selection. The first and most critical aspect of using the induced membrane technique is that the patient has a healthy stable soft tissue envelop over the area of skeletal defect. It the soft tissue envelop is compromised or poor, other techniques to restore the skeleton are likely better served in this situation (eg, distraction osteogenesis, vascularized fibula transfer). As previously discussed, this technique can be used to restore bone lost due to acute trauma, nonunion with devitalized bone, and chronic osteomyelitis associated with union and nonunion. Patients need to understand that there will likely be multiple surgeries, but the end goal is a functional, skeletally healed limb. The technique has and allows for subtle nuances/changes that pertain specifically to each case; however, the overall treatment algorithm should be fairly standardized in the approach.

The first portion of the procedure should begin with an adequate and thorough surgical débridement; this includes both the bone and overlying soft tissue envelop. A systematic approach should be taken starting with the skin and soft tissues before débridement of the underlying bone. For the procedure to be successful, an adequate soft tissue envelope must be present and therefore may require the use of local or free flaps to obtain adequate soft tissue coverage. In the face of infection or draining wound, the débridement must be aggressive enough to remove any draining sinus or infected soft tissues as persistent infection will negatively affect the outcome of the procedure. The use of the "SPY" (Stryker product: SPY-PHI Portable Handheld Imaging System) can help discern the vascularity of some of the soft tissue edges that are in question.[25] The SPY imaging system uses no ionizing radiation and a fluorescent imaging agent injected intravenously with a very short half-life (indocyanine green). This allows surgeons to use repeat intraoperative perfusion assessment multiple times if needed. Bone débridement is performed following the soft tissue. It is important to identify what bone is viable. In the traumatic setting, bone fragments that are completely stripped of soft tissue attachment should be removed if contaminated. Other loose fragments that are easily removed by pulling on it with a Kocher clamp may be removed if contaminated. If a fragment cannot be easily removed, retention of some or all of it should be considered.[26]

In the setting of nonunion with infection, all fibrous tissue should be removed. The area of further bone débridement/removal should be performed back to bone that is healthy with adequate blood flow. The soft tissue débridement and bony débridement should be performed without a tourniquet to be able to assess the viability of the structures with punctate or capillary bleeding. This can be determined by drilling into the bone with a 2.5-mm drill bit and observing bleeding.[27] The bone is then cut with an oscillating saw under adequate irrigation to cool the bone edge being cut often in an en bloc fashion. The authors then recommend débridement of the intramedullary canal in the face of infection. That can be performed with flexible reamers or RIA. The authors preferentially use the RIA to help clear any intramuscular sepsis that might be remote from the actively infected cortical bone. After the completion of the débridement but before the irrigation, multiple wound cultures are taken of both the soft tissue and the bone to direct systemic intravenous antibiotic treatment postoperatively. The wound bed should be irrigated with normal saline and gravity irrigation tubing. Highly contaminated wounds may require more than one débridement, and in those cases, each subsequent débridement should be approached in a similar fashion.

Skeletal fixation is the next step in the process. In cases of contamination or a tenuous soft tissue envelope, external fixation is used during initial débridement. This can be transitioned to internal fixation when the wound is clean and ready for instrumentation. The authors often take a final culture at the time of instrumentation and closure of the wound. In the case of acute trauma, while internal fixation can be performed with plates and/or intramedullary devices, there is recent evidence that has shown that the induced membrane technique seems to be more successful with intramedullary fixation, at least in the lower extremity long bones.[28]

Morwood et al[28] showed that patients treated with IMN (intramedullary nail[ing]) had faster union, fewer grafting procedures, and fewer reoperations for all causes (femur or tibia defect) than those treated with plates, with differences more evident in the femur.

After the bone and soft tissue have been adequately débrided, the next step in the process is the placement of the PMMA cement spacer. As previously discussed, antibiotics can be added to the cement for the treatment of infection without compromise to the development of a membrane. In fact, some antibiotics have been shown to cause a more robust bioactive membrane and therefore potentially a better environment to induce bone in-growth in the defect. The current mixology of antibiotics is to add 3 g of vancomycin to each pack of 40 mg gentamicin-infused PMMA packet. However, if sensitivities are known for a specific pathogen, the appropriate antibiotic can be mixed with the cement, with the caveat that the molecule is heat stable. Studies have shown that tobramycin can be used to treat gram-negative infection, and meropenem powder can be added for the treatment of anaerobic coverage.[29]

Mixing of the cement should be done in a mixing bowl by the hand. It is important to mix the cement without the addition of a vacuum seal to the increase of porosity of the cement leading to a larger elution of antibiotics into the surrounding tissue. It has become more routine in the authors' practice now to mix a small amount of methylene blue to the cement mixture to help delineate the hardened cement from bone at the time of the secondary procedure. The cement should be mixed until "doughy" and no longer sticky. At this time, the cement can be molded and placed in the defect. However, surgeons must remember that PMMA undergoes an exothermic reaction when curing, so it is important to be mindful of neurovascular structures adjacent to any defect to prevent thermal injury. A malleable ribbon or the plastic mixing device that comes with the cement can be used to protect the surrounding structures. Irrigation with normal saline should not be performed as the cement is curing so as to prevent the early elution of the antibiotics within the cement.

An alternative to placing the cement within the defect in one large piece, the cement can be placed piecemeal using multiple smaller pieces to fill the wound bed. This makes removal more efficient, but there will be some membrane around each piece of cement that will likely be removed. When placing cement around a nail, it can be created into two half circle and inserted after it has cured. This makes placement much easier and assures adequate space for bone graft around the intramuscular nail.

When placing the cement in the defect, it is important to overlap the ends of the adjacent bone. This technique promotes induced membrane over the bone ends that can help facilitate bone ingrowth in this area upon placement of the bone graft. This will help prevent seam nonunion that can occur with graft "creep" or movement of the graft that can occur when the patient becomes mobile and the effect of gravity on the graft is felt. New research into helping prevent graft creep or displacement is underway in the form of a resorbable graft cage that can been custom made to fit into the patient's defect (as seen on computed tomography scan). This technology is very new, and the efficacy and cost analysis are not known. If the decision is made to insert a drain into the wound bed, make sure the cement is fully cured so that the tubing does not adhere to the cement.

The second stage of the procedure involves removal of the cement spacer and bone grafting of the defect. As discussed earlier, the timing for optimal biology is between 4 and 8 weeks. However, this timeline can be adjusted depending on the quality of the soft tissue and confirmation that any previously present infection has been eradicated. In the authors' practice, they often wait at least 8 weeks after the initial procedure. This allows the patient to be off intravenous antibiotics for 2 weeks and trending of inflammatory markers while off antibiotics. With down trending markers, the authors proceed to the second stage.

A careful surgical approach is taken to expose the membrane. If there is low suspicion for infection, the authors do not recommend routinely taking cultures. If the concern for infection remains high, the authors will open the membrane, remove the spacer, obtain new cultures of the intramedullary region of the bone, and the overlying soft tissues. The authors then place a new antibiotic spacer, close the wound, and wait for the new cultures before harvesting and potentially wasting autologous bone graft. When opening the membrane, a longitudinal incision is used and carried onto each bone end and periosteum to preserve the membrane overlap on the outer cortex. Removal of the spacer can be done en bloc or piecemeal depending on how the cement was placed. Removal in pieces if facilitated using an osteotome with the additional of drill holes placed in the block. Placing a moist lap or Ray-Tec sponge over in the wound to prevent cement particles from becoming airborne potentially contaminating the field. The authors try to collect all the bone cement that is removed in order to measure the defect size, especially for large defect areas. This is where the use of methylene blue can be helpful. The authors take the cement and place it in a container with a known amount of saline. By doing this, the authors can use the displacement as a measure/estimate for the volume of graft that is needed to fill the defect.

With the membrane exposed, and the cement removed, the wound bed is irrigated and prepared for placement of bone graft. Autograft bone graft is the gold standard. The authors have elected to use RIA bone graft from the femur as the primary source for obtaining graft. If the femur is not available, the authors will now use RIA from the tibia with the RIA-2 as it allows for a 10-mm harvest. If this is not an option, or the authors need considerably more graft, the authors will move to the posterior iliac crest. Several adjuncts can be added to the graft before placement, and this may be tailored to specific patient factors, such as advanced age, immunocompromised states, or medical comorbidities. It has been shown that RIA can reliably obtain 40 to 50 mL of graft with one pass from a single femur.[21] If additional volume is needed, the authors can harvest from the other femur when available but will often add cancellous allograft chips (small 1-4 mm in size) to increase the graft volume. This serves several purposes; it helps expand the graft volume and helps "aerate" the RIA graft (making it less dense) and inviting easier vascular ingrowth making it more favorable for incorporation. In addition, it is osteoconductive and can provide some scaffolding, which can help inhibit "creep" (gravity-induced settling of the graft). The ratio should be kept at 2:1 for autograft versus allograft.[30]

When packing graft into the membrane, focus on starting in the areas that are less exposed from the surgical site, usually posterior and on the opposite side of the fixation from the incision. When possible, close the membrane over the packed graft and suture in place with an absorbable monofilament suture.

With consideration to permanent fixation, it is the authors' recommendation to use intramedullary nailing whenever possible. As previously stated, this improves the likelihood of graft incorporation and bony union. When additional fixation is needed, the nail plate combination can also be utilized.[28] When fixation allows, the patients are encouraged to weight bearing as tolerated after surgery. If plates are utilized, the authors often weight 10 to 12 weeks for some radiographic evidence of graft consolidation before weight bearing, especially in large defects.

SPECIAL CONSIDERATIONS

The second stage and graft implantation often does not occur during the ideal time frame of 4 to 8 weeks. This can be from patient compliance, continued infection, or the soft tissue envelope has not healed. It has been shown that over time the vascularization of the membrane is diminished as is the bioactivity. To increase vascularity at the time of grafting for delayed second stage, the authors recommend pie crusting of the membrane or scraping the membrane with an elevator to invite new blood flow. For cases of infection where the bone is stabilized with a plate in the first stage of grafting, the authors will often exchange the plate (sometimes for a nail or even a nail/plate) during the second stage to help decrease the chance of continued infection related to retained hardware and help with potential earlier weight bearing.

The use of graft cages may enhance to constructs by adding an osteoconductive substate holding autogenous graft. Ongoing clinical studies and cost-benefit analyses will be necessary to help discern the graft cage's utility. Laboratory data on the use of the graft cage in the defect model of sheep showed faster time to union with more robust and stronger callus.[31]

OUTCOMES

Indications for Use in Acute Fracture

Case

A 28-year-old male suffered a type IIIA open tibia after a motorcycle accident. He emergently had a débridement and irrigation followed by an external fixator. Bone loss occurred during this initial débridement, but no spacer was placed. After the soft tissues stabilized, the patient was taken back for definitive fixation with an intramedullary nail. At the time of the definitive fixation, a cement spacer was placed in the defect to manage the bone loss. The patient was brought back 8 weeks later for RIA bone graft from the ipsilateral femur. This patient went on to successful union of his tibia several months later.

In the setting of acute fracture with bone loss, the decision to commit the patient to two stage Masquelet can often be difficult. Large segmental defects without any cortical contact make it easier to move to a staged management of the bone defect. Often, however, the defect is much more subtle, with an area of bone loss but perhaps some cortical contact. In these circumstances, the surgeon must make the decision intraoperatively whether to stage a bone graft or give the fracture a chance to unite primarily. The nonunion risk determination score is one tool that has been presented to aid surgeons to predict tibia nonunion. It uses seven factors to create a score that increases the likelihood of nonunion. These factors include flap placement, compartment syndrome, patient comorbidities, open fracture, male gender, ASA scores, and percentage of cortical contact.[32] With a high likelihood of nonunion, consideration for Masquelet in the acute setting is reasonable. Additionally, a recent study is helping to quantify the size of the defect to help determine the chances of union.[1] Prior data have suggested even defects up to 2 cm in the tibia can heal about 50% of the time without intervention.[2] Using that size and the recent nonunion risk determination score should make it easier to predict or decide patients who would benefit with early use of the Masquelet technique. Several case series have been published demonstrating the results of this technique in the acute setting.

Hatashita et al[33] reported their results of the Masquelet technique in patients with bone defects in the acute setting. Their retrospect series included seven patients with lower extremity injuries. Their injuries were classified using the Gustilo-Anderson classification and include three IIIA and one IIIB open femur fractures and two IIIB and one IIIC open tibia fractures. Further they described their bone defect as either partial (apposition of at least one cortex) or segmental (no cortical apposition). Their spacers were removed at an average of 8 weeks, and iliac crest bone graft was used in all cases. Of their seven patients, five went on to bone union without the need for further surgery. Of the two patients who did not heal, one was reported to have a deep infection, and one required additional fixation and bone grafting to obtain union.[33] In another publication by Giotikas et al,[34] 14 open tibias were reported. Unfortunately, they did not meet with the same degree of success as the prior study, achieving union after the initial bone grafting in only eight patients (57%). Five of the remaining patients (35%) required additional grafting procedures to achieve union.[34] Publications presenting this treatment option for acute fractures is limited, consist of a small series and retrospective in nature. These data cloud the picture of the actual success rate when Masquelet is used in the acute setting.

The Treatment of Nonunion or Infected Nonunion With Bone Loss

Case

A 45-year-old male with open distal femur fracture (IIIA). Treated initially with operative débridement and external fixation. The patient subsequently underwent ORIF with a lateral locking plate. At 6 months postoperatively, the patient was having continued pain and no visible bridging callus on radiograph. The decision was made to repair his nonunion and rule out deep infection. He was taken back to the OR for débridement of the nonunion, deep cultures, and placement of antibiotic spacer. Cultures at the time were negative for infection. The second stage procedure was performed around 6 weeks post spacer placement. RIA bone graft was obtained from the contralateral femur and an intramedullary nail was added to the fixation construct prior to bone grafting. The patient went on to successful union.

Masquelet et al[5] published the landmark paper in 2000 demonstrating his technique. He treated 31 patients with defects ranging from 5 to 25 cm. He reported 87% union rate at 4 months after the second stage bone grafting. In the time since his initial publication, multiple retrospective case series and case reports have been published each containing variables such as defect size, presence of infection, and anatomic location of bone defect.[5]

An additional study published by Karger et al[35] in 2011 looked retrospectively at 84 patients with bone defects treated with the Masquelet technique. The location of the defect was in the tibia in 61 cases, the femur in 13 cases, the humerus in 6 cases, and within the forearm in 4 cases. The average number of prior procedures was 4.5 per patient. The average time to treatment of the bone defect with the Masquelet technique was 8 months. Despite these variables, they reported union in 76 out of 84 patients (90%).[35] The largest study at a single treatment center was published by Giannoudis et al[36] in 2016 where they treated 43 bone defects. A difference in their treatment was that 2 g of vancomycin was added to the cement spacer. The overall rate of union in their study was 93% with a mean time to union of 5.4 months.[36] In a recent review published by Masquelet et al[37] in 2019, they compiled the data from 12 different studies and found an overall success rate of 86%. It should be noted that there is a paucity of high-level evidence for this technique and a multicenter prospective study should be pursued.

Finally, largest study to date has been performed by Morwood et al.[28] They examined retrospectively a cohort of 121 patient who were treated with the Masquelet technique. Their study consisted of 56 tibia and 65 femur nonunions. They further examined the fixation construct in each patient. A plate was used in 64 patients, and an intramedullary nail was used in 57 patients. They reported that the rate of union was 89.5% in patients who were treated with intramedullary rod and 85.9% in patient treated using plate fixation, which was not statistically significant. They did find that patient treated with a plate often underwent multiple grafting procedures prior to union and additionally had a significantly higher reoperation rate. In their discussion, they advocate for the use of intramedullary nails over plates. They theorize that the nail helps in the creation of a new medullary canal within the bone graft and that the nature of the load sharing construct helps create a neocortex of the implanted graft.[28] Further investigation is warranted but the authors believed that an intramedullary nail seems to offer advantages over plate fixation in the Masquelet technique and the authors preferred to use this type of fixation whenever possible.

Even with the lack of high-level evidence, the use of this technique has gained significant popularity within the orthopedic trauma world (Table 10.1). Patients with these catastrophic injuries are often complicated, treatment is not always successful, resource utilization is high, and they strain the health care system and certainly can be extremely costly. A recent analysis by Norris et al[4] examined 904 patients with large segmental defects. They reported hospital costs ranged from $86,453 to $156,818. Additionally, success was not guaranteed with the Masquelet technique as the amputation rate was as high as 14.5% when treating large defects complicated with chronic osteomyelitis.[4]

TABLE 10.1 Clinical Series (With >15 Cases) Describing the Use of the Masquelet Technique

Study (Year)	Study Design	Level of Evidence	No. of Patients/ No. of Defects	Anatomical Site (No. of Defects)	Size of the Defect	Etiology	Time to Union	Outcomes and Complications	Comments
Qiu et al (2017)	Retrospective case-control series	III	40/40	Tibia (40)	Mean, 40 cm^3 (range, 15-70 cm^3)	Posttraumatic osteomyelitis	90% at a mean of 7.5 mo (SD, 1.8 mo) after second stage	6 recurrences of infection; 12 superficial pin-site infections	PMMA spacer with antibiotics (22) vs PMMA beads (18); both groups with gentamicin and vancomycin; fixation was ext. fix. (27) and plating (13); ICAG used in all cases with the addition of allograft in 11
Masquelet et al (2000) and Masquelet (2003)	Retrospective case series	IV	31/31	Tibia (23), femur (2), and upper limb (6)	>10 cm in 65% (range, 5-25 cm)	Septic NU, aseptic NU, or tumor	87% at 4 mo after second stage	4 refractures (2 at 6 mo and 2 at 2 yr); unaided mobilization at 8.5 mo; no recurrence of infection	PMMA without antibiotics; fixation included ext. fix. and plating; ICAG was used in all cases, with the addition of xenograft when defect was >15 cm
Apard et al (2010)	Retrospective case series	IV	12/12	Tibia (12)	Mean, 8.7 cm (range, 6-15 cm)	Acute trauma, septic NU, or aseptic NU	92% at 4 mo after second stage	1 recurrence of infection (wk after second stage); 4 recurrences of infection after union of bone (at 8-24 mo); 1 implant failure (at 13 mo)	PMMA with antibiotics (gentamicin); fixation was nailing (12); ICAG was used in all cases, with the addition of TCP in 4
Stafford and Norris (2010)	Retrospective case series	IV	25/27	Tibia (19) and femur (8)	Mean, 5.8 cm (range, 1-25 cm)	Septic NU or aseptic NU	70% at 6 mo; 90% at 12 mo after first stage	3 NUs persisted and 1 recurrence of infection	PMMA with antibiotics (gentamicin and vancomycin); fixation was nailing (6), plating (15), and nailing and plating (6); RIA graft used in all cases and composite graft (RIA and BMP-allograft) used in 85% of cases

(continued)

TABLE 10.1 Clinical Series (With >15 Cases) Describing the Use of the Masquelet Technique (*continued*)

Study (Year)	Study Design	Level of Evidence	No. of Patients/ No. of Defects	Anatomical Site (No. of Defects)	Size of the Defect	Etiology	Time to Union	Outcomes and Complications	Comments
Karger et al (2012)	Retrospective case series	IV	84/84	Tibia (61), femur (13), humerus (6), and forearm (4)	>5 cm in 57%; mean, 7.1 cm (range, 2-23 cm)	Acute trauma, septic NU, or aseptic NU	90% at a mean of 14 mo after first stage	8 failures were all open tibial fractures; 15 malunions; 4 patients had amputation (2 for NU and 2 for functional reasons)	PMMA without antibiotics; fixation was ext. fix. (30), nailing (8), plating (8), elastic nailing (1); primary fixation was preserved in remaining patients; ICAG was used in all, with bone substitutes in some, with vascularized graft in 7, and with an "intertibiofibular" graft in 15
El-Alfy and Ali (2016)	Prospective case series	IV	17/17	Tibia (13) and femur (4)	Mean, 7 cm (range, 4-11 cm)	Septic NU or chronic osteomyelitis	82% at a mean of 10 mo after second stage	2 NUs, 2 recurrences of infection; 6 cases had secondary procedures (regrafting in 5 and fibular osteotomy in 1)	PMMA without antibiotics; fixation was circular fixators (at first stage in 13 cases and at second stage in 4); ICAG was used at the second stage
Azi et al (2016)	Retrospective case series	IV	33/34	Tibia (19) and femur (15)	Mean, 6.7 cm (range, 1.8-15.5 cm)	Acute trauma, septic NU, or aseptic NU	79% at a mean of 8.5 mo after second stage	4 required further surgery to unite; 7 of 23 recurrences of infection; 4 donor-site complications	PMMA with antibiotics (gentamicin and vancomycin); fixation was ext. fix. (13), nailing (11), and plating (10); ICAG used in all
Giannoudis et al (2016)	Retrospective case series	IV	43/43	Tibia (11), femur (14), forearm (15), and foot (3)	Mean, 4.2 cm (range, 2-12 cm)	Acute trauma, septic NU, or aseptic NU	93% at a mean of 5.4 mo (range, 2-12 mo) after second stage	1 persistent nonunion/ failure of treatment; 6 secondary procedures	PMMA with antibiotics (gentamicin and vancomycin); fixation was circular fixator (1), nailing (11), and plating (32); composite grafting used in all but 4 (these had only iliac crest autologous bone graft) and included RIA (34), BMAC (36), BMP-7 (34), xenograft (10), and allograft (1)

Moris et al (2016)	Retrospective case series	IV	18/30	Hands intermediate phalanx (11), proximal phalanx (10), and metacarpal (9)	Mean, 2 cm (range, 0.5-4 cm)	Acute trauma, septic NU, or aseptic NU	90% at a mean of 4 mo (range, 2-12 mo) after second stage	2 NUs; 2 of 18 recurrences of infection	PMMA without antibiotics; fixation was ext. fix. (2), Kirschner wire pinning (25), plating (3); ICAG used in 8 patients, and ABG from radius in 10; 2 patients had additional synthetic graft inserted
Cho et al (2017)	Prospective case series	IV	21/21	Tibia (11), femur (8), and humerus (2)	Mean, 8.9 cm (range, 2-12 cm)	Acute trauma, septic NU after trauma, osteomyelitis, or chronic osteomyelitis	86.7% at a mean of 9.1 mo (range, 6-12 mo) after first stage	2 donor site complications; 3 patients required secondary surgeries	PMMA with antibiotics (gentamicin and vancomycin); fixation was single plating (8), dual plating (7), nail and plating (3), nailing (3); ICAG or ABG from proximal part of tibia; gelatin sponge used as core to the grafted defect during the second stage
Siboni et al (2018)	Retrospective case series	IV	18/19	Tibia (19)	Mean, 5.24 cm (range, 1.1-18 cm)	Septic NU	89% at a mean of 16 mo (SD, 10.8 mo) after second stage	4 recurrences of infection; 11 cases required secondary surgeries	PMMA spacer with gentamicin; fixation was ext. fix. (6), plating (8), and plaster casting (5); ICAG used in all cases with the addition of allograft in 9

NU, nonunion; ICAG, iliac crest autologous graft; PMMA, polymethylmethacrylate; TCP, tricalcium phosphate; RIA, reamer irrigator aspirator; BMP, bone morphogenetic protein; BMAC, bone marrow aspirate concentrate; SD, standard deviation.

Adapted with permission from Masquelet A, Kanakaris NK, Obert L, Stafford P, Giannoudis PV. Bone repair using the Masquelet technique. *J Bone Joint Surg Am.* 2019;101(11):1024-1036, Table 2.

REFERENCES

1. Tetsworth KD, Burnand HG, Hohmann E, Glatt V. Classification of bone defects: an extension of the orthopaedic trauma association open fracture classification. *J Orthop Trauma.* 2021;35(2):71-76. doi:10.1097/BOT.0000000000001896. PMID:32639397.
2. Haines NM, Lack WD, Seymour RB, Bosse MJ. Defining the lower limit of a "critical bone defect" in open diaphyseal tibial fractures. *J Orthop Trauma.* 2016;30(5):e158-e163. doi:10.1097/BOT.0000000000000531. PMID:27101166.
3. Schemitsch EH. Size matters: defining critical in bone defect size! *J Orthop Trauma.* 2017;31(Suppl 5):S20-S22. doi:10.1097/BOT.0000000000000978. PMID:28938386.
4. Norris BL, Vanderkarr M, Sparks C, Chitnis AS, Ray B, Holy CE. Treatments, cost and healthcare utilization of patients with segmental bone defects. *Injury.* 2021;52(10):2935-2940. doi:10.1016/j.injury.2021.01.016. PMID:33514450.
5. Masquelet AC, Fitoussi F, Begue T, Muller GP. Reconstruction des os longs par membrane induite et autogreffe spongieuse [Reconstruction of the long bones by the induced membrane and spongy autograft]. *Ann Chir Plast Esthet.* 2000;45(3):346-353. French. PMID: 10929461.
6. Patel J, Gudehithlu KP, Dunea G, Arruda JA, Singh AK. Foreign body-induced granulation tissue is a source of adult stem cells. *Transl Res.* 2010;155(4):191-199. doi:10.1016/j.trsl.2009.08.010. PMID: 20303468.
7. Anderson JM, Rodriguez A, Chang DT. Foreign body reaction to biomaterials. *Semin Immunol.* 2008;20(2):86-100. doi:10.1016/j.smim.2007.11.004. PMID: 18162407; PMCID: PMC2327202.
8. Pelissier P, Masquelet AC, Bareille R, Pelissier SM, Amedee J. Induced membranes secrete growth factors including vascular and osteoinductive factors and could stimulate bone regeneration. *J Orthop Res.* 2004;22(1):73-79. doi:10.1016/S0736-0266(03)00165-7. PMID: 14656662.
9. Wang X, Wei F, Luo F, Huang K, Xie Z. Induction of granulation tissue for the secretion of growth factors and the promotion of bone defect repair. *J Orthop Surg Res.* 2015;10:147. doi:10.1186/s13018-015-0287-4. PMID: 26381122; PMCID: PMC4574139.
10. Aho OM, Lehenkari P, Ristiniemi J, Lehtonen S, Risteli J, Leskelä HV. The mechanism of action of induced membranes in bone repair. *J Bone Joint Surg Am.* 2013;95(7):597-604. doi:10.2106/JBJS.L.00310 PMID:23553294.
11. Gruber HE, Ode G, Hoelscher G, Ingram J, Bethea S, Bosse MJ. Osteogenic, stem cell and molecular characterisation of the human induced membrane from extremity bone defects. *Bone Joint Res.* 2016;5(4):106-115. doi:10.1302/2046-3758.54.2000483. PMID: 27056768; PMCID: PMC5009235.
12. Tang Q, Tong M, Zheng G, Shen L, Shang P, Liu H. Masquelet's induced membrane promotes the osteogenic differentiation of bone marrow mesenchymal stem cells by activating the Smad and MAPK pathways. *Am J Transl Res.* 2018;10(4):1211-1219. PMID: 29736214; PMCID: PMC5934580.
13. Fischer C, Doll J, Tanner M, et al. Quantification of TGF-ß1, PDGF and IGF-1 cytokine expression after fracture treatment vs. non-union therapy via Masquelet. *Injury.* 2016;47(2):342-349. doi:10.1016/j.injury.2015.11.007. PMID:26775211.
14. Nau C, Seebach C, Trumm A, et al. Alteration of Masquelet's induced membrane characteristics by different kinds of antibiotic enriched bone cement in a critical size defect model in the rat's femur. *Injury.* 2016;47(2):325-334. doi:10.1016/j.injury.2015.10.079. PMID: 26652225.
15. Shah SR, Smith BT, Tatara AM, et al. Effects of local antibiotic delivery from porous space maintainers on infection clearance and induction of an osteogenic membrane in an infected bone defect. *Tissue Eng Part A.* 2017;23(3-4):91-100. doi:10.1089/ten.TEA.2016.0389. PMID: 27998243; PMCID: PMC5312600.
16. Sen MK, Miclau T. Autologous iliac crest bone graft: should it still be the gold standard for treating nonunions? *Injury.* 2007;38(Suppl 1):S75-S80. doi:10.1016/j.injury.2007.02.012. PMID: 17383488.
17. Dhawan A, Kuklo TR, Polly DW Jr. Analysis of iliac crest bone grafting process measures. *Am J Orthop (Belle Mead NJ).* 2006;35(7):322-326. PMID: 16927657.
18. Westrich GH, Geller DS, O'Malley MJ, Deland JT, Helfet DL. Anterior iliac crest bone graft harvesting using the corticocancellous reamer system. *J Orthop Trauma.* 2001;15(7):500-506. doi:10.1097/00005131-200109000-00007. PMID: 11602833.
19. Goulet JA, Senunas LE, DeSilva GL, Greenfield ML. Autogenous iliac crest bone graft. Complications and functional assessment. *Clin Orthop Relat Res.* 1997;339:76-81. doi:10.1097/00003086-199706000-00011. PMID: 9186204.
20. McCall TA, Brokaw DS, Jelen BA, et al. Treatment of large segmental bone defects with reamer-irrigator-aspirator bone graft: technique and case series. *Orthop Clin North Am.* 2010;41(1):63-73; Table of Contents. doi:10.1016/j.ocl.2009.08.002. PMID: 19931054.
21. Stafford PR, Norris BL. Reamer-irrigator-aspirator bone graft and bi Masquelet technique for segmental bone defect nonunions: a review of 25 cases. *Injury.* 2010;41(Suppl 2):S72-S77. doi:10.1016/S0020-1383(10)70014-0. PMID:21144933.
22. Dimitriou R, Mataliotakis GI, Angoules AG, Kanakaris NK, Giannoudis PV. Complications following autologous bone graft harvesting from the iliac crest and using the RIA: a systematic review. *Injury.* 2011;42(Suppl 2):S3-S15. doi:10.1016/j.injury.2011.06.015. PMID:21704997.
23. Henrich D, Nau C, Kraft SB, et al. Effect of the harvest procedure and tissue site on the osteogenic function of and gene expression in human mesenchymal stem cells. *Int J Mol Med.* 2016;37(4):976-988. doi:10.3892/ijmm.2016.2489. PMID: 26935410; PMCID: PMC4790676.

24. Schmidmaier G, Herrmann S, Green J, et al. Quantitative assessment of growth factors in reaming aspirate, iliac crest, and platelet preparation. *Bone.* 2006;39(5):1156-1163. doi:10.1016/j.bone.2006.05.023. PMID: 16863704.
25. Zenn MR. Evaluation of skin viability in nipple sparing mastectomy (NSM). *Gland Surg.* 2018;7(3):301-307. doi:10.21037/gs.2018.04.04. PMID: 29998079; PMCID: PMC6006020.
26. Paul S, Brent N, Azad D, Mark C. Femoral bone defects managed with the induced-membrane technique. *Tech Orthopaedics.* 2016;31(1):42-50. doi:10.1097/BTO.0000000000000164
27. Mauffrey C, Hake ME, Chadayammuri V, Masquelet AC. Reconstruction of long bone infections using the induced membrane technique: tips and tricks. *J Orthop Trauma.* 2016;30(6):e188-e193. doi:10.1097/BOT.0000000000000500. PMID: 26618666.
28. Morwood MP, Streufert BD, Bauer A, et al. Intramedullary nails yield superior results compared with plate fixation when using the Masquelet technique in the femur and tibia. *J Orthop Trauma.* 2019;33(11):547-552. doi:10.1097/BOT.0000000000001579. Erratum in: *J Orthop Trauma.* 2020;34(8):e290. PMID: 31403558.
29. Schmid M, Steiner O, Fasshold L, Goessler W, Holl AM, Kühn KD. The stability of carbapenems before and after admixture to PMMA-cement used for replacement surgery caused by Gram-negative bacteria. *Eur J Med Res.* 2020;25(1):34. doi:10.1186/s40001-020-00428-z. PMID: 32811560; PMCID: PMC7433091.
30. Hoit G, Kain MS, Sparkman JW, et al. The induced membrane technique for bone defects: basic science, clinical evidence, and technical tips. *OTA Int.* 2021;4(Suppl 2):e106(1-5). doi:10.1097/OI9.0000000000000106. PMID: 37608856; PMCID: PMC10441675.
31. Teixeira CR, Rahal SC, Volpi RS, et al. Tibial segmental bone defect treated with bone plate and cage filled with either xenogeneic composite or autologous cortical bone graft. An experimental study in sheep. *Vet Comp Orthop Traumatol.* 2007;20(4):269-276. PMID:18038002.
32. O'Halloran K, Coale M, Costales T, et al. Will my tibial fracture heal? Predicting nonunion at the time of definitive fixation based on commonly available variables. *Clin Orthop Relat Res.* 2016;474(6):1385-1395. doi:10.1007/s11999-016-4821-4. PMID: 27125823; PMCID: PMC4868164.
33. Hatashita S, Kawakami R, Ejiri S, et al. 'Acute Masquelet technique' for reconstructing bone defects of an open lower limb fracture. *Eur J Trauma Emerg Surg.* 2020;47:1153-1162. doi:10.1007/s00068-019-01291-2. PMID: 31894350.
34. Giotikas D, Tarazi N, Spalding L, Nabergoj M, Krkovic M. Results of the induced membrane technique in the management of traumatic bone loss in the lower limb: a cohort study. *J Orthop Trauma.* 2019;33(3):131-136. doi:10.1097/BOT.0000000000001384. PMID: 30562247.
35. Karger C, Kishi T, Schneider L, Fitoussi F, Masquelet AC. French Society of Orthopaedic Surgery and Traumatology (SoFCOT). Treatment of posttraumatic bone defects by the induced membrane technique. *Orthop Traumatol Surg Res.* 2012;98(1):97-102. doi:10.1016/j.otsr.2011.11.001. PMID: 22244249.
36. Giannoudis PV, Harwood PJ, Tosounidis T, Kanakaris NK. Restoration of long bone defects treated with the induced membrane technique: protocol and outcomes. *Injury.* 2016;47(Suppl 6):S53-S61. doi:10.1016/S0020-1383(16)30840-3. PMID: 28040088.
37. Masquelet A, Kanakaris NK, Obert L, Stafford P, Giannoudis PV. Bone repair using the Masquelet technique. *J Bone Joint Surg Am.* 2019;101(11):1024-1036. doi:10.2106/JBJS.18.00842. PMID: 31169581.

11 Systemic Agents in Fracture Healing

Kelly Krohn

INTRODUCTION

Currently there are no systemic drugs that are approved for fracture healing. Drugs that suppress bone turnover are known as antiresorptive. Examples are bisphosphonates, estrogen, and denosumab. These drugs do not enhance fracture healing, and some clinicians worry about the negative impact upon fracture healing especially for bisphosphonates. In general, it may make sense to delay staring an antiresorptive until the fracture healing has progressed for several weeks. If the patient has high risk for future fractures, these drugs may be important to reduce that risk. If the patient is already on an oral or intravenous bisphosphonate, the drug is bound to the surface of bone and likely will not be gone for many months so there is no real reason to abruptly stop these drugs at the time of fracture. The authors will focus on the anabolic drugs approved for osteoporosis, which stimulate bone formation since they have potential to enhance fracture healing.

PTH 1-34, PTH 1-84, AND PTHRP 1-34

The biology of pulsatile parathyroid hormone (PTH) has been well worked out with over 20 years of experience in the treatment of osteoporosis. There is an increased recruitment and maturation of mesenchymal stem cells into both young chondrocytes and osteoblasts. There is reduced apoptosis of existing osteoblasts resulting in more bone formation. PTH encourages remodeling, which has been shown to be the primary biology of the anabolic effect. While there is increased bone resorption and an increase in bone resorption markers like serum C-terminal telopeptide, this occurs in a setting of increased bone formation. The effect is remodeling with a net increase in new bone.[1]

This biology of PTH is very much in parallel to the biology of fracture healing and therefore led to the early empirical use of PTH 1-34 (aka teriparatide TPTD) to assist in fracture healing in settings of delayed or nonunion. While TPTD is not Food and Drug Administration (FDA) approved for fracture healing, the use in aiding the healing of a nonunion or perhaps speeding up the healing of some fractures in the older adults or elite athletes has become common place in clinical practices that handle large volume of patients with fractures. The authors will highlight some of the studies in fracture healing with TPTD. It is important to consider that the anatomical site of the fracture, the pattern of the fracture, the patient's underlying medical conditions, other drugs the patients are using, the proper fixation of the fracture, and other factors all impact the fracture healing process, and it is not appropriate to completely assume that if TPTD will help in isolation in all scenarios.

The use of TPTD to rescue delayed or nonunions was initially reported, and there is a growing body of research illustrating the potential benefit of TPTD in this setting. Bukata and Puzas[2] shared their early experience in posters from the University of Rochester Department of Orthopaedics. They had a strong anecdotal experience that TPTD treatment was able to assist in the healing of several fractures including odontoid and tibia fractures that were classified as nonunion. Difficult painful nonunions including a sternum traumatic fracture that did not heal have been described to heal with TPTD treatment.[3]

Based upon the large anecdotal experience with fracture healing, the manufacturers of TPTD (Eli Lilly & Co.) went forward with a phase 2 distal radius fracture healing study. These were all simple distal radius fractures which did not require surgical reduction and fixation. The statistical plan assumed that 40 μg/d dosage would work better than the approved 20 μg dose that had been used by many clinicians for fracture healing. The primary outcome was cortical bridging of three out of four cortices using standard AP and lateral forearm x-rays. The patients were treated with placebo, 20 μg TPTD or 40 μg TPTD in a blinded fashion for 8 weeks. The statistical plan mandated that the 40-μg dose needed to be positive before the team could look at the 20-μg dose group. Interestingly, the 40-μg dose group was not different than placebo, which internally made the study a failure. However, when the 20-μg dose group was analyzed, there was cortical bridging statistically sooner than placebo. There was no functional difference since all patients wore a cast for the same duration. While a valuable study, these results initiated some confusion and corporate pause in the progress of investigating TPTD for fracture healing.[4]

Holzer and co-workers performed a clinical trial in Austria with older adult patients who had suffered a pelvic fracture. They used PTH 1-84, which was available in Europe at that time. While not a classical randomization, every third patient was treated with PTH 1-84. They showed significantly more rapid fracture healing by CT scans, and perhaps more importantly, they showed more rapid functional recovery as measured by the Timed Up and Go testing. Given the importance of getting older adult patients back to normal ambulation, this more rapid functional recovery is likely clinically significant. Since most of these older adult patients had severe osteoporosis that put them at risk for the pelvic fracture, this study is supportive of treating older adult patients with severe osteoporosis/pelvic fractures with TPTD to reduce future fractures and likely hasten their healing and improve their functional recovery and ambulation.[5]

Aspenberg et al developed a study comparing bone mineral density (BMD) changes with TPTD and oral risedronate in patients who had suffered a pertrochanteric (aka intertrochanteric) fracture of the proximal femur. The BMD changes were predictably better with TPTD compared to oral risedronate. Secondary outcomes looked at functional outcomes and return to ambulation. The TPTD patients had more rapid Timed Up and Go times once again suggesting that in fractures in older adult patients with osteoporosis, the use of TPTD may hasten recovery and return to ambulation as well as reduce the risk of future fractures.[6]

The manufacturer of TPTD (Eli Lilly & Co.) and an orthopedic device company (Synthes) conducted a phase III fracture healing registration trial. After negotiation with the Food and Drug Administration (FDA), it was decided to move forward with a femoral neck fracture healing study with a complicated composite outcome that included rate of revision surgery to a total or hemiarthroplasty, which was a marker for potential failure of healing and sometimes osteonecrosis of the femoral head (which likely would not be improved by TPTD), pain, and function. The priori power analysis determined that 600 patients in the placebo arm and 600 in the treatment arm were necessary. FDA demanded two identical studies for a total of 2,400 older adult patients who needed to be followed for 3 years. At the end of over a year of vigorous recruitment effort, only approximately 160 patients were enrolled worldwide. Families were hesitant to allow older adult patients to enroll, and many patients had too much dementia to meet enrollment criteria. The sponsors terminated the study due to futility. The patients enrolled completed the trial, and there was no difference in rates of revision arthroplasty; however, caution must be used in the interpretation of this incomplete data set that did not reach an enrollment to achieve the power to see a difference in treatments. The results were published, but this basically stopped the fracture healing program by the sponsors.[7]

Clinicians continue to use TPTD for delayed and nonunions and of course in some elite athletes. The literature continues to grow with small case series. While these are not level I evidence, the experience to date has been frustrating for researchers attempting to complete randomized controlled trial with TPTD. A recent study from Europe enrolled 32 patients with nonunion at several anatomical sites. The average time since the fracture to the initiation of TPTD was

24 months. Patients were treated with TPTD for an average of 7.3 weeks. The success rate for successful fracture healing in this very complex group of patients was 94%. The authors nicely summarize their experience with the following quote: "Meanwhile, in otherwise hopeless situations of aseptic nonunions, in patients with normal vitamin D levels, when the usual therapeutic options are exhausted, the treatment with PTH should be considered as a viable alternative."[8]

The new anabolic drug abaloparatide lacks both clinical trial data and anecdotal experience for fracture healing. There is some preclinical data that suggest improved healing in a rat femur model. The bone biopsies done in the phase III study show more "cortical porosity" in abaloparatide-treated patients than in placebo patients, which is suggestive of a biology that promotes remodeling in the setting of an anabolic response. This is similar to TPTD, and it is possible that abaloparatide may have some similar biology with fracture healing and spine fusion, but the authors will need more evidence before they are able to consider abaloparatide in these orthopedic uses.[9]

ANTISCLEROSTIN ANTIBODY

The antisclerostin antibody romosozumab has been approved for treating postmenopausal menopause with reduction in fractures similar to the PTH/PTHrP (parathyroid hormone–related protein) molecules. The primary biology of romosozumab is anabolism with modeling rather than remodeling biology. The drug may also reduce bone resorption. Based upon this biology, it might be predicted that romosozumab would not be an ideal choice for fracture healing since the biology of fracture healing is very dependent upon bone remodeling. Recent published studies of hip fractures (femoral neck and intertrochanteric) and tibia fractures failed to show any difference in radiographic healing or functional outcomes. Systemic inhibition of sclerostin with romosozumab does not appear to enhance fracture healing based upon clinical series and consideration of its mechanism of action.[10,11]

NUTRITION

Whether the patient is a young athlete or an older adult patient with osteoporosis, it is important to supply adequate nutrition for bone formation. While many nutrients and trace elements are part of a comprehensive bone health strategy, the focus is mainly on calcium and vitamin D due to their key and critical roles. The daily needs for the mature skeleton are around 1,000 to 1,200 mg of elemental calcium per day. When calculating the patient's calcium in the diet, the authors generally estimate about 250 to 350 mg of elemental calcium per serving of dairy (any type of milk, yogurt, cottage cheese). Most people do not have enough dairy in their diet to reach 1,000 to 1,200 mg/d of elemental calcium. There are many calcium supplements with differing calcium salt and percentages of elemental calcium and inconsistent labeling. Tums (antacid medication) 1,000 mg is a calcium carbonate supplement that contains 400 mg of elemental calcium. More expensive calcium supplements may contain a variety of additional ingredients. The gut can only absorb 600 mg of calcium at a time, so it is usually divided into two daily doses.

In general, patients are advised to separate calcium supplements from vitamin D_3 supplements to allow for individual dosing and due to differing absorption characteristics. Usually, the amount of vitamin D_3 in calcium supplements is not adequate for the goal of reaching the 25-OH vitamin D level of 40 to 60 ng/mL, which is generally accepted as the correct goal for 25-OH vitamin D levels. Often a dose of around 2,000 IU vitamin D_3 is a good starting dose with the potential to adjust after 3 to 4 months checking a new 25-OH vitamin D level. Vitamin D can rarely be toxic, and excessive high doses can lead to hypercalcemia and potentially kidney stones. D_2 is a plant-based vitamin D and can be given every few weeks. However, most experts feel that daily vitamin D_3 is more physiologic, and the best way to replete vitamin D deficiency.

Adequate caloric and protein intake are important especially in the older adults. A dietician consult may be valuable to ensure that the patient is getting adequate nutrition, which may sometimes be improved with supplements.

CONCLUSION

Anabolic agents like TPTD and possibly abaloparatide may be of some value for fracture healing. It is unlikely that either molecule will be FDA approved for on-label use for fracture healing in the near future. Further reports by clinicians utilizing these agents in practice are necessary to help guide clinical judgment on appropriate use to enhance fracture healing in acute and delayed scenarios.

REFERENCES

1. Dempster DW, Zhou H, Ruff VA, Melby TE, Alam J, Taylor KA. Longitudinal effects of teriparatide or zoledronic acid on bone modeling- and remodeling-based formation in the SHOTZ study. *J Bone Miner Res.* 2018;33(4):627-633.
2. Bukata SV, Puzas JE. Orthopedic uses of teriparatide. *Curr Osteoporos Rep.* 2010;8(1):28-33.
3. Chintamaneni S, Finzel K, Gruber B. Successful treatment of sternal fracture nonunion with teriparatide. *Osteoporos Int.* 2010;21(6):1059-1063. doi:10.1007/s00198-009-1061-4
4. Aspenberg P, Genant HK, Johansson T, et al. Teriparatide for acceleration of fracture repair in humans: a prospective, randomized, double-blind study of 102 postmenopausal women with distal radial fractures. *J Bone Miner Res.* 2010;25(2):404-414.
5. Peichl P, Holzer LA, Maier R, Holzer G. Parathyroid hormone 1-84 accelerates fracture-healing in pubic bones of elderly osteoporotic women. *J Bone Joint Surg Am.* 2011;93(17):1583-1587.
6. Aspenberg P, Malouf J, Tarantino U, et al. Effects of teriparatide compared with risedronate on recovery after pertrochanteric hip fracture: results of a randomized, active-controlled, double-blind clinical trial at 26 weeks. *J Bone Joint Surg Am.* 2016;98(22):1868-1878.
7. Bhandari M, Jin L, See K, et al. Does teriparatide improve femoral neck fracture healing: results from a randomized placebo-controlled trial. *Clin Orthop Relat Res.* 2016;474(5):1234-1244.
8. Kastirr I, Reichardt M, Andresen R, et al. Therapy of aseptic nonunions with parathyroid hormone. *Eur J Orthop Surg Traumatol.* 2018;29(1):169-173.
9. Moreira C, Fitzpatrick L, Wang Y, Recker R. Effects of abaloparatide-SC (BA058) on bone histology and histomorphometry: the ACTIVE phase 3 trial. *Bone.* 2017;97:314-319.
10. Schemitsch E, Miclau T, Karachalios T, et al. A randomized, placebo-controlled study of romosozumab for the treatment of hip fractures. *J Bone Joint Surg Am.* 2020;102(8):693-702.
11. Bhandari M, Schemitsch E, Karachalios T, et al. Romosozumab in skeletally mature adults with a fresh unilateral tibia diaphyseal fracture: a randomized phase-2 study. *J Bone Joint Surg Am.* 2020;102(16):1416-1426.

12 Future Directions in Biologics

Michael Beebe, Mark Cinque, Christopher M. LaPrade, and Henry Goodnough

INTRODUCTION

During complex fracture care and posttraumatic reconstruction, the surrounding soft tissue remains one of the most critical and challenging aspects of fracture management. Failure to adequately address soft tissue compromise will inevitably lead to treatment failure. Appropriate management and reconstruction of the soft tissue envelope is a complex matter based on the reconstructive ladder. This chapter will focus on innovative options relating to reconstruction and healing promotion. While bone devoid of periosteum, in most cases, will require coverage in the form of a rotational or free flap, many other wounds, even those with exposed periosteum or tendon, may be amenable to delayed autologous split-thickness skin grafting (STSG), or even closure by secondary intention through use of these techniques.

Autologous STSG remains the gold standard for superficial coverage of open wounds; however, not all wounds are amenable to immediate STSG, and failure to adequately prepare the application site may result in failure, or worse, infection of the complex reconstruction performed below. Often, exposed structures at the open wound site require stimulation of granulation tissue before STSG. This is frequently completed through the application of a skin substitute. The ideal skin substitute should act as a bacterial barrier, withstand hypoxia, be nonantigenic, prevent dehydration, resist shear, prevent excess hypertrophy, be easy to secure, restore both dermal and epidermal components, conform to wounds, hold durability, be immediately available off the shelf, retain a long shelf life, and be inexpensive.[1] Unfortunately, this does not describe the currently available nonautologous skin substitutes; however, significant advances continue to improve the available products and outcomes.

CLASSIFICATIONS

Skin substitutes do not have a standardized classification that is universally recognized; however, the classification proposed by Kumar[2] is likely the most widely recognized. Class I consists of temporary impervious materials in this classification. These materials do not have any epidermis-like layer with no in-growth of cells and, therefore, act like an impervious mechanical barrier to prevent bacterial invasion, reduce evaporative water loss, and help to produce a moist environment for better healing (ie, Aquacel Ag).

Class II materials are single-layer durable skin substitutes recreating either the dermal or epidermal layers but not both (ie, ACell). Class III products have a composite bilayer constitution (ie, Integra) for reproducing the epidermal and dermal layers. In most cases, the epidermal layer is a barrier to dehydration and is not a permanent supplement.

Davison-Kotler et al[3] described a potentially more helpful classification. Their classification is broken down by five descriptive factors of the substitute: cellularity (acellular or cellular), layering (single or bilayer), replaced region (epidermis, dermis, or both), the material used (natural, synthetic, or both), and permanence (temporary or permanent). Due to its ease of understanding and improved compartmentalization of similar products, this is the classification the authors will use in this chapter (Table 12.1).

TABLE 12.1 Commonly Utilized Skin Substitutes[a]

Product	Base Composition	Company	Cellularity	Layering	Replaced Region	Materials Used	Permanence
Cadaveric Skin	Biological	N/A	Acellular	Single layer	Dermis only	Natural acellular dermis	Temporary
Integra Dermal Regeneration Template	Biological	Integra LifeScience Corp, Plainsboro, NJ	Acellular	Bilayer	Epidermis and dermis	Silicone, bovine collagen type I, and chondroitin-6-sulfate	Temporary once the silicone film is removed
ACell Cytal Wound Matrix	Biological	ACell Inc., Columbia, MD	Acellular	Single layer	Dermis only	Porcine urinary bladder matrix with intact epithelial basement membrane	Temporary
NovoSorb Biodegradable Temporizing Matrix	Synthetic	PolyNovo, LLC, Carlsbad, CA	Acellular (synthetic)	Bilayer	Epidermis and dermis	Silicone and open cell polyurethane matrix	Temporary once the silicone film is removed
Restrata	Synthetic	Acera Surgical, Inc., St. Louis, MO	Acellular (synthetic)	Single layer	Epidermis and dermis	Electrospun polyglactin 910 poly and polydioxanone nanofiber matrix	Temporary

[a]As classified by Davison-Kotler et al and modified with the addition of a composition classification by the current authors.

Modified with data from Davison-Kotler E, Sharma V, Kang NV, Garcia-Gareta E. A universal classification system of skin substitutes inspired by factorial design. *Tissue Eng Part B Rev*. 2018;24(4):279-288.

TEMPORARY SKIN SUBSTITUTES

Temporary skin substitutes are most often utilized as a provisional dressing of wounds or coverage of partial-thickness injuries. In orthopedics, their application can decrease pain, decrease the frequency of dressing changes, limit bacterial colonization, and decrease the desiccation of vital structures such as exposed tendons or bone. Temporary substitutes can be divided into biological and synthetic products.

Biologics Temporary Skin Substitutes

Little has changed regarding biological temporary substitutes, such as amniotic membranes, allografts, and xenografts. The human amniotic membrane has been a cheap and readily available option for wound coverage for over 100 years.[4,5] The first described use of allogeneic skin grafting was described in 1881 by Girdner and became increasingly popular for treating extensive burns through the early 20th century.[6,7] The first use of a xenograft, in the form of sheepskin, predates even allograft by nearly a century.[8,9] Xenograft functions like cryopreserved allograft in that it does not vascularize and will inevitably be rejected. Most contemporary xenografts are composed of preparations of porcine epidermis and dermis, although acellular fish skin, such as Kerecis Omega3 (Kerecis, Isafjordur, Iceland) harvested from the North Atlantic Cod, is an evolving alternative.[10] The most significant benefit of these three options is the low cost and wide availability, making it an essential choice for areas with less access to more expensive and difficult-to-store commercial alternatives.

Synthetic Temporary Skin Substitutes

Synthetic temporary skin substitutes consist of advanced wound dressings designed to protect the dermal layer during the healing of the epidermis. However, these are commonly utilized in orthopedics for postsurgical wounds. The most contemporary are those of advanced silver-impregnated dressings. Acticoat is a three-layered dressing impregnated with silver in a nanocrystalline metallic form. The silver crystals are activated upon hydrating the product with sterile water or wound drainage. Acticoat requires the application of a soft dressing over the top when used for postsurgical windshield held.[11] One of the more employed options is Mepilex Ag. This antimicrobial foam dressing consists of a soft silicone wound contact layer containing silver and activated carbon and a second layer of absorbent polyurethane foam layer.[12] Aquacel Ag is a similar dressing consisting of a sodium carboxymethylcellulose Hydrofiber impregnated with silver ions, which converts to a hydrogel upon contact with liquid.[11] In a randomized trial of the three dressings, Mepilex was shown to be the most cost-effective but not significantly more than Aquacel. Both were markedly cheaper than Acticoat. However, the overall effectiveness of any of the three was similar in final wound healing.[13]

Despite favorable results in multiple studies, a Cochrane review on topical silver-containing dressings and creams identified 26 randomized controlled trials (n = 2,066) and collectively found insufficient evidence of their use as they did not promote wound healing or prevent wound infections compared to more standard dressings.[14] However, most of the included trials were small, with many demonstrating a high or uncertain risk of bias.

PERMANENT SKIN SUBSTITUTES

When the area of concern involves loss of both the epidermal and the dermal layer, which is the case in most orthopedic reconstructive or posttraumatic cases, treatment requires recreating both the epidermal layer and regrowth of a robust dermal layer. Regarding innovation, this is the area where the most energy and funding have been focused. Permanent substitutes, like temporary substitutes, can be divided into biologics and synthetics.

Biologic Permanent Skin Substitutes

Collagen-Chondroitin Silicone Bilayer (Integra)

In the 1970s, the first engineered skin substitute, Integra (Integra LifeScience Corp, Plainsboro, NJ, USA), was developed. Burke et al[15] initially published Integra's success in 1981; however, it was not until 1996 that the Food and Drug Administration approved its use in the United States.[7,15] It was initially employed as a biologic dressing and graft extender for treating burns. However, its success has been translated to many non–burns-related soft tissue injuries. Although a thicker monolayer option is available, the most utilized option is a bilayer matrix. The "dermal" layer comprises cross-linked bovine tendon collagen and chondroitin-6-sulfate, whereas the "epidermal" layer consists of a semipermeable silicone sheet, protecting against dehydration.[16,17]

The dermal regeneration follows four distinct phases during incorporation,[18] imbibition, fibroblast migration, endothelial migration, and maturation. In the final phase, after applying a skin graft, the recruited fibroblasts replace the Integra's collagen with host collagen. Eventually, the neodermis collagen becomes histologically comparable to the patient's native dermal layer. Ideally, this creates a more durable graft with increased pliability and improved scar mobility and elasticity.

The success of Integra for traumatic wounds has shown great promise. One of the first publications in orthopedic trauma, by Violas et al.[19] displayed its use for the coverage of traumatic pediatric wounds, including those with exposed bone. Although their series only covered three patients, it paved the way for a more extensive series.

The Walter Reed Army Medical Center staff published one of the first small series on its use for traumatic wound coverage in adults.[16] Their case series covered a total of 16 wounds from blast-related injuries in a variety of sites over the upper and lower extremities. The only failures reported were in those patients with exposed cortical bone devoid of periosteum. The repeated application was successful in two of the three failures, while the third was healed by secondary intention. The authors note that fluid accumulation under the Integra resulted in one of the failures. This continues to be a problem with the silicone epidermal layer but can be managed through fenestration of the layer or using a premeshed version of the product. Surgeons should note that the premeshed product comes at an increased cost, but passing the product through a standard meshing unit can quickly destroy the relatively fragile dermal layer, so fenestration with a scalpel is recommended.

Barnett and Shilt[20] published a similar series of Gustilo and Anderson type IIIB open lower extremity injuries in pediatric patients and successfully treated seven patients without free flap coverage in injuries that would have otherwise required tissue transfer. However, they had one patient develop a nonunion and another going on to malunion. Their discussion of internal fixation strategies needs to be improved. Thus, care must be taken when applying this option to patients with acute fractures or reconstructions requiring bony healing, as the lack of vascularized muscle may decrease bony healing.

More recently, Alet et al[21] prospectively followed patients with either open fractures or full-thickness skin wounds involving exposure of tendons without paratenon, bones without periosteum, or joints without articular capsules. At 18 months, only one patient had a recalcitrant wound, and no patient required amputation or tissue transfer.

Application methods are variable, with bolster dressing or negative pressure wound therapy (NPWT) devices being the most common. Jeschke et al[22] published a small series of patients randomized to either conventional bolster application or NPWT closure with the underlying application of fibrin glue. They showed that using fibrin glue and an NPWT device decreased the time for skin grafting from 24 ± 3 days to 10 ± 1 day while increasing the subsequent STSG take rate from 78% ± 8% to 98% ± 2% (Figure 12.1).

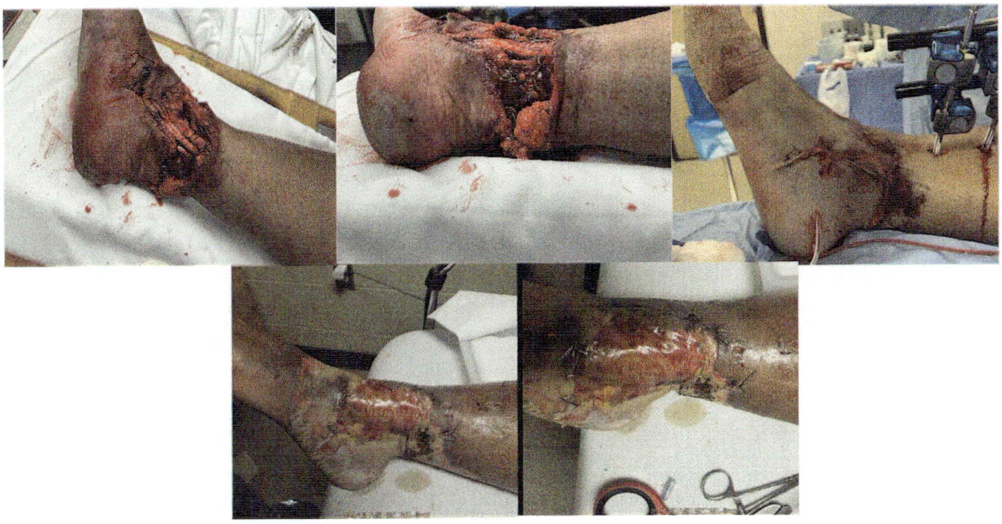

Figure 12.1. Traumatic wounds were treated with initial primary closure followed by the application of Integra. The patient went on to further dermal necrosis, requiring excision and a second application of Integra before skin grafting.

Urinary Bladder Matrix: Extracellular Matrix

One of the most utilized Urinary Bladder Matrix-Extracellular Matrix (UBM-ECM) products is ACell (ACell Inc., Columbia, MD, USA). ACell utilizes porcine urinary bladder matrix processed to remove cellular content but preserve the collagen structure and associated proteins of the extracellular matrix (ECM). The structure consists of an intact epithelial basement membrane to promote cellular migration and proliferation and the associated lamina propria to promote neovascularization.[23] The function is overall like the dermal layer of Integra, but unlike Integra, the monolayer ACell does require a secondary covering to prevent evaporative losses. It has shown great promise for treating open wounds, especially in those patients who are not flap candidates.

Geiger et al[24] reported on the use of ACell on 13 patients with distal third lower extremity wounds with an exposed tendon. All patients were deemed unsuitable for free flap coverage, and wounds were not amenable to rotational flap coverage. In all cases, the product was retained in the wound with sutures or staples, and a polyurethane sheet dressing was placed over the wound to keep the product moist. After the UBM-ECM product placement, subsequent wound care was determined by the amount of wound drainage and the need to keep the tendon moist. The time to complete healing ranged from 6 to 78 weeks (average, 33 weeks), with 5 patients requiring delayed skin grafting and 7 of 13 undergoing more than one application of ACell, with most secondary applications occurring in the clinic setting. Seventy-seven percent of patients had culture-positive, but not grossly infected, wounds, which did not appear to affect the healing potential.

The same group reported on the second series of 9 patients with 11 open fractures.[25] Two patients had failed previous application of Integra. Six patients had exposed implants within the wound bed at the time of application, and 90% of wounds were culture-positive at the time of initial application. One patient died from unrelated causes, and one patient required secondary bone grafting, while all living patients healed their wounds at an average of 26.5 weeks (range, 16-42). This study displayed the potential for obtaining coverage over exposed implants.

Parry et al[26] reported on a similar and more recent series of 17 patients with traumatic wounds having exposed tendons, bones, or implants. Like Kraemer et al,[25] they successfully obtained secondary healing over exposed implants, bone, and tendon in all patients. However,

29% of patients had complications due to infection or graft failure, and the average number of procedures to obtain a healed wound was 1.5 per wound. However, this remains a guarded success in patients with no viable alternatives. The same group later compared a slightly larger group of UBM-ECM–treated patients (n = 26) to those who underwent flap coverage (n = 26; 9 propellers, 16 pedicled, 1 free).[27] The UBM-ECM group had a higher average American Society of Anesthesiologists (ASA) physical status score, more foot/ankle wounds, and were more likely to be colonized, but overall, they had more minor defects. While UBM-ECM took longer to obtain healing (6 vs 2 months), the group required less time in the hospital (2 vs 14 days, $P < .0001$). Both groups had comparable rates of coverage failure, complications, and returns to the operating room. It should be noted, however, that all three acute traumatic wounds undergoing UBM-ECM grafting concurrently with fracture fixation experienced graft failure and osteomyelitis.

Unlike Integra, which is contraindicated for use in a region of known infection, ACell has shown promise in application over colonized but not grossly infected areas. This may be due to ECM degradation products' inherent antimicrobial properties against gram-positive and gram-negative bacteria (Figure 12.2).[28]

From experience, all authors recommend the application of powdered UBM-ECM to fill gaps and crevices in native tissue with the overlying application of a multilayer sheet to keep the powder in place. Overtop of the UBM-ECM sheet, a nonadherent dressing is applied with gel lubricant followed by either an impervious polyurethane dressing or an NPWT device. Parry et al[26] recommended that the overlying nonadherent dressing be stapled down. Only qualified individuals should remove the overlying NPWT device, as multiple patients in their group had the UBM-ECM removed during NPWT removal by home health wound care personnel.

Acellular Bovine Dermal Matrix

The bovine dermis is another common source for collagen scaffolds closely mimicking the human dermal layer. MatriDerm (MedSkin Solutions Dr. Suwelack AG, Billerbeck, Germany) is one of the more common options with numerous supporting studies. MatriDerm is an acellular matrix composed of collagen types I, III, and V sourced from the bovine dermis and elastin from the bovine nuchal ligament. The collagen layer is not chemically cross-linked, resulting in an increased biocompatibility.[29] The product may be applied in a single stage with immediate STSG applied over the top or as a two-stage procedure with application of the product and delayed STSG at around 3 weeks after application.

In the setting of posttraumatic wounds, single-stage application of MatriDerm with immediate STSG increased the epithelization rate of wounds compared to STSG alone (95% vs 80%).[30] In a prospective study of donor site treatment after free tissue transfer, MatriDerm with STSG improved cosmesis, skin plasticity, and sensory compared to full-thickness skin grafting.[31]

Synthetic Permanent Skin Substitutes

NovoSorb Biodegradable Temporizing Matrix

Biodegradable temporizing matrix (BTM) (PolyNovo, LLC., Carlsbad, CA, USA) is a fully synthetic product containing no human or animal material. It comprises a 2-mm synthetic dermal template of biodegradable polyurethane open-cell foam bonded to a superficial transparent nonbiodegradable polyurethane sealing membrane to prevent evaporative loss. It was initially trialed as an NPWT device interface to prove biocompatibility and later applied as a skin substitute in burn patients.[32] Histologic studies show that BTM may improve application sites' inflammatory response and neovascularization compared to Integra in animal models.[33] In a series by Wu et al,[34] the percentage of skin graft failure was significantly higher in the Integra group (23.1%) when

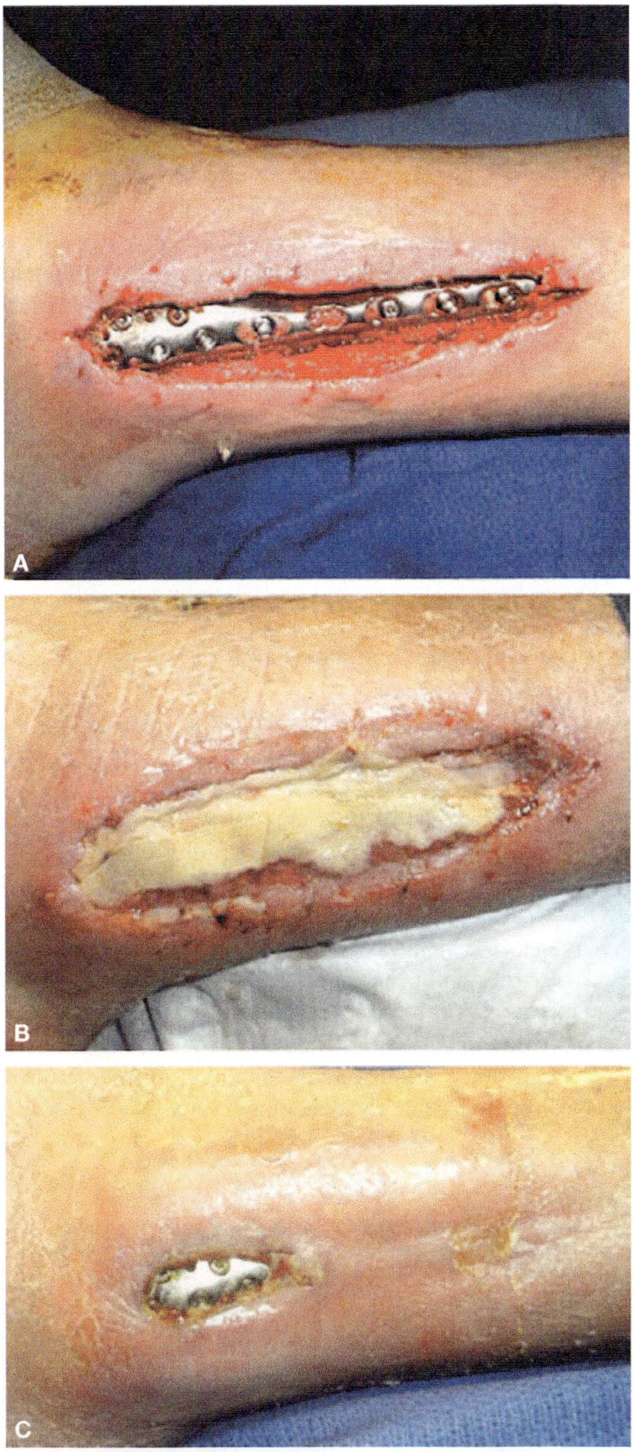

Figure 12.2. Open lateral ankle wound. **A.** Initial wound appearance prior to treatment with the powder form and multilayer sheets. **B.** Wound and product appearance as the wound healed. **C.** The wound at the time the fracture had sufficiently healed, allowing plate removal at 31 weeks. Wound care for the first month was negative pressure wound therapy and then polyurethane sheet dressings changed weekly. (Courtesy of J. Tracy Watson, MD.)

compared with the BTM subset (3.6%), resulting in more secondary procedures as well. BTM use in trauma is limited to small case series. Still, it has shown promise as a cheaper alternative to a collagen-chondroitin silicone (CCS) bilayer (Integra) with equivalent or improved results. The cost of BTM, when compared to a CCS bilayer, may be less than 1/3, with one author reporting the price of a CCS bilayer at $3,150 per 100 cm^2 and BTM at $850 per 100 cm^2.[34]

Restrata

Restrata (Acera Surgical, Inc., St. Louis, MO, USA) is an alternative new fully synthetic skin substitute consisting of a hybrid-scale fiber matrix with architecture resembling human ECM aimed at supporting cell ingrowth, retention, and differentiation like that of native ECM. The fibers are deposited through the hydro spinning of two synthetic polymers, polyglactin 910 poly (lactic-co-glycolic acid) (10:90) and polydioxanone, both of which are Food and Drug Administration approved and commonly utilized in resorbable suture material.[35] Unlike BTM or CCS bilayer, the product is a single layer designed to degrade through hydrolysis after infiltration and neovascularization. Like UBM-ECM, this allows implantation under closed but threatened skin to improve wound healing. It has commendable handling characteristics and is water permeable, which prevents the requirement of fenestration to prevent fluid buildup. However, if desired for expansion, Restrata is amenable to meshing by all commercially available meshers. However, this requires the product to be protected from dehydration by a nonadherent dressing followed by either an impervious polyurethane dressing or an NPWT device. Unfortunately, comparative studies have not yet been published and show the efficacy of Restrata compared to available alternatives (Figure 12.3).

Application of Skin Substitutes and Subsequent Grafting

The authors' preferred method for the two-stage application of a skin graft substitute is to apply the chosen substitute with the placement of a nondurable, disposable NPWT device for 1 week, followed by applying a bolster dressing until grafting. If the selected substitute has a silicon layer, such as Integra, the NPWT is applied directly over the substitute. If the substitute is a single layer, a nonadherent petroleum gauze is applied over the top and stapled along the periphery with the NPWT device applied over the top of the gauze. The NPWT device is removed and replaced with a bolster dressing in 1 week. In the case of a single-layer substitute, the nonadherent gauze is left in place before applying the bolster dressing. Once the wound is shown to have a healthy vascular granulation layer, as noted through a red coloration under the silicon or nonadherent gauze layer, the patient is brought back to the operating theater to apply an STSG. In the authors'

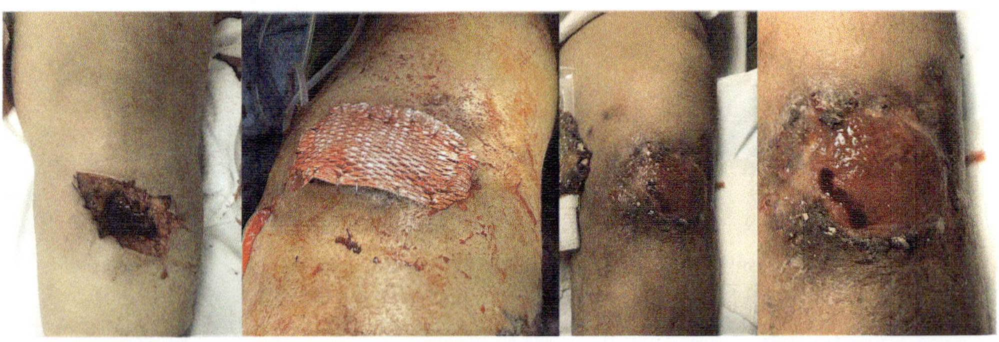

Figure 12.3. A large caliber exit wound near the tibial tubercle required a gastrocnemius rotational flap and application of Restrata for exposed fascia. Follow-up images at 3 weeks after 2 weeks of negative pressure wound therapy and 1 week of bolster dressing.

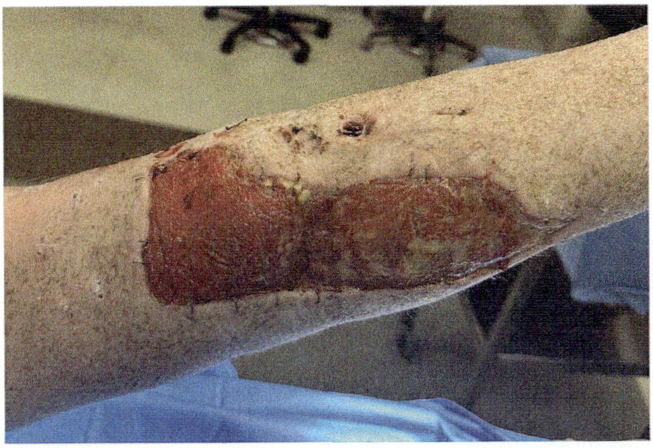

Figure 12.4. One week after the application of Integra for coverage of a lateral fasciotomy wound with the exposed tendon. The disposable negative pressure wound therapy device was removed at 1 week, exposing the silicone top layer. The granulation process has begun, decreasing the exposure of the underlying tendon; however, the visible white areas at the central and distal aspects of the wound show that the wound is not yet ready for grafting. A bolster dressing was applied directly over the silicon layer, and the patient was successfully grafted 3 weeks after the initial application.

experience, a rule of 3 weeks is generally optimal for most patients. If, at the 3-week point, granulation tissue is not fully formed, a second application is performed before the application of an STSG. It is common for a thin layer of fibrinous material to form over the healthy, viable granulated base. This is débrided during the STSG procedure with care taken to avoid débriding the vascular granulated base. Applying a fibrin glue or strict hemostasis of the débrided base layer with epinephrine-soaked sponges after light débridement will minimize the risk of hematoma formation under the STSG. Like the application of the substitute, a nondurable NPWT device is then applied for 1 week with removal in the clinic and application of a bolster dressing until the graft site is healed (Figures 12.4 and 12.5).

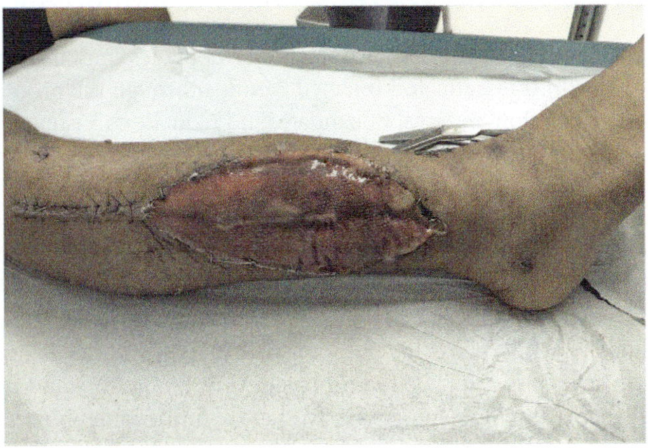

Figure 12.5. Three weeks after application of Restrata for coverage of a gastrocnemius and soleus flap for a type IIIB open tibia. Complete granulation is noted with a thin layer of fibrinous material. The fibrinous layer is lightly débrided to expose a healthy vascular base during split-thickness skin grafting application.

CONTEMPORARY WOUND AND INFECTION MANAGEMENT PRODUCTS

Hydrogels

Hydrogels are formed by cross-linking of natural or synthetic hydrophilic polymers and have been recognized as a potential for biological use since 1960.[36] Initially, only natural hydrogels were utilized; however, this advanced to creating synthetic gels with application-specific modifications to provide optimum support for the ingrowth of cells while acting as a barrier to bacteria.[37] More recently, these products have been modified to allow the delivery of antimicrobials, proteins, peptides, growth factors, and enzyme inhibitors.[38] The newest forms are stimuli-responsive hydrogels, designed to react to changes in pH, temperature, light, shear stress, or localized enzyme presence. These modifications can be used to improve the release of active compounds when it is most critical. This same technology can monitor wound healing through sensor-active, self-reporting gels indicating when bacteria-specific enzymes are present.[39] Hydrogels have been widely available for quite some time; however, the authors have only begun to explore their true potential.

Antimicrobial Peptides

As traditional antibiotics become less effective against ever-increasing bacterial resistance, clinical trials of antimicrobial peptides have rapidly increased in the last decade. Antimicrobial peptides (AMPs) are part of the human innate response, formed from small groups of positively charged amino acid chains.[40] Some AMPs function by killing bacteria directly, while others modulate the immune response. The most known AMP is polymyxin, which, like many AMPs, disrupts the bacterial cell wall. It is commonly used for external application but only intravenously as a last resort for drug-resistant infections caused by gram-negative pathogens. While more than 2,000 AMPs have been discovered, there are significant limitations to delivery, and thus, those currently on the market are mostly limited to external applications. This is mainly related to low oral bioavailability due to enzymatic degradation and a short half-life due to rapid enzymatic breakdown in the blood.[41] Despite this, several AMP-based drugs are undergoing clinical trials and may be available for patients within the next few years.

Negative Pressure Wound Therapy With Instillation and Dwell Time

NPWT has been a staple for managing open wounds in orthopedics since its introduction in 1997. It has significant benefits in traumatic and infected wounds through the promotion of perfusion and granulation tissue formation, removal of exudate, and reduction in edema.[42] While appropriate débridement is still necessary, newer negative pressure wound therapy technology with instillation and dwell time (NPWTi-d) allows the surgeon to provide automated cleansing of the wound surface between débridements. NPWTi-d has been shown to significantly decrease bioburden in infected wounds compared to NPWT, which may increase the bioburden between débridements. In contrast, wounds treated with NPWT had an increase in bioburden over the 7 days.[43,44] Clinical experts recommend an instillation time of 10 minutes, and multiple fluids may be utilized, including normal saline, hypochlorous acid solution, sodium hypochlorite solution (dilute Dakins solution 0.125% or quarter strength), acetic acid solution (0.25%-1.0%), and polyhexamethylene biguanide (0.1%) + betaine (0.1%).[45] Unfortunately, there is limited literature in orthopedic management utilizing NPWTi-d. In one series, 131 patients were treated by NPWTi-d, with 42% failing to respond to traditional NPWT, and 98% of patients could be closed successfully through skin graft, flap, or primary closure. Despite limited evidence, the potential for NPWTi-d use in orthopedic shows excellent promise. Combination with other modalities, such as AMP therapy, may drastically change the management of open wounds in the coming years.

CONCLUSIONS

In recent years, the understanding and application of orthobiologics in fracture healing and soft tissue management have greatly expanded. Growth factors and cell-based therapies appear to be the future of orthobiologics in fracture healing. A growing body of literature supports using growth factors and cell-based therapies in fracture care and nonunion management. Improvement in synthetic applications for wound dressings and skin substitutes has provided significant advances in the past decade. Moreover, unconventional management with advancing technologies such as environment-responsive drug delivery hydrogels and new and more selective applications of antimicrobial peptides may drastically change the treatment of infection management during reconstruction. As technology advances, the surgeon's armamentarium increases to provide optimal care for fracture management and soft tissue reconstruction.

REFERENCES

1. Shores JT, Gabriel A, Gupta S. Skin substitutes and alternatives: a review. *Adv Skin Wound Care.* 2007;20(9 Pt 1): 493-508; quiz 509-510.
2. Kumar P. Classification of skin substitutes. *Burns.* 2008;34(1):148-149.
3. Davison-Kotler E, Sharma V, Kang NV, Garcia-Gareta E. A universal classification system of skin substitutes inspired by factorial design. *Tissue Eng Part B Rev.* 2018;24(4):279-288.
4. Kesting MR, Wolff KD, Hohlweg-Majert B, Steinstraesser L. The role of allogenic amniotic membrane in burn treatment. *J Burn Care Res.* 2008;29(6):907-916.
5. Davis J. Skin transplantation with a review of 550 cases at the Johns Hopkins Hospital. *Johns Hopkins Med J.* 1910;15:307-396.
6. Girdner JH. Skin-grafting with grafts taken from the dead subject. *Medical Record (1866-1922).* 1881;20(5):119.
7. Liu HF, Zhang F, Lineaweaver WC. History and advancement of burn treatments. *Ann Plast Surg.* 2017;78(2 Suppl 1): S2-S8.
8. Baronio G. Degli innesti animali: dalla stamperia e fonderia del Genio 1804.
9. Schlottmann F, Bucan V, Vogt PM, Krezdorn N. A Short history of skin grafting in burns: from the gold standard of autologous skin grafting to the possibilities of allogeneic skin grafting with immunomodulatory approaches. *Medicina (Kaunas).* 2021;57(3):225. doi:10.3390/medicina57030225. PMID: 33801228; PMCID: PMC7998351.
10. Alam K, Jeffery SLA. Acellular fish skin grafts for management of split thickness donor sites and partial thickness burns: a case series. *Military Med.* 2019;184(Suppl 1):16-20.
11. Verbelen J, Hoeksema H, Heyneman A, Pirayesh A, Monstrey S. Aquacel® Ag dressing versus Acticoat dressing in partial thickness burns: a prospective, randomized, controlled study in 100 patients. Part 1: burn wound healing. *Burns.* 2014;40(3):416-427.
12. Davies P, McCarty S, Hamberg K. Silver-containing foam dressings with Safetac: a review of the scientific and clinical data. *J Wound Care.* 2017;26(Sup6a):S1-S32.
13. Aggarwala S, Harish V, Roberts S, et al. Treatment of partial thickness burns: a prospective, randomized controlled trial comparing four routinely used burns dressings in an ambulatory care setting. *J Burn Care Res.* 2021;42(5):934-943.
14. Storm-Versloot MN, Vos CG, Ubbink DT, Vermeulen H. Topical silver for preventing wound infection. *Cochrane Database Syst Rev.* 2010;(3):CD006478.
15. Burke JF, Yannas IV, Quinby WC Jr, Bondoc CC, Jung WK. Successful use of a physiologically acceptable artificial skin in the treatment of extensive burn injury. *Ann Surg.* 1981;194(4):413-428.
16. Helgeson MD, Potter BK, Evans KN, Shawen SB. Bioartificial dermal substitute: a preliminary report on its use for the management of complex combat-related soft tissue wounds. *J Orthop Trauma.* 2007;21(6):394-399.
17. Rosenbaum AJ, Banerjee S, Rezak KM, Uhl RL. Advances in wound management. *JAAOS.* 2018;26(23):833-843.
18. Moiemen NS, Staiano JJ, Ojeh NO, Thway Y, Frame JD. Reconstructive surgery with a dermal regeneration template: clinical and histologic study. *Plast Reconstr Surg.* 2001;108(1):93-103.
19. Violas P, Abid A, Darodes P, Galinier P, de Gauzy JS, Cahuzac JP. Integra artificial skin in the management of severe tissue defects, including bone exposure, in injured children. *J Pediatr Orthop B.* 2005;14(5):381-384.
20. Barnett TM, Shilt JS. Use of vacuum-assisted closure and a dermal regeneration template as an alternative to flap reconstruction in pediatric grade IIIB open lower-extremity injuries. *Am J Orthop.* 2009;38(6):301-305.
21. Alet JM, Weigert R, Castede JC, Casoli V. Management of traumatic soft tissue defects with dermal regeneration template: a prospective study. *Injury.* 2014;45(7):1042-1048.
22. Jeschke MG, Rose C, Angele P, Fuchtmeier B, Nerlich MN, Bolder U. Development of new reconstructive techniques: use of Integra in combination with fibrin glue and negative-pressure therapy for reconstruction of acute and chronic wounds. *Plast Reconstr Surg.* 2004;113(2):525-530.

23. Brown B, Lindberg K, Reing J, Stolz DB, Badylak SF. The basement membrane component of biologic scaffolds derived from extracellular matrix. *Tissue Eng.* 2006;12(3):519-526.
24. Geiger SE, Deigni OA, Watson JT, Kraemer BA. Management of open distal lower extremity wounds with exposed tendons using porcine urinary bladder matrix. *Wounds.* 2016;28(9):306-316.
25. Kraemer BA, Geiger SE, Deigni OA, Watson JT. Management of open lower extremity wounds with concomitant fracture using a porcine urinary bladder matrix. *Wounds.* 2016;28(11):387-394.
26. Parry JA, Shannon SF, Strage KE, et al. Urinary bladder matrix grafting: a simple and effective alternative to flap coverage for wounds in high-risk orthopaedic trauma patients. *J Orthop Trauma.* 2022;36(4):e152-e157.
27. Mundra LS, Tucker NJ, Parry JA. Urinary bladder matrix grafting versus flap coverage for acute or infected wound defects in patients with orthopaedic trauma. *J Orthop Trauma.* 2022;36(10):e374-e379.
28. Brennan EP, Reing J, Chew D, Myers-Irvin JM, Young EJ, Badylak SF. Antibacterial activity within degradation products of biological scaffolds composed of extracellular matrix. *Tissue Eng.* 2006;12(10):2949-2955.
29. Cervelli V, Lucarini L, Cerretani C, et al. The use of Matriderm and autologous skin grafting in the treatment of diabetic ulcers: a case report. *Int Wound J.* 2010;7(4):291-296.
30. Cervelli V, Brinci L, Spallone D, et al. The use of MatriDerm® and skin grafting in post-traumatic wounds. *Int Wound J.* 2011;8(4):400-405.
31. Watfa W, di Summa PG, Meuli J, Raffoul W, Bauquis O. Matriderm decreases donor site morbidity after radial forearm free flap harvest in transgender surgery. *J Sex Med.* 2017;14(10):1277-1284.
32. Wagstaff MJ, Driver S, Coghlan P, Greenwood JE. A randomized, controlled trial of negative pressure wound therapy of pressure ulcers via a novel polyurethane foam. *Wound Repair Regen.* 2014;22(2):205-211.
33. Cheshire PA, Herson MR, Cleland H, Akbarzadeh S. Artificial dermal templates: a comparative study of NovoSorb Biodegradable Temporising Matrix (BTM) and Integra® Dermal Regeneration Template (DRT). *Burns.* 2016;42(5):1088-1096.
34. Wu SS, Wells M, Ascha M, Gatherwright J, Chepla K. Performance of biodegradable temporizing matrix vs collagen-chondroitin silicone bilayer dermal regeneration substitutes in soft tissue wound healing: a retrospective analysis. *Wounds.* 2022;34(4):106-115.
35. MacEwan MR, MacEwan S, Kovacs TR, Batts J. What makes the optimal wound healing material? A review of current science and introduction of a synthetic nanofabricated wound care scaffold. *Cureus.* 2017;9(10):e1736.
36. Wichterle O, LÍM D. Hydrophilic gels for biological use. *Nature.* 1960;185(4706):117-118.
37. Drury JL, Mooney DJ. Hydrogels for tissue engineering: scaffold design variables and applications. *Biomaterials.* 2003;24(24):4337-4351.
38. Francesko A, Petkova P, Tzanov T. Hydrogel dressings for advanced wound management. *Curr Med Chem.* 2018;25(41):5782-5797.
39. Sadat Ebrahimi MM, Voss Y, Schonherr H. Rapid detection of *Escherichia coli* via enzymatically triggered reactions in self-reporting chitosan hydrogels. *ACS Appl Mater Interfaces.* 2015;7(36):20190-20199.
40. Fox JL. Antimicrobial peptides stage a comeback. *Nat Biotechnol.* 2013;31(5):379-382.
41. Mahlapuu M, Hakansson J, Ringstad L, Bjorn C. Antimicrobial peptides: an emerging category of therapeutic agents. *Front Cell Infect Microbiol.* 2016;6:194.
42. Orgill DP, Manders EK, Sumpio BE, et al. The mechanisms of action of vacuum assisted closure: more to learn. *Surgery.* 2009;146(1):40-51.
43. Goss SG, Schwartz JA, Facchin F, Avdagic E, Gendics C, Lantis JC 2nd. Negative pressure wound therapy with instillation (NPWTI) better reduces post-debridement bioburden in chronically infected lower extremity wounds than NPWT alone. *J Am Coll Clin Wound Spec.* 2012;4(4):74-80.
44. Ludolph I, Fried FW, Kneppe K, Arkudas A, Schmitz M, Horch RE. Negative pressure wound treatment with computer-controlled irrigation/instillation decreases bacterial load in contaminated wounds and facilitates wound closure. *Int Wound J.* 2018;15(6):978-984.
45. Kim PJ, Attinger CE, Constantine T, et al. Negative pressure wound therapy with instillation: international consensus guidelines update. *Int Wound J.* 2020;17(1):174-186.

Index

Note: Page numbers followed by '*f*' indicate figures and '*t*' indicates tables.

R